NONSURGICAL
SPORTS MEDICINE

NONSURGICAL SPORTS MEDICINE

Preparticipation Exam through Rehabilitation

N. Nichole Barry, M.D.

Michael F. Dillingham, M.D.

James L. McGuire, M.D.

THE JOHNS HOPKINS UNIVERSITY PRESS
Baltimore & London

Note to the Reader: This book discusses the treatment of sports-related injuries in general. *It is not intended to provide medical or legal advice regarding specific cases.*

Drug dosage: The authors and publisher have made reasonable efforts to determine that the selection and dosage of drugs discussed in this text conform to the practices of the general medical community. The medications described do not necessarily have specific approval by the U.S. Food and Drug Administration for use in the diseases and dosages for which they are recommended. In view of ongoing research, changes in governmental regulations, and the constant flow of information relating to drug therapy and drug reactions, the reader is urged to check the package insert of each drug for any change in indications and dosage and for warnings and precautions. This is particularly important when the recommended agent is a new and/or infrequently used drug.

© 2002 The Johns Hopkins University Press
All rights reserved. Published 2002
Printed in the United States of America on acid-free paper
9 8 7 6 5 4 3 2 1

The Johns Hopkins University Press
2715 North Charles Street
Baltimore, Maryland 21218-4363
www.press.jhu.edu

Library of Congress Cataloging-in-Publication Data

Barry, N. Nichole.
    Nonsurgical sports medicine : preparticipation exam through rehabilitation /
N. Nichole Barry, Michael F. Dillingham, James L. McGuire.
        p. cm.
    Includes bibliographical references and index.
    ISBN 0-8018-6894-7 (hbk. : alk. paper) — ISBN 0-8018-6896-3 (pbk. : alk. paper)
    1. Sports medicine.   I. Dillingham, Michael F. II. McGuire, James L. III. Title.
    RC1210 B286 2002
    617.1′027—dc21

                                                                2001004065

A catalog record for this book is available from the British Library.

Illustrations by Jacqueline Schaffer

To our late colleague and friend James McGuire,
whose inspiration and vision is reflected in this book.

N. N. B.
M. F. D.

CONTENTS

TABLES AND FIGURES

TABLES

FIGURES

NONSURGICAL
SPORTS MEDICINE

INTRODUCTION

The field of nonoperative sports medicine has reached proportions unimaginable just a decade ago. Impressive orthopedic achievements in the correct diagnosis of injury and in operative interventions have vastly improved outcomes for injured athletes. These orthopedic advances have been paralleled by an expansion of the whole field of clinical medicine in general, resulting in a health promotion movement that encourages regular lifelong exercise for everyone.

Certain advances in sports medicine have produced therapies that permit a rapid return to the previous level of play in the same season, especially for the elite or Olympic athlete. These impressive advances reflect the ability to diagnose more accurately, to intervene early when appropriate, and to rehabilitate the athlete through intensive, individualized programs. The result may be high-quality but costly care, directly affecting the approach to sports medicine for all levels of athletes, not just the elite or Olympic athlete. A compromised approach to the issues of acute and overuse injuries has developed that reflects the constraints of a cost-controlled health care environment. Nevertheless, early and accurate diagnosis that results in appropriate therapy and better outcomes is critically important for the athlete's overall health.

The advances in sports medicine, which have yielded dramatic recoveries from athletic injuries while minimizing joint dysfunction and osteoarthritic sequelae, comprise three broad areas: technology, clinical approach, and rehabilitation. First, the ability to image soft tissue and bone, especially with magnetic resonance imaging (MRI), has significantly advanced the study of structure and function. Arthroscopic technologies allow confirmation of diagnosis by direct visualization. For instance, although a tear of the rotator cuff may be imaged by an arthrogram, the MRI has the advantage of not only providing evaluation of the rotator cuff but also allowing visualization of the associated soft tissue structures.

Second, the use of arthroscopy in clinical evaluation of joint injuries has prolonged many athletic careers. As late as the 1970s, surgical procedures on the knee required a large disruption of the joint capsule to permit adequate visualization and repair, which prevented early rehabilitation and further complicated the extent of muscle atrophy. Surgical repair of the knee using arthroscopy spans the spectrum from anterior cruciate ligament (ACL) transplantation to meniscal suturing. The next phase of arthroscopic therapies has involved such technologies as laser ablation and cutting, a variety of controlled thermal-insult procedures to provide joint stability, and multiple techniques for articular surface repair.

Third, physical medicine and rehabilitation has provided a nonoperative approach to the diagnosis and treatment of spine and nerve problems with aggressive acute programs that allow the athlete to progress to pain-free, full-strength performance levels equal to pre-injury levels. Also reflecting the technology and clinical approach is the success of bracing, as in treating knee injuries. An athlete with a complete ACL tear, once a career-ending injury, can now (depending on the extent of other injured structures in the knee) receive a diagnosis by MRI, undergo repair by arthroscopy, undergo successful rehabilitation—and return to play in the same season.

One of the most important considerations in sports medicine is the decision to take an aggressive or a conservative approach to the sports injury. An aggressive approach that results in better function and less disability could justify the higher up-front costs of imaging and surgery. For example, studies have shown that a torn meniscus left in place may enlarge, contributing significantly to an earlier development of osteoarthritis. Early management of a torn meniscus may delay progression of osteoarthritis, decreasing long-term disability. Unfortunately, no cost comparisons are available for aggressive versus conservative treatments. Hopefully, data will soon be available to assist in these decisions.

Internists and family practitioners can be part of a medical team that includes specialists in orthopedics and physical medicine and rehabilitation. Other health care providers may have specific roles as well: for example, the pediatrician for growth and development of the young athlete, the physical therapist for implementation of the rehabilitation program, the psychologist or psychiatrist for individuals' stress reactions and team dynamics, and occasionally the chiropractor for providing physical therapy. The involvement of various members of the medical team at the appropriate time is crucial to a cost-effective approach that begins with the correct diagnosis.

Emphasis on the musculoskeletal exam, specifically tailored for sports medicine, requires the development of confidence and skill with orthopedic examination maneuvers designed to evaluate the integrity of various crucial joint and muscular structures. This skill begins with the preparticipation exam. In this exam, the physician determines the integrity of the joints and periarticular structures, which may have been injured or are at risk for injury depending on the particular sport. Internists and family practitioners are already well acquainted with the neuromuscular examination and play an important role on the sports medicine team in diagnosing and managing any medical problems or conditions that may be affected by exercise and athletic performance. They also need to be familiar with the unique management and implications of some medical conditions in athletes that may differ from those for inactive individuals.

Physicians and their allied health professional partners are increasingly being asked to interpret the wide range of social and legal implications of sports. Drug use for performance enhancement, the risk of HIV transmission in contact sports, sudden cardiac death in otherwise healthy athletes, the association of amenorrhea and osteoporosis in female athletes with low body fat, and regular exercise and its potential to cause osteoarthritis are just a few of the common topics facing the medical professional. Clearly, a background in internal medicine provides the optimal platform for addressing these public concerns.

The legal issues of sports medicine are also growing. Here again, a complete preparticipation physical exam, often accompanied by a signed waiver, can define and document preexisting injuries, cardiac risk, and potential illicit drug use. Although initially developed for professional athletes, waivers are now required for most pre-elite and collegiate athletes, and even some high school athletes.

Sports physicians should have a contract with any organization for which they provide coverage, even if the care is provided without compensation. The contract can be brief, and probably should be, but it serves as a basis should any legal difficulty arise. Malpractice is rare in sports medicine, but certain cases involving elite athletes have made the headlines, especially a missed diagnosis or a career-shortening injury. Unfortunately, some athletes have used these legal suits or threats to sue during contract negotiations.

The physician who takes on responsibility for a community's school athletic program may have a great opportunity to influence the health of teenagers in terms of nutrition and exercise. Coverage of specific sports usually carries little risk of legal problems, provided the appropriate medical equipment and emergency medical transportation are available. For any sport, the physician needs to be aware of the most common musculoskeletal injuries and the potential for serious cardiac or neurological problems.

Internists and family practitioners are the appropriate physicians to provide care in two major areas of preventive sports medicine. First, they should monitor athletes for osteoporosis and bone health. Adequate calcium intake must be ensured, especially in teenage girls as they go through a period of increasing bone density that is dependent on sufficient calcium absorption and adequate estrogen levels. Of major concern is the early detection of amenorrhea or dysmenorrhea, which may lead to secondary osteoporosis. Attention to eating disorders and the low body weight and size associated with certain sports is also critical. Second, the risk of developing osteoarthritis is a common concern among athletes, especially those who have incurred lower-extremity injuries. The risk of secondary osteoarthritis resulting from a meniscal tear is less if the tear is sutured, even though not all tears can be repaired. Hypermobility of injured joints leading to subluxation, especially in the knee and shoulder, can produce a series of traumatic events that result in various degenerative syndromes. In the near future, the repair of articular cartilage defects by transplantation or by manipulation of chondrocytes or articular cartilage may be able to stabilize or repair what is currently an irreversible cartilage loss.

As a component of many preparticipation physical exams, the physician is asked about the risk of osteoarthritis following a regular jogging routine. Usually the answer includes testimony about the many long-term long-distance runners with no evidence of osteoarthritis, but each answer must be individualized based on the person's running technique, weight, and preexisting injuries and the presence of any osteo-arthritis prior to an exercise program based on running.

The specialty of sports medicine has evolved to cover multiple non-surgical musculoskeletal syndromes and injuries as well as unique management of medical problems. Internists or family practitioners function as nonoperative sports medicine physicians, working closely with orthopedists to provide complete, optimal care for the athlete.

THE PREPARTICIPATION
PHYSICAL EXAMINATION

Starting at the scholastic or collegiate level, a physical examination for the athlete before participation in a competitive sport is often a requirement. Many medical associations, including the American College of Sports Medicine, the American Heart Association, and the American College of Pediatrics, recommend that prior to a new sport or season, all potential athletes, both competitive and recreational, should have a physical examination performed by a physician who is familiar with the demands of exercise and sports.

The physician performing this physical exam (the "preparticipation exam") needs not only to be aware of the stress that exercise places on various body systems, especially cardiovascular, musculoskeletal, and psychological, but also to be able to take a comprehensive history and recognize the signs and symptoms of various types of heart disease (1). The preparticipation exam differs from a general physical exam and is not intended to replace it. It should focus both on the athlete's general health and on detecting any defects or preexisting conditions that may limit or worsen with sports participation, as well as any conditions that may predispose the athlete to injury (2). The ultimate goal is to allow athletes to reach their optimal performance level safely and with reasonable risk. For the athlete involved in organized sports, at the high school, collegiate, or professional level, the preparticipation exam is usually necessary to fulfill legal and insurance requirements as well (3). Preexisting conditions must be documented to protect the athlete and the institution. The risk of injury and the responsibility of each party should be clearly written out in the form of a contract between the athlete and the organization.

During the preparticipation exam, careful attention must be paid to the athlete's past medical history, such as previous injuries and focal musculoskeletal weaknesses. The exam should also be as "sport specific" as possible—for instance, the focus should be on the knee and ankle for soccer. For the purpose of the exam, based on the differing risks for heart disease, athletes are divided into three groups according to age: pediatric, younger than 16 years old; young adult, ages 16–30 years; and adult, ages 31 years and older (4). The young adult group generally includes high school and college athletes participating in organized sports, as well as most elite athletes. The adult group tends to be composed mainly of recreational athletes. Many individuals in this group exercise for health benefits or participate sporadically in sports activities. Medical history is as important for these athletes as for the younger groups, and their individual exercise program needs to be reviewed to help avoid any acute or overuse injuries (4). These individuals are more likely to have preexisting medical conditions, which generally do not prevent them from participating in an exercise program but may require changes in medical management, such as the optimal antihypertensive medication.

The general preparticipation exam for all ages should include the following:

1. Check of vital signs
2. Measurement of height and weight (any unusual variance or drastic change from previous exams may suggest Marfan's syndrome, steroid use, hypo- or hyperthyroidism, eating disorders, gastrointestinal disorders, or depression)
3. Vision testing
4. Cardiovascular exam
5. Quick skin survey (especially for any possible contagious conditions, such as herpes, ringworm, impetigo)
6. Physical exam for organomegaly
7. Musculoskeletal exam, with particular attention to the symmetry and gross strength of each major muscle group, the range of motion (active) of all joints including the spine, and the stability of the major joints (4). The musculoskeletal exam is designed to detect and document any preexisting injuries, including those that the athlete

has not reported. It can also elicit any muscle weakness or structural abnormality that might place the athlete at a higher risk of injury and thus allow preventive management (such as a strengthening program).

The history can be very helpful as a screening tool and can be tailored to be sensitive and specific. A standardized, easy to understand form will ensure that all relevant questions are addressed for each athlete. Individuals should complete the forms before the physical exam, so the physician can review them and ask more detailed questions if necessary. These forms may vary somewhat among different institutions, but all should include questions on the following topics:

–episodes of exercise-induced syncope
–family history of any major illnesses, especially heart attack before the age of 50 years
–loss of consciousness or concussion, including dates of these incidents
–any present illness and previous injuries or surgeries
–present medications
–allergies (including environmental, such as to insect bites)
–date of last tetanus injection
–use of any mouth, eye, or ear appliance (which will be relevant if the athlete becomes unconscious) (4)
–menstrual irregularities

The timing of the examination is important, especially for seasonal sports. When feasible, it should occur at least 4–6 weeks before the beginning of the season to allow enough time for any necessary rehabilitation. If the exam is performed too long before the beginning of the season, a new injury may develop in the interval, which may not be evaluated appropriately (4).

For assessing the cardiac risk of younger athletes, the American College of Cardiology and the American Heart Association recommend screening for heart disease in high school athletes every two years (although a detailed interim history should be performed) (6). For collegiate athletes, a comprehensive history and physical exam should be performed in the first year, with an interim history and blood pressure measurement in subsequent years. Yearly screening and evaluation of interim musculoskeletal injuries is critical and should be included as well. Routine urine or blood tests have not proved a useful part of the screening evaluation (5).

Athletes over 40 years of age should have a general physical exam, including vision testing and a musculoskeletal exam. Routine blood and urine tests for these individuals are not unreasonable, especially to establish baseline values. Serum cholesterol levels might be included to evaluate the possible risk of coronary artery disease and help determine whether an exercise stress test is necessary.

For routine screening of large numbers of individuals, use of an organized team with multiple stations is often the most efficient approach. Each station evaluates a particular aspect of the entire exam, such as registration, vital signs, visual acuity, and general examination. An exit station to verify that all aspects of the exam have been performed and documented and any follow-up actions have been arranged is essential to ensure completeness. Nonmedical persons such as coaches or student trainers may perform some of the evaluations, such as vital signs and vision testing with eye charts, but only with appropriate training and with instruction to report any abnormal findings or questions to the physician in charge. A physician or nurse practitioner should perform the medical (i.e., cardiac) exam, and a trainer or physical therapist may assist with the musculoskeletal evaluation (6). The recreational athlete and any athlete with specific medical or orthopedic problems should have an individual or office-based examination.

The physician is the only person who should ultimately make decisions about the eligibility of an individual for a particular sport. A general guideline has been set up for assessing the eligibility of athletes with certain medical problems for particular types of sports (table 1.1). At the completion of the exam, the physician has the option of clearing the athlete, either without limitation or with limitation to specific activities and sports, or deferring clearance until certain medical or musculoskeletal conditions are further evaluated or treated. Complete disqualification of an athlete from all sports on medical grounds is relatively rare (4).

The Mayo Clinic conducted a long-term study of the successes and

Table 1.1. Disqualifying Conditions

	Absolute Contraindications		Relative Contraindications	
	Contact	Noncontact	Contact	Noncontact
Seizure within past year	X	X*	—	X
Concussions with consciousness loss	X	—	—	—
Large postsurgical cranial defect	X	—	—	X
Solitary functioning eye	X	—	—	—
Retinal detachment history	X	X	—	—
Congenital glaucoma	X	X	—	—
Pulmonary infection, including tuberculosis	X	X	—	—
Pyelonephritis	X	X	—	—
Bone infection	X	X	—	—
Systemic infection	X	X	—	—
Cardiomegaly	X	—	—	X
Aortic or mitral stenosis	X	—	—	X
Cyanotic heart disease	X	—	—	X
Active myocarditis/pericarditis	X	—	—	X
Major visceromegaly (liver, kidneys, spleen)	X	—	—	X
Solitary functional kidney	X	—	—	X
Testis overlying pubic ramus	X	—	—	—
Unhealed fracture	X	—	—	X
Spondyolisthesis with back pain	X	X	—	—
Painful hip disease	X	X	—	—
Spinal epiphysitis	X	X	—	—
Blood coagulation defect	X	—	—	X
Uncontrolled asthma	—	—	X	X
Skin infection, including herpes	X†	—	X	X
Active otitis media	—	X‡	—	—
Uncontrolled diabetes mellitus	—	—	X	X
Recurrent shoulder subluxation	—	—	X	X
Uncontrolled hypertension	—	—	X	X

Source: Reprinted by permission of W. B. Saunders from: McKeag DB: Preparticipation screening of the potential athlete. Clin Sports Med 8(3):394, 1989. Adapted from Hara JH, Puffer JC: The preparticipation physical examination. *In* Mellion MB (ed): Office Management of Sports Injuries and Athletic Problems. Philadelphia, Hanley and Belfus, 1988.

*Diving, swimming, high bar, and rings.
†Herpes simplex in wrestlers.
‡Swimming and diving.

deficiencies of the station setup for the preparticipation physical exam for collegiate athletes. The authors concluded that the station method was the most optimal mode for these types of exams, at least in collegiate athletes. They also found that musculoskeletal abnormalities and injuries were the most common reason for restriction or recommended follow-up (7). The most frequent abnormalities, however, were hypertension and visual problems, a finding supported by other studies (8). Most of these problems are easily dealt with in follow-up and rarely result in complete restriction from participation in sports.

CONDUCTING THE CARDIOVASCULAR EXAMINATION

Evaluation of the cardiovascular system deserves specific attention. The individual's medical history can be quite helpful in determining risk factors for cardiac problems, which may indicate the need for further evaluation. Certain questions have been recommended by the American College of Sports Medicine, among other professional medical associations (9). These include questions about any episodes of syncope, dizziness, chest pain either during or after exercise, history of high blood pressure or a heart murmur, dyspnea or a persistent tendency to tire more quickly than colleagues during exercise, and any palpitations or "skipped beat" during exertion. A history of any recent viral illness or use of drugs (such as cocaine or anabolic steroids) is also relevant (10), as is the presence of the usual cardiac risk factors: obesity, elevated cholesterol, diabetes mellitus, and a family history of cardiac disease and sudden death before 50 years of age. These questions can easily be added to the general history form.

The cardiac exam is particularly important. It should include blood pressure, palpation of femoral pulses, auscultation of the heart, and evaluation of possible stigmata of Marfan's syndrome (6). In general, normal blood pressure is 125/75 for individuals younger than 12 years and 135/85 for individuals 12 years of age and older. If higher values are found, blood pressure should be rechecked at least twice, perhaps in a quieter, more relaxed atmosphere. If it remains above 125/75 (under 12 years old) or 135/85 (12 years and older), further evaluation should be considered (10). The femoral artery pulses should be palpated to assess the possibility of coarctation of the aorta.

Auscultation of the heart differs from the usual examination. The athlete should sit or stand so as to eliminate any benign murmur and accentuate the splitting of the second heart sound (S2) (10). The first heart sound (S1) should be auscultated at the left sternal border; S2 should be auscultated with particular attention to the splitting, which normally occurs only during inspiration. Splitting that does not disappear during expiration suggests a delay in the closure of the pulmonic valve, possibly indicating pulmonary stenosis, atrial septal defect, mitral valve regurgitation, or right ventricular failure (11). An extra sound or "click" in systole can occur with mitral valve prolapse (MVP) (10). Auscultation of the heart at the left sternal border while the athlete changes position from squatting for 15 seconds to standing will accentuate the murmur associated with hypertrophic cardiomyopathy. This quick maneuver is useful and is advisable for all athletes, especially those younger than 30 years. Any diastolic murmur is significant and usually indicates heart disease, and this requires further evaluation (10). A systolic murmur is often considered functional if it is short and in early systole rather than holosystolic and faint (11–14).

An electrocardiogram (ECG) or echocardiogram (echo) for every athlete below the age of 30 is not cost effective, since these athletes are generally healthy and positive test results are infrequent (6). The use of an ECG for screening in asymptomatic athletes is not generally advocated, although the issue is still not resolved (15–17). An ECG is relatively inexpensive, but, on a large scale, the cost of follow-up for abnormal findings can be considerable (1). The usefulness of echo, even limited echo studies, for mandatory screening in the same population has also been explored (18–21). Abnormal test results were found in up to 10% of athletes, but further evaluation revealed no significant findings (such as hypertrophic cardiomyopathy) that would lead to restriction of exercise or involvement in sports. Older athletes (over 30 years) have different risk factors and should be screened for cardiac disease more closely, with a focus on coronary artery disease.

A general physical exam and extensive history often produce a low yield of significant cardiac abnormalities. Most of these findings are made on the basis of history (7). Nevertheless, a low threshold for further cardiac evaluation is recommended, since even the low probability of preventing a sudden cardiac event outweighs the cost (1,7).

Although the preparticipation physical exam is quite effective for discovery and management of many injuries and disorders (e.g., musculoskeletal), whether it can decrease the incidence of sudden cardiac death in athletes is unclear. One series of studies examining sudden cardiac death in athletes found that 97% of athletes who died suddenly had undergone preparticipation exams, and 14% overall were found to have cardiac abnormalities (22). Only 1% of athletes who died suddenly eventually had been restricted or disqualified from sports as a result of findings in the preparticipation exam.

EVALUATION OF CARDIAC SYMPTOMS

Syncope

Fainting, or syncope, is defined as a brief loss of consciousness, usually following a sudden decrease in cerebral blood flow. Other less common causes of syncope include hypoglycemia, seizures, or hypoxia. One of the most common causes of syncope in the athlete is dehydration and hyperthermia resulting from prolonged exercise in extreme heat. These cases can be managed with hydration and lowering body temperature (see Chapter 11).

To determine the significance of a reported episode(s) of syncope, the physician must be aware of multiple factors: the environmental conditions (temperature), the athlete's condition (last meal, hydration state), any associated symptoms, previous episodes, and whether it occurred during or after activity was completed. Chest discomfort, palpitations, or occurrence during exercise are suggestive of a possible cardiac etiology and indicate the need for further evaluation (23,24). The occurrence of multiple episodes of syncope over long periods of time is often benign, but recurrent syncope over short periods of time has a much higher possibility of association with organic heart disease (25).

Palpitations

Palpitations are usually due to premature (ectopic) beats or a bradyarrhythmia or tachyarrhythmia. Palpitations are a common symptom in the general population, including athletes. Many palpitations are benign, most commonly described as a "skipped beat," which is due to one ectopic beat. A rapid heart rate that does not resolve with rest may signify a serious tachyarrhythmia such as atrial flutter or fibrillation, supraventricular tachyarrhythmia, or ventricular tachycardia. Evaluation should include an ECG to rule out an abnormal conduction or pre-excitation. Exercise tolerance testing is often very helpful as well. Cardiac event monitoring, with patient activation during an event, is also useful (1).

Athletic Heart Syndrome

The physician who performs preparticipation exams and cares for athletes should be aware that regular exercise training often results in certain physiological changes or adaptations in the cardiovascular system that may affect the findings in the cardiac exam. In response to the increased demands (volume and pressure), the left ventricle dilates and wall thickness increases (1,26). The mass-to-volume ratio, however, does not change (21). These changes are referred to as the athletic heart syndrome (AHS) (10).

On physical examination, a heart rate of 40–60 is not uncommon in the athlete with AHS, due to a higher systolic volume. Ectopic beats or a sinus arrhythmia may also occur, but these often disappear on expiration. A questionable or significant arrhythmia should always suggest the need for further evaluation (10). During auscultation, S1 is generally normal, but S2 may remain split during expiration, with a shorter split than during inspiration (27). A third heart sound may occur, considered to be the result of a greater diastolic filling rate, as well as a fourth, the significance of which remains unclear (28). A benign systolic murmur at the base of the heart is present in up to 50% of trained athletes (29). This type of murmur should be less than a grade III/VI and should not become louder with a change in position from squatting to standing or with a Valsalva maneuver (30).

A wide range of normal variation can be seen on the ECGs of athletes with AHS. As already mentioned, sinus bradycardia and sinus arrhythmia may be present, as well as first-degree atrioventricular block and Mobitz type I atrioventricular block (Wenckebach phenomenon). Atrial arrhythmias may also occur, which may disappear upon exertion (31).

These variations are considered secondary to a physiological vagotonia, reduced sympathetic tone, and hypertrophy with training (10). Changes suggestive of left ventricular hypertrophy are common, and ST segment elevation and T-wave inversion (probably due to early repolarization) have been reported in more than 80% of endurance athletes (32). ST segment elevation and narrow T waves have been documented in up to 50% of ECGs in athletes (31,33).

The left ventricle will hypertrophy dynamically in an athlete; muscle mass may increase with training and decrease upon cessation of training after several weeks (34). Hypertrophy is symmetric, with reported increases in mass of up to 45% and wall thickness of up to 20% (35). The thickness of the ventricular wall is usually less than 13 mm, with the ratio of septal to posterior wall thickness less than 1.3:1 (35). Multiple studies have demonstrated that exercise-induced hypertrophy has no adverse effects on cardiac function (36–39). Endurance athletes tend to develop an increased chamber size of the left ventricle; power athletes (weight lifters or shot putters) may develop more wall hypertrophy from repeated isometric contractions (35). AHS may also be associated with "globular" hearts as revealed by chest radiographs (10).

MANAGEMENT OF CARDIAC CONDITIONS

Certain preexisting medical conditions in the athlete need to be addressed in order to guarantee optimal benefit from exercise with minimal risk of injury. Management of some conditions differs when dealing with an athlete rather than a more inactive person.

Many preexisting cardiac (usually valvular) abnormalities may be asymptomatic before the individual starts an exercise program, but they may pose significant risk when additional stress is placed on the heart. The 26th Bethesda Conference report (40) summarizes the present recommendations for exercise by individuals with specific cardiac or valvular defects, which will be reviewed below.

The issue of possible sudden cardiac death (SCD) in athletes often arises. Sudden death during exercise is extremely rare. Among the 25 million competitive athletes in the United States, it is estimated that only four cases of SCD occur per 1 million athletes per year (13). Sports

associated with higher levels of exertion, such as track, running, basketball, soccer, and football, have been associated with the highest incidence of sudden death in young athletes (22). The major causes of SCD
in athletes are age dependent. In athletes under 30 years, death tends to
be related to structural, usually congenital, cardiovascular anomalies
such as hypertrophic cardiomyopathy and coronary artery or valvular
abnormalities. Exercise and exertion can evoke symptoms related to
these defects. Changes in sympathetic and adrenergic stimulation during exercise alter the electrical environment of the heart, facilitating
conduction and enhancing arrhythmias. In older athletes (over 30
years), coronary artery disease is the most common cause of SCD. Intense exercise can lead to the rupture of atherosclerotic plaques, producing ischemia and electrical instability (1). Estimates of the incidence
of SCD in older athletes involved in intense activity range from 1 in
15,000 to 1 in 18,000 (41,42). The most common mechanism of SCD
may be a lethal arrhythmia, which has been demonstrated in most cardiac defects and coronary artery disease or ischemia (14,43,44). Certain
drugs, both ergogenic (anabolic steroids) and recreational (cocaine),
can also be associated with cardiac dysfunction. The danger of these
needs to be emphasized to athletes who might be involved in their use.

Hypertrophic Cardiomyopathy

In individuals between 14 and 21 years of age, 30% of all sudden, non-
traumatic deaths are cardiac related (45). One report examining exercise-related sudden deaths in a group of 29 trained athletes between 13
and 30 years of age found structural cardiac abnormalities in 97%; 14
of the athletes had hypertrophic cardiomyopathy (HCM). Other defects
included coronary artery disease, ruptured aorta, anomalous origin of
the left coronary artery, and idiopathic concentric left ventricular hypertrophy (LVH) (46).

The leading cause of SCD during exercise in the athlete under the age
of 30 years is HCM (47). The prevalence in the general population is
1 in 500 (1). HCM is a primary cardiac disease, often familial. The hallmark of HCM is a thickened left ventricular wall, greater than 13 mm,
with a normal cavity size. It may be difficult to differentiate between

mild hypertrophic cardiomyopathy and the normal left ventricular hypertrophy often found in highly conditioned athletes (48), but left ventricular wall thickness of greater than 13 mm is very uncommon in athletes. HCM presents a diagnostic challenge for the physician, since affected individuals are often asymptomatic and have normal findings on cardiac examination and ECG. The only tip-off may be a family history of sudden death at an early age.

The preparticipation exam should always include questions about the presence of symptoms associated with HCM, which include exertional dyspnea, fatigue, chest discomfort, dizziness, or history of syncope. Auscultation of the heart may be normal or reveal a systolic murmur, loudest at the left lower sternal border. The murmur intensifies with a Valsalva maneuver or with the individual's position change from squatting to standing (conversely, it softens upon squatting) (40,47). These maneuvers decrease left ventricular blood volume and thus increase the outflow obstruction resulting from HCM. Either or both of these maneuvers are useful additions to the preparticipation cardiac exam of the athlete.

No particular ECG pattern or finding is characteristic of HCM, but certain variations may be seen. These include evidence of LVH, anterior displacement of electrical forces, the absence of normal septal Q waves or presence of deep Q waves, and deeply inverted T waves (32). Of note, none of these ECG changes is associated with athletic heart syndrome. No relation exists between the ECG pattern and the prognosis.

Diagnosis is based on an echocardiograph. Criteria are hypertrophy of the left ventricle without associated dilation (although the left ventricular cavity size may be diminished) and an intraventricular or left ventricular free-wall thickness of greater than 15 mm (40). If wall thickness is between 13 and 15 mm, other criteria are needed to make the diagnosis of HCM, such as asymmetric septal or nonseptal areas of hypertrophy and possible ventricular muscle disarray (46). Diastolic dysfunction and impaired filling may be present.

Hypertrophic cardiomyopathy may present as sudden cardiac death. HCM is associated with a mortality rate of 2–4% in young adults (1). The mechanism of sudden death remains unclear but is thought to be related to primary ventricular arrhythmias, supraventricular arrhythmias with or without an accessory atrioventricular pathway, and conduction abnormalities triggered by an exertional tachycardia (47,49, 50). Obstruction of the left ventricular outflow tract or myocardial ischemia due to small intramural vessels may potentiate these arrhythmias (10). Medical treatment is recommended for any patient with symptomatic HCM, with or without documented arrhythmias. However, treatment for patients with asymptomatic HCM is still controversial. There are no conclusive data on the efficacy of drug treatment in asymptomatic patients, but some cardiologists recommend calcium channel blockers or beta-blockers for asymptomatic patients with a positive family history of premature sudden death and evidence of marked left ventricular wall thickening or subaortic obstruction revealed by echo (47).

The 26th Bethesda Conference report recommends disqualification from competitive sports of all athletes with HCM and one or more of the following characteristics:

–marked LVH (>20 mm)
–evidence of significant left ventricular outflow obstruction, revealed by cardiac catheterization or echo
–significant ventricular or atrial arrhythmia evident on ambulatory ECG
–history of SCD in a relative, especially before 50 years of age
–history of syncope

The report strongly discourages all individuals with HCM from participating in competitive sports and recommends activities such as walking, biking, swimming, and golf, if the workload is kept reasonably light (40).

Interestingly, studies have found an incidence of HCM in sudden cardiac death in young competitive athletes of up to 30% in the United States (22,46,51,52). A recent Italian study reported a low prevalence of HCM in sudden cardiac death in the same type of athletes, only 2%. The lower incidence was attributed to successful preparticipation screening, which has been implemented in Italy for more than 20 years. This study also reported the overall incidence of HCM detected in athletes during preparticipation screening as 0.07%, accounting for 3.5% of the disqualifications due to cardiovascular abnormalities. The majority of cardiovascular-based disqualifications were due to rhythm and conduction abnormalities (38.3%), followed by systemic hypertension (53).

Mitral Valve Prolapse

Mitral valve prolapse is the most common cardiac valve disorder, present in approximately 5% of the general population (54). It has been reported in up to 17% of young females (55). Although it is infrequently a cause of cardiac death in the general population, the direct association of MVP with SCD remains unclear. It has been implicated as a cause in only 60 reported cases according to one report (54). However, a later report claimed that up to 5% of cases of SCD were attributable to MVP (56).

Mitral valve prolapse is generally described as an abnormal superior and posterior displacement of the mitral valve leaflets from the left ventricle into the left atrium during systole. The distensibility of the valve leaflets is related to abnormalities in the connective tissue. Recent data support an association of MVP with overall connective tissue abnormalities in the body, including Marfan's and Ehlers-Danlos syndromes (57,58).

Auscultation may be normal or reveal a characteristic mid-systolic click (due to a tightening of the leaflets) followed by a late systolic murmur of mitral regurgitation (MR). If present, the murmur tends to soften or disappear upon squatting, which increases left ventricular volume (59). Most individuals with MVP are asymptomatic, but some may complain of chest pain, fatigue, dyspnea, or episodes of syncope.

Any individuals suspected of having MVP should undergo further evaluation. Definitive diagnosis is by echo, which also helps to classify the risk of possible complications, including thickening of the leaflets and annulus, and the extent of mitral regurgitation (59). Although an ECG is not diagnostic of MVP, it is useful to determine any conduction disturbances. The ECG may reveal primary biphasic or inverted T waves in the inferior limb leads or arrhythmias (10). Ventricular and atrial arrhythmias have been associated with MVP, although reports of the incidence vary from 23% (60) to 75% (61). Evaluation of symptomatic individuals may also include use of a Holter monitor, graded exercise stress test, or angiogram.

The 26th Bethesda Conference classified sports by both static and dynamic demands (table 1.2) and recommended certain criteria for exercise participation by individuals with MVP with or without MR (40, 62). Individuals with MVP and any of the following should participate in only low-intensity competitive sports (class 1A: low static, low dynamic):

–syncope associated with documented arrhythmia
–moderate to marked mitral regurgitation
–repetitive forms of sustained and nonsustained supraventricular arrhythmias, especially if accentuated with exercise
–family history of sudden death associated with MVP
–any prior embolic event (40,62)

Recommendations for athletes with MVP and associated MR vary. Athletes with MVP and mild MR, in normal sinus rhythm and with normal left ventricular size and function, may participate in all competitive sports. Athletes with mild left ventricular enlargement, even with normal ventricular function at rest and only mild MR, in sinus rhythm or atrial fibrillation, should participate only in low to moderate static and low to moderate dynamic sports (classes 1A, 1B, 2A, 2B; see table 1.2). Some of these athletes may also participate in high dynamic sports (class C), but they should avoid high static sports (class 3) (62,63). Exercise stress testing in athletes with atrial fibrillation can evaluate ventricular response rate to exercise. Individuals with any definitive left ventricular enlargement or impairment of ventricular function should not engage in any competitive sports. And individuals undergoing chronic anticoagulation treatment should avoid all contact sports (59).

Marfan's Syndrome

Marfan's syndrome is also associated with mitral valve prolapse. However, as a diffuse connective tissue disease, it is also associated with exercise-related sudden death secondary to ascending aortic dissection and rupture and/or arrhythmia. Marfan's syndrome should always be considered when evaluating athletes participating in basketball, which attracts tall individuals. Other skeletal abnormalities may be present,

Table 1.2. Classification of Sports by Static and Dynamic Demands

	A. Low Dynamic	B. Moderate Dynamic	C. High Dynamic

1. Low Static	Billiards
	Bowling
	Cricket
	Curling
	Golf
	Riflery
		Baseball
		Softball
		Table tennis
		Tennis (doubles)
		Volleyball
			Badminton
			Cross-country skiing
			  (classic technique)
			Field hockey*
			Orienteering
			Race walking
			Racquetball
			Running (long
			  distance)
			Soccer*
			Squash
			Tennis (singles)

2. Moderate Static	Archery
	Auto racing*†
	Diving*†
	Equestrian*†
	Motorcycling*†
		Fencing
		Field events
		  (jumping)
		Figure skating*
		Football (American)*
		Rodeo*†
		Rugby*
		Running (sprint)
		Surfing*†
		Synchronized
		  swimming†
			Basketball*
			Cross-country skiing
			  (skating technique)
			Football (Australian
			  rules)*
			Ice hockey*
			Lacrosse*
			Running (middle
			  distance)
			Swimming
			Team handball

3. High Static	Bobsledding*† Field events (throwing) Gymnastics*† Karate/Judo* Luge*† Rock climbing*† Sailboarding*† Sailing Waterskiing*† Weight lifting*†	Body building*† Downhill skiing*† Wrestling*	Boxing* Canoeing/Kayaking Cycling*† Decathlon Rowing Speed skating

Source: Reprinted with permission from: Mitchell JH, Haskell WL, Raven PB: 26th Bethesda Conference: recommendations for determining eligibility for competition in athletes with cardiovascular abnormalities. Classification of sports. Med Sci Sports Exerc 26(10, suppl):S242–S245, 1994.

*Danger of body collision.
†Increased risk if syncope occurs.

including unusually long limbs and slender fingers, hypermobile joints, and sternal deformities (63). Additional manifestations that may support the diagnosis include cutaneous striae, a high, arched palate, and myopia (due to an increased ocular globe length) (64). (Recommendations regarding exercise for those with Marfan's syndrome are made in the 26th Bethesda Conference [40,62].)

Myocarditis

Myocarditis, inflammation of the myocardium, is often associated with a viral infection, of which Coxsackie B, echovirus, adenovirus, and influenza viruses are the most common causative agents. The Coxsackie B virus has been associated with up to 50% of cases of myocarditis (13% of these cases may progress to a dilated cardiomyopathy) (65). Although SCD secondary to myocarditis is relatively rare, in one report reviewing 10 cases of myocarditis-associated SCD, exercise was considered directly related in 9 cases (66). When dealing with a younger population, the physician needs to be aware of myocarditis as a complication; this diagnosis has serious implications and should lead to at least temporary abstention from exercise (10).

Unfortunately, myocarditis can be difficult to diagnose, and restricting all individuals with a viral infection or low-grade fever from exercise is unreasonable. Most individuals with myocarditis have a subclinical disease and are relatively asymptomatic. Symptoms that should raise suspicion are a recent viral illness or fever associated with the onset of dyspnea, orthopnea, cough, or nonresolving exercise intolerance (10). Auscultation may reveal an S3 gallop or new, soft apical systolic murmur. In more compromised cases the exam may reveal evidence of left ventricular failure or a pulsus alternans. A sinus tachycardia at rest or low-voltage complexes may be present on the ECG, and the chest x-ray may show an enlarged cardiac silhouette (10). Definitive diagnosis is provided by an endocardial biopsy, but this does not need to be performed in all suspected cases. Treatment with rest, nonsteroidal anti-inflammatory drugs (NSAIDs), and occasionally steroids is often sufficient. The individual with a normal ECG, no significant arrhythmia, and normal ventricular function at rest and with exertion may be cleared to return to exercise; however, an exercise stress test, Holter monitor, or echo may be needed to make the final assessment (50). Of note, individuals with healed myocarditis may be at risk of SCD, since electrical instability may develop from scarred tissue (40). Prolonged inflammation may lead to cardiomyopathy and weakness of cardiac tissue.

Aortic Stenosis

Aortic stenosis (AS) is not considered to be a major cause of SCD, but it is a risk factor. This condition is often congenital and caused by a bileaflet valve. A harsh systolic murmur on auscultation that increases with squatting and Valsalva (the opposite of the findings in MVP and HCM) is suggestive of AS (11). An increase in left ventricular pressure during exertion can result in chest pressure or pain, dizziness, syncope, or dyspnea (1). An echo is needed to make the definitive diagnosis and determine the individual's eligibility for various forms of exercise. Individuals with mild AS and normal left ventricular function may participate in all forms of activity; those with asymptomatic moderate AS should be restricted to low-intensity exercise activities. Any individual with severe AS or symptomatic AS should avoid competitive and high-intensity exercise (67).

Aortic Regurgitation

Aortic regurgitation is a less common valvular disorder. Common causes include congenital bicuspid aortic valve, rheumatic heart disease, infectious endocarditis, and diseases associated with aortic root dissection (e.g., Marfan's syndrome) (1). However, since this disorder can be asymptomatic for decades, auscultation may be the only means of early detection. A diastolic murmur should always raise the suspicion of aortic regurgitation. Due to the decrease in the total peripheral resistance and the diastolic filling time that occurs with exercise conditioning, initially the affected athlete experiences a greater increase in the cardiac output than would be expected (68). Continued large regurgitant volumes eventually lead to left ventricular dilation, which can be irreversible. The individual becomes symptomatic when the cardiac output can no longer fulfill the blood flow demands of the body.

The 26th Bethesda Conference recommends that any individual with symptomatic aortic regurgitation, regardless of the severity of the regurgitation and left ventricular dimension, should not participate in competitive sports. Individuals with mild to moderate regurgitation and moderate ventricular enlargement may be allowed to participate in moderate static and low to high dynamic sports. Individuals with mild or moderate regurgitation and mild ventricular enlargement (which is often present in conditioned athletes) may participate in any competitive sport (69).

The decision regarding the timing of valve replacement should be based on the same criteria used for the general population, although the level of competition at which the athlete would like to participate may be a significant consideration. The type of sport may also become an issue, since athletes taking oral anticoagulation medication are discouraged from engaging in contact sports (70). Individuals who are rated at functional class 1 level following valve replacement have not been found to experience prosthetic valve dysfunction or increased hemolysis as a direct result of vigorous exercise (at 60–80% of the individual's maximal heart rate; see Chapter 2) (70). After aortic valve replacement, athletes should limit their exercise to forms rated as moderate static and low to moderate dynamic (69). They should also undergo exercise stress testing at the anticipated level of exercise intensity, as well as serial echocardiograms (68). The cardiologist should actively participate in the evaluation and decision regarding clearance for athletic activity of any individual with aortic valve regurgitation or valve replacement.

Congenital Heart Disease

Atrial septal defect, an opening in the atrial wall, produces a shunt that results in a systolic ejection murmur, best auscultated at the base of the heart. A fixed split of S2 is also characteristic. This defect may be asymptomatic during childhood, but if not corrected can result in pulmonary hypertension or arrhythmias that limit exercise tolerance. The degree of the shunt and presence of pulmonary hypertension, as well as possible arrhythmia, are best evaluated by an ECG and echo, which then determines eligibility to participate in sports (71).

Ventricular septal defect, an opening in the ventricular wall, produces a shunt, the severity of which is rated as small, moderate, or large. It produces a holosystolic murmur in the midparasternal region. With normal heart size and pulmonary artery pressure, exercise does not need to be limited (71). If a larger defect is suspected or pulmonary arterial pressure is elevated, further evaluation is necessary.

Abnormalities of the Cardiac Conducting System

Wolff-Parkinson-White syndrome is one of the more common causes of arrhythmias. It is still relatively rare, with an incidence of 15 in 10,000 in the general population. It also has a very small association with SCD (less than 0.1%) (72). In Wolff-Parkinson-White syndrome, an extra electrical pathway in the conducting system can give rise to a rapid tachycardia, which is usually symptomatic. Symptoms include palpitations, lightheadedness, and syncope. An ECG at rest reveals a slurred QRS complex upstroke, known as a delta wave. Sudden cardiac death can occur only if ventricular fibrillation occurs as a result of atrial fibrillation with rapid ventricular response. Athletes with an ECG suggestive of Wolff-Parkinson-White syndrome should be further evaluated with exercise testing and 24-hour arrhythmia monitoring (73).

Long QT syndrome is a congenital abnormality of the conducting system that is associated with a high risk of SCD. It is characterized by prolonged repolarization of the ventricle leading to life-threatening arrhythmias, usually a polymorphic tachycardia, during emotional stress and physical activity (74,75). Long QT interval, which may also lead to life-threatening arrhythmia, can also be associated with various medications and medical conditions, such as anorexia nervosa or starvation, hypothyroidism, and hypokalemia (76).

Some cardiomyopathies can also be arrhythmogenic, but many of the arrhythmias associated with SCD are idiopathic.

REFERENCES

1. Basilico FC: Cardiovascular disease in athletes. Am J Sports Med 27(1): 108–121, 1999

2. Allman FL, McKeag DB, Bodner LM: Prevention and emergency care of sports injuries. Fam Pract Recert 5:141–163, 1983

3. Lombardo JA: Pre-participation physical examination. Prim Care Clin 11:3–21, 1984

    4. McKeag DB: Preparticipation screening of the potential athlete. Clin Sports Med 8:373–397, 1989

    5. Runyan DK: The preparticipation examination of the young athlete. Clin Pediatr (Phila) 22:674–679, 1983

    6. Maron BJ, Thompson PD, Puffer JC, et al: Cardiovascular preparticipation screening examination of competitive athletes. Circulation 94:850–856, 1996

    7. Smith J, Laskowski ER: The preparticipation physical examination: Mayo Clinic experience with 2,739 examinations. Mayo Clin Proc 73:419–429, 1998

    8. Magnes SA, Henderson JM, Hunter SC: What conditions limit sports participation? Experience with 10,540 athletes. Physician and Sportsmedicine 20(5):143–158, 1992

    9. Strong WB, Steed D: Cardiovascular evaluation of the young athlete. Prim Care Clin 11:61–75, 1984

    10. Rich BSE: Sudden death screening. Med Clin North Am 78:267–288, 1994

    11. Bates B: The cardiovascular system. In A Guide to Physical Examination and History Taking. Philadelphia, JB Lippincott, 1987, 253

    12. Coyle EF: Fat metabolism during exercise. Sports Science Exchange 8:1–6, 1995

    13. Ades PA: Preventing sudden death. Physician and Sportsmedicine 20(9):75, 1992

    14. Amsterdam EA, Laslett L, Holly R: Exercise and sudden death. Cardiol Clin 5:337, 1987

    15. Fuller CM, McNulty CM, Spring DA, et al: Prospective screening of 5,615 high school athletes for risk of sudden cardiac death. Med Sci Sports Exerc 29:1131–1138, 1997

    16. LaCorte MA, Boxer RA, Gottsfield IB, et al: EKG screening program for school athletes. Clin Cardiol 12:42–44, 1989

    17. Ryan MP, Cleland JG, French JA, et al: The standard electrocardiogram as a screening test for hypertrophic cardiomyopathy. Am J Cardiol 76:689–694, 1995

    18. Feinsteing RA, Colvin E, Oh MK: Echocardiographic screening as part of a preparticipation examination. Clin J Sport Med 3:149–152, 1993

    19. Lewis JF, Maron BJ, Diggs JA, et al: Preparticipation echocardiographic screening for cardiovascular disease in a large, predominantly black population of collegiate athletes. Am J Cardiol 64:1029–1033, 1989

    20. Murry PM, Cantwell JD, Heath DL, et al: The role of limited echocardiography in screening athletes. Am J Cardiol 76:849–850, 1995

    21. Weidenbener EJ, Krauss MD, Waller BF, et al: Incorporation of screening echocardiography in the preparticipation exam. Clin J Sport Med 5:86–89, 1995

    22. Maron BJ, Sharani J, Poliac LC, et al: Sudden death in young competitive athletes: clinical, demographic, and pathological profiles. JAMA 276:199–204, 1996

23. Kapoor WN: Evaluation and management of the patient with syncope. JAMA 268:2553–2560, 1992

24. Manolis AS, Linzer M, Salem D, et al: Syncope: current diagnostic evaluation and management. Ann Intern Med 112:850–863, 1990

25. Calkins H, Shyr Y, Frumin H, et al: The value of the clinical history in the differentiation of syncope due to ventricular tachycardia, atrioventricular block, and neurocardiogenic syncope. Am J Med 98:365–373, 1995

26. Huston TP, Puffer JC, Rodney WM: The athletic heart syndrome. N Engl J Med 313:24–32, 1985

27. Harvey WP, Knowlan DM: Techniques of clinical cardiovascular evaluation, with special emphasis on examination of athletes. *In* Waller BF, Harvey WP (eds): Cardiovascular Evaluation of Athletes: Toward Recognizing Young Athletes at Risk of Sudden Death. Newton, NJ, Laennec Publishing, 1993, 31

28. George KP, Wolfe LA, Burggraf GW: The "athletic heart syndrome." Sports Med 11:300, 1991

29. Huston TP, Puffer JC, Rodney WM: The athletic heart syndrome. N Engl J Med 313:24, 1985

30. Cantwell JD: The athlete's heart syndrome. Int J Cardiol 17:1–6, 1987

31. Wight JN Jr, Salem D: Sudden cardiac death and the "athlete's heart." Arch Intern Med 155:1473–1480, 1995

32. Zeppilli P: The athlete's heart: differentiation of training effects from organic heart disease. Pract Cardiol 14:61, 1988

33. Zehender M, Meinertz T, Keul J, et al: ECG variants and cardiac arrhythmias in athletes: clinical relevance and prognostic importance. Am Heart J 119:1378–1391, 1990

34. Martin WH III, Coyle EF, Bloomfield SA, et al: Effects of physical deconditioning after intense endurance training on left ventricular dimensions and stroke volume. J Am Coll Cardiol 7:982–989, 1986

35. Maron BJ: Structural features of the athlete heart as defined by echocardiography. J Am Coll Cardiol 7:190–203, 1986

36. Finkelhor RS, Hanak LJ, Bahler RC: Left ventricular filling in endurance-trained subjects. J Am Coll Cardiol 8:289–293, 1986

37. Granger CB, Karimeddini MK, Smith V-E, et al: Rapid ventricular filling in left ventricular hypertrophy. I. Physiologic hypertrophy. J Am Coll Cardiol 5:862–868, 1985

38. Colan SD, Sanders SP, MacPherson D, et al: Left ventricular diastolic function in elite athletes in physiological cardiac hypertrophy. J Am Coll Cardiol 6:545–549, 1985

39. Maron BJ: Sudden death in young athletes: lessons from the Hank Gathers affair. N Engl J Med 329:55–57, 1993

40. Maron BJ, Isner JM, McKenna WJ: Task Force 3: hypertrophic cardiomyopathy, myocarditis and other myopericardial diseases and mitral valve prolapse. *In* Maron BJ, Mitchell JH (eds): 26th Bethesda Conference: recom-

mendations for determining eligibility for competition in athletes with cardio-vascular abnormalities. J Am Coll Cardiol 24:880–885, 1994

41. Siscovick DS, Weiss NS, Fletcher RH, et al: The incidence of primary cardiac arrest during vigorous exercise. N Engl J Med 311:874–877

42. Thompson PD, Funk EJ, Carleton RA, et al: Incidence of death during jogging in Rhode Island from 1975 through 1980. JAMA 247:2535–2538, 1982

43. Lown B: Sudden cardiac death: the major challenge confronting contemporary cardiology. Am J Cardiol 43:313, 1979

44. Maron BJ, Epstein SE, Roberts WC: Causes of sudden cardiac death in competitive athletes. J Am Coll Cardiol 7:204, 1986

45. Oppenheim EB: Sudden cardiac death: what primary care providers need to know. Residents and Staff Physicians 35:97, 1989

46. Maron BJ, Roberts WC, McAllister HA: Sudden death in young athletes. Circulation 62:218, 1980

47. Maron BJ: Hypertrophic cardiomyopathy in athletes. Physician and Sportsmedicine 21(9):83–91, 1993

48. Maron BJ, Pelliccia A, Spirito P: Cardiac disease in young trained athletes: insights into methods for distinguishing athlete's heart from structural heart disease, with particular emphasis on hypertrophic cardiomyopathy. Circulation 91:1596–1601, 1995

49. Fananapazir L, Chang AC, Epstein SE, et al: Prognostic determinants in hypertrophic cardiomyopathy. Circulation 86:730, 1992

50. Maron BJ, Fananapazir L: Sudden cardiac death in hypertrophic cardiomyopathy. Circulation 85:1–57, 1992

51. Burke AP, Farb A, Virmani R, Goodin J, Smialek JE: Sports-related and non-sports related sudden cardiac death in young adults. Am Heart J 121:568–575, 1991

52. Van Camp SP, Bloor CM, Mueller FO, Cantu RC, Olson HG: Non-traumatic sports death in high school and college athletes. Med Sci Sports Exerc 27:641–647, 1995

53. Corrado D, Basso C, Schiavon M, Thiene G: Screening for hypertrophic cardiomyopathy in young athletes. N Engl J Med 339:362–369, 1998

54. Jeresaty RM: Mitral valve prolapse: definition and implications in athletes. J Am Coll Cardiol 7:231, 1986

55. Savage DD, Garrison RJ, Devereux RB, et al: Mitral valve prolapse in the general population. 1. Epidemiologic features: the Framingham Study. Am Heart J 106:571–576, 1983

56. Deveraux RB: Mitral valve prolapse. J Am Med Women's Assoc 49:192–196, 1994

57. Pocock WA, Bosman CK, Chester E, et al: Sudden death in primary mitral valve prolapse. Am Heart J 107:378–382, 1984

58. Boudoulas H, Kolibash AJ Jr, Baker P, et al: Mitral valve prolapse and the

mitral valve prolapse syndrome: a diagnostic classification and pathogenesis of symptoms. Am Heart J 118:796–818, 1989

59. Joy E: Mitral valve prolapse in active patients. Physician and Sportsmedicine 24(7):78–86, 1996

60. Kavey RW, Sondheimer HM, Blackman MS: Detection of dysrhythmia in pediatric patients with mitral valve prolapse. Circulation 62:582–587, 1980

61. Winkle RA, Lopes MG, Fitzgerald JW, et al: Arrhythmias in patients with mitral valve prolapse. Circulation 52:73–81, 1975

62. Mitchell JH, Haskell WL, Raven PB: 26th Bethesda Conference: recommendations for determining eligibility for competition in athletes with cardiovascular abnormalities. Classification of sports. Med Sci Sports Exerc 26:S242–S245, 1994

63. Maron BJ: Structural features of the athlete heart as defined by echocardiography. J Am Coll Cardiol 10:1214, 1987

64. Fahrenbach MC, Thompson PD: The preparticipation sports examination. Cardiol Clin 10:319–328, 1992

65. Bresler MJ: Acute pericarditis and myocarditis. Emerg Med 24:35, 1992

66. McCaffrey FM, Braden DS, Strong WB: Sudden cardiac death in young athletes. Am J Dis Child 145:177, 1991

67. Cheitlin MD, Bonow RO, Parmley WW, et al: Task Force II: acquired valvular heart disease. J Am Coll Cardiol 6:1209, 1985

68. O'Connor FG, Levy WS, Oriscello RG, Wilder RP: Asymptomatic aortic insufficiency in a runner. Physician and Sportsmedicine 23(10):32–42, 1995

69. Cheitlin MD, Douglas PS, Parmley WW: Task Force 2: acquired valvular heart disease. In Maron BJ, Mitchell JH (eds): 26th Bethesda Conference: recommendations for determining eligibility for competition in athletes with cardiovascular abnormalities. J Am Coll Cardiol 24:874–880, 1994

70. Landry F, Habel C, Desaulniers D, et al: Vigorous physical training after aortic valve replacement: analysis of 10 patients. Am J Cardiol 53:562–566, 1984

71. Graham TP Jr, Bricker JT, James FW, et al: Task Force 1: congenital heart disease. In Maron BJ, Mitchell JH (eds): 26th Bethesda Conference: recommendations for determining eligibility for competition in athletes with cardiovascular abnormalities. J Am Coll Cardiol 24:867–873, 1994

72. Wight JN Jr, Salem D: Sudden death in athletes. Sports Med 18:375–383, 1994

73. Zipes DP, Garson A Jr: Task Force 6: Arrhythmias. In Maron BJ, Mitchell JH (eds): 26th Bethesda Conference: recommendations for determining eligibility for competition in athletes with cardiovascular abnormalities. J Am Coll Cardiol 24:892–899, 1994

74. Tan HL, Hou CJ, Lauer MR, et al: Electrophysiologic mechanisms of the long QT interval syndromes and torsades de pointes. Ann Intern Med 122:701–714, 1995

75. Ackerman MJ: The long QT syndrome: ion channel diseases of the heart. Mayo Clin Proc 73:250–269, 1998

76. Moss AJ, Behnorin J: QT interval prolongation: basic considerations and clinical consequences. *In* Braunwald E (ed): Heart Disease: A Textbook of Cardiovascular Medicine—Updates. Philadelphia, WB Saunders, 1993, 1–9

Chapter 2

PREEXISTING
MEDICAL CONDITIONS

CORONARY ARTERY DISEASE

In athletes older than 30 years, coronary artery disease (CAD) is the most common cause of sudden cardiac death (SCD). Other less frequent causes include valvular defects, conduction system disease, and hypertrophic cardiomyopathy (1). Data combining the results of several studies demonstrated the presence of CAD in 80% of cases of sudden exercise-induced death in athletes older than 35 years (2). One report found that a significant number of the individuals were aware of their disease or had experienced symptoms before their deaths. Clearly, for individuals over the age of 30 years who actively exercise, educating them about prodromal symptoms of CAD is one of the most important functions of the sports physician.

Screening of these older athletes is more complicated than the screening of high school and collegiate athletes. Many clinicians recommend at least a resting ECG in all individuals older than 35 years who plan to exercise. Cardiac risk factors, such as high cholesterol level, hypertension, history of smoking, obesity, postmenopause (for women), and a strong family history of cardiac disease, should be evaluated in the context of the planned exercise regimen. The American College of Sports Medicine specifically recommends an exercise stress test for any individual with one or two risk factors, for all men over 40 and women over 50 years old who do not seem to have any risk factors, and for any individuals with cardiac, pulmonary, or metabolic disease (3). Many cardiologists would also add to this list individuals with an abnormal ECG, especially if they have any personal history of chest discomfort during exertion, nausea, dizziness, or general fatigue (1). In addition, the physician should reassess these risk factors or assess the onset of new symptoms yearly and should repeat exercise stress tests for patients with significant risk factors, perhaps every other year for those under the age of 55 years and every year for older patients (1).

Not all cardiologists agree with performing an exercise stress test on individuals solely on the basis of age. The high rate of false-positive results in exercise stress tests, which may be as high as 10% in physically active individuals, must always be taken into account in interpreting test results (4). The predictive value is also often questionable for individuals without symptoms or risk factors, since long-term studies have not always found a correlation between positive results on exercise tests and myocardial infarctions or SCD (5,6). A positive test result should be followed by an exercise thallium scintigraphy test to detect any myocardial perfusion defect (7).

For individuals with documented ischemic disease, the exercise stress test can be an important noninvasive means of assessing the extent of underlying disease and the extent to which it might limit exercise intensity or duration. Variables associated with more severe disease or a worse prognosis include the presence of ischemic ST depression at a low workload, limitation of exercise duration by symptoms, and hypotension during exercise (8). The 16th Bethesda Conference recommends that individuals with ischemic heart disease and any of the following conditions engage in only low-intensity exercise:

–reduced systolic left ventricular capacity at rest
–ventricular tachycardia during or after exercise
–reduced systolic blood pressure during exercise testing
–decreased exercise tolerance (depending on age) (9)

Individuals with ischemic cardiac disease and with the following findings on the exercise stress test are considered at lower risk and able to participate in low-intensity competitive sports (but they should avoid high-intensity sports):

–normal left ventricular function and normal exercise capacity
–no ischemia during exercise or only with a high level of exercise
–no evidence of ventricular tachycardia during the stress test (9)

The exercise stress test can also be useful for evaluating possible arrhythmias. Certain arrhythmias are not uncommon in athletes, such as ventricular premature beats, sinus arrhythmias, and first-degree atrioventricular block, and thus do not require further evaluation in otherwise healthy and asymptomatic individuals (10,11). Individuals who presently exercise or plan on starting an exercise program and have a history of symptoms such as syncope, near-syncope, or dizziness should have a thorough workup, probably including an exercise stress test, to help evaluate the possibility of exercise-induced arrhythmia (12).

The risk of cardiac death in the general population may be reduced by an appropriate exercise program. Individuals in their 50s who have previously been sedentary can improve their cardiovascular health by participating in aerobic exercise. They should begin with brisk walking and slowly progress (over several months) to jogging. Swimming and bicycling are alternative forms of exercise to improve cardiovascular fitness. Sports involving intermittent bursts of strenuous activity, such as racquetball, tennis, or basketball, may not be appropriate for the individual with possible cardiac disease. Regardless of the form of exercise, one simple means of maintaining appropriate cardiovascular conditioning is to maintain a heart rate between 65% and 85% of the maximal heart rate. The maximal heart rate is more accurately determined by an exercise stress test, but a rough estimate can be obtained by subtracting the age in years from 220. This equation is not accurate for well-conditioned individuals. An exercise heart-rate monitor is an excellent and affordable tool that allows athletes of all levels to optimize their conditioning programs.

Individuals with documented cardiac disease should not be completely discouraged from exercise. They should exercise under supervised conditions initially, possibly with continuous cardiac monitoring, and slowly increase their workload until the physician can clear them to exercise on their own. Any individual who has several risk factors and has previously been sedentary may benefit from a cardiac rehabilitation program (1).

HYPERTENSION

Diagnosis and Nonpharmacological Management

Hypertension is the most common cardiovascular disorder in competitive athletes (13). It is present in 1–2.5% of all teenagers (14), and the incidence increases exponentially with age to almost one-third of individuals over 65 years of age (15). Although hypertension may be associated with SCD and arrhythmias, if managed properly it should not be an absolute contraindication to exercise. The World Hypertension League advocates the use of exercise alone or with an antihypertensive medication (16).

The sports physician should measure blood pressure in all athletes during their yearly or preparticipation physical exam. Blood pressure above 125/75 for children under 12 years and 135/85 for individuals 12 years of age and older is generally considered abnormal. Measurements above these levels (unless already controlled by an antihypertensive medication) need to be documented three times before a diagnosis of hypertension is made. Blood pressure between 135 and 150 systolic and 85 and 95 diastolic is considered borderline hypertension and should be monitored (it may decrease with exercise). Individuals with persistent hypertension should be evaluated for any secondary causes and end-organ damage.

Although the vast majority (almost 95%) of patients with hypertension have essential hypertension, secondary causes, especially in the younger population, must be considered. These include hyperthyroidism, renal artery stenosis, renal disease, and pheochromocytoma, among others. The physician should keep in mind that external factors may also be present, including the use of an androgen or growth hormone, erythropoietin, excessive alcohol, or illicit drugs (e.g., cocaine, amphetamines) (17). The examination should include a thorough history and physical exam, urinalysis, a resting ECG, and blood tests including glucose, creatinine, electrolytes, hematocrit, and serum cholesterol (13). Any abnormality requires referral for further workup. Additional testing, such as an echocardiogram or exercise stress test, is not necessarily indicated unless the patient has symptoms of ischemia or other cardiac risk factors. As always, this decision needs to be made on an individual basis.

In normotensive individuals, the initiation of exercise produces a rapid heart rate due to a reduction in vagal tone, followed by an increase in sympathetic tone (which may already be present from the initial "anticipation" of exercise) and in circulating catecholamines (18). All these factors combine to increase the systolic blood pressure by 50–70 mm Hg, while the diastolic blood pressure remains constant or may decrease by 4–8 mm Hg. The cardiac output, 5–6 liters per minute (L/min) at rest, increases to as high as 20–25 L/min during peak exercise, depending on the workload and the exercise demand (18). With static exercise (unlike dynamic exercise), no change in peripheral resistance occurs. Regular exercise results in left ventricular hypertrophy, but this does not affect diastolic function and cardiac output (19–21).

At rest, the cardiovascular system of hypertensive patients exhibits an above-normal total peripheral resistance (TPR) and normal or below-normal stroke volume. During exercise, TPR increases further, leading to a subnormal increase in both heart rate and stroke volume (22). The result is a limited cardiac output and a lower anaerobic threshold (23–27). The standard measure for describing maximal exercise performance is the maximal oxygen consumption (Vo_{2max}), defined as the maximal oxygen utilization that occurs just before metabolism switches to anaerobic energy sources. It reflects the efficiency of energy utilization. The limiting factor in an individual's Vo_{2max} is the cardiovascular component of the body's oxygen-transport system (28). An abnormally elevated TPR may also contribute to a lower anaerobic threshold at the level of the muscle cell by further limiting the oxygen delivery (29). Estimates suggest a reduction in exercise capacity of up to 30% in hypertensive individuals compared with age-matched controls (25,27,30–32). The pathological left ventricular hypertrophy that may develop over time with regular exercise also contributes to a lower cardiac output, because of stiff, noncompliant left ventricular walls (17). Interestingly, although the exercise blood pressure in untreated hypertensive individuals may be much higher than in normotensive individuals, the absolute change in blood pressure between resting and exercise is similar (30).

On average, long-term cardiovascular or endurance training can result in a reduction of 10 mm Hg in resting systolic and diastolic blood pressure in cases of mild hypertension, with reductions of up to 25 mm Hg in systolic blood pressure in some individuals (16). Although the antihypertensive effect of endurance training is well accepted, the hemodynamic mechanism remains to be established (16). These data have led the American College of Sports Medicine to recommend endurance training as a nonpharmacological means of reducing the incidence of hypertension in susceptible individuals. Cases of newly diagnosed mild or borderline hypertension, without evidence of target-organ damage, can be initially managed nonpharmacologically with an appropriate cardiovascular exercise program (see below) and dietary changes for weight loss and salt restriction. Whether to add medication depends on the success of these blood-pressure control measures.

Hypertensive individuals should be encouraged to start or continue exercise; it is safe and has a beneficial effect on blood pressure. For individuals with moderate hypertension, the choice of the antihypertensive agent is key. The goal is not only to control the blood pressure both at rest and during exercise but also to prevent any adverse effect on physical performance. Antihypertensives that work by decreasing TPR seem to have the least effect on exercise performance (table 2.1).

Pharmacological Control of Hypertension

Calcium Channel Blockers

Calcium channel blockers are antihypertensive agents that work primarily by reducing TPR without diminishing the cardiac index, making them a good choice for the hypertensive athlete (22). These agents are associated with a mild negative inotropic effect, but this effect is not usually clinically important to the non-elite athlete at the usual doses used to manage essential hypertension (33). Verapamil and diltiazem are generally preferred over nifedipine, because they are better at reducing systolic blood pressure and increasing cardiac index during exercise, most likely due to less sympathetic stimulation (22,34). Some of the newer calcium channel blockers may prove superior for the athlete, but the data are not yet conclusive.

Angiotensin-Converting Enzyme Inhibitors

Angiotensin-converting enzyme (ACE) inhibitors also reduce TPR. Captopril and enalapril have been shown to decrease blood pressure without an associated increase in sympathetic activity or tachycardia, allowing for a more normalized response to exercise (22,35). One study demonstrated a 12% reduction in submaximal endurance-exercise performance in hypertensive patients treated with enalapril (36). This may be an undesirable side effect in the competitive endurance athlete. Data on the effect of the selective ACE II inhibitors on exercise are not available, although the better side-effect profile is attractive.

Alpha-Inhibitors and Diuretics

Alpha-1-adrenergic blocking agents (alpha-inhibitors; alpha-agonists) have not been studied very extensively in the hypertensive athlete, although one study of doxazosin illustrated a moderate decrease in maximal oxygen consumption and thus in physical endurance capacity (37), and a study of prazosin did not show any change in endurance parameters (38). Presently there are no data on the long-term effect of treatment with diuretics in the athlete. Short-term treatment with diuretics was shown to decrease both the maximal exercise capacity and the duration of prolonged submaximal exercise (39). In comparisons of clonidine with atenolol in acute exercise response and overall conditioning, clonidine was shown to produce a minimal effect on endurance time and an overall improvement in Vo_{2max} (as expected) with conditioning and therefore was considered better than atenolol for controlling hypertension in athletes (40).

Beta-Blockers

Beta-adrenergic blocking agents (beta-blockers; beta-agonists) are notorious for their unfavorable negative inotropic and chronotropic ef-

Table 2.1. A Profile of Common Antihypertensive Medications: Mechanism of Action, Adverse Effects, and Effects on Aerobic Capacity

Class	Agents	Mechanism of Action	Adverse Effects	Effects on Aerobic Capacity
Angiotensin-converting enzyme (ACE) inhibitors	Benazepril hydrochloride Captopril Enalapril maleate Lisinopril Quinapril hydrochloride	Prevent production of angiotensin II, a potent vasoconstrictor	Cough, renal dysfunction, hyperkalemia	None
Calcium channel blockers	Amlodipine Diltiazem hydrochloride Isradipine Verapamil hydrochloride Nifedipine	Decrease vascular smooth muscle contractility; cause negative inotropic and chronotropic effects on myocardium	Bradycardia, constipation, peripheral edema; for short-acting dihydropyridines, increased cardiac mortality	None
Alpha-1-receptor blockers	Doxazosin mesylate Terazosin Prazosin	Cause decreased vascular contractility by blocking alpha-1 receptors in smooth muscle	Orthostatic hypotension, tachycardia	None
Central alpha-receptor antagonists	Clonidine hydrochloride	Act on CNS alpha-2 receptors to block sympathetic stimulation	Many CNS effects, including dry mouth, dizziness, sedation; postexercise hypotension	None, but poor first-line choice because of CNS effects and risk of post-exercise hypotension

Beta-blockers*			
Nonselective	Propranolol hydrochloride Nadolol	Block cardiac beta-receptors, leading to decreased heart rate, myocardial contractility, and cardiac output	Bradycardia, depression, exacerbation of asthma, and impotence	Decreased aerobic capacity
Cardioselective	Atenolol Metoprolol Labetalol hydrochloride	Same as above (except labetalol has beta-1, beta-2, and alpha-1 blocking activity)	Bradycardia, depression, and impotence	None
Diuretics[†]	Hydrochlorothiazide Furosemide	Decreased circulatory volume	Hypokalemia, hyponatremia, volume depletion, dehydration	None directly, but adverse effects are accentuated by athletic activity
Angiotensin receptor blockers	Losartan potassium Valsartan	Block angiotensin II receptor size, preventing vasoconstriction	Renal dysfunction, hyperkalemia. (No cough, however.)	None

Source: Used with permission of McGraw-Hill, Inc., from: MacKnight JM: Hypertension in athletes and active patients. Physician and Sportsmedicine 27(4):35–44, 1999.

*Beta-blockers are banned by the International Olympic Committee (IOC) and the National Collegiate Athletic Association (NCAA) for competitors in archery and riflery.
[†]Diuretics are banned by the IOC and NCAA; in addition to being used in rapid weight loss, they have been implicated in attempts to enhance the renal clearance of anabolic steroids.

fects, especially during exercise. When exercise is prolonged, even at a submaximal level, endurance time and aerobic power (or Vo_{2max}) are reduced by up to 50% (16). These agents may also predispose the athlete to dehydration and hyperthermia (41). Several studies have shown that beta-1-selective agents, such as atenolol, diminish these effects, probably allowing greater blood flow to exercising muscles (since beta-2 receptors mediate peripheral arteriolar vasodilation and glycogenolysis) (41–46). One study even found no significantly different effect on exercise capacity between atenolol and diltiazem-SR (a calcium channel blocker) (47).

Although beta-blockers are not considered the preferred antihypertensive agents for athletes, individuals who have coronary artery disease and are treated with beta-blockers can still improve their cardiorespiratory fitness with exercise (41). The negative inotropic and chronotropic effects of beta-blockers, by diminishing myocardial oxygen requirements, may actually enhance the exercise tolerance in individuals with effort-induced ischemia.

Athletes with hypertension are generally advised that the preferred endurance activities for improving cardiovascular status are running, cycling, swimming, and cross-country skiing (16). Training intensity can be monitored either by perceived exertion (e.g., conversation is possible during mild and moderate exercise) or by measuring heart rate (16). Hypertensive individuals have usually been discouraged from participating in weight lifting or weight training, because of the possibility that an exaggerated rise in blood pressure in the already hypertensive athlete increases the risk of stroke or arrhythmia (48). Although weight lifting does subject an individual to repeated peaks of elevated pressure (possibly up to 320/250 [49]), no evidence suggests an increased cardiac morbidity among these athletes (30). Strength training may lead to an overall decrease in blood pressure (16), fewer ischemic events, and fewer ECG changes in patients with coronary artery disease (50–55). In fact, circuit training may be a good option for hypertensive individuals who are just beginning exercise. Circuit training is a form of strength training in which the athlete performs multiple weight-lifting exercises with moderate weight loads and frequent repetitions. The athlete moves quickly from one exercise to the next, which promotes increased muscle strength and cardiovascular endurance—an attractive combination for many individuals (49). Resistance training can decrease blood pressure if performed regularly using weights of 40–50% of a one-repetition maximum (56–58).

Individuals who have mild to moderate hypertension without any evidence of target-organ damage or concomitant heart disease do not need to limit the type of exercise they perform (13). The blood pressure should be remeasured every 2–4 months to monitor the effect of the exercise. Individuals with severe hypertension should avoid high static and competitive sports. In the absence of any target-organ damage, these athletes should be allowed to participate in competitive sports without restriction, once blood pressure is controlled by lifestyle modification or medication. For individuals with hypertension and cardiac disease or other organ involvement or disease, the eligibility for competitive sports is usually based on the type and severity of the other conditions (13).

DIABETES MELLITUS

Diabetes mellitus, both insulin-dependent (IDDM; type I) and non-insulin-dependent (NIDDM; type II), is another common preexisting condition the sports physician must manage. Individuals who are diabetic should be encouraged to exercise, since the benefits far outweigh the risks. Athletes with diabetes must be willing to take an active role in the management of their disease, working closely with the physician.

In both healthy and diabetic individuals, exercise increases body sensitivity to insulin in proportion to the level of physical fitness. This is most likely a result of several factors, including enhanced blood flow; increased activity of muscle enzymes, including glycogen synthetase; and a change in body composition, with a shift from adipose tissue to muscle protein (59).

Even healthy subjects are not always able to achieve euglycemia during exercise, although trained athletes more easily maintain a steady blood glucose (60). The metabolic effects of insulin include inhibition of liver glycogenolysis, gluconeogenesis, and lipolysis, basic metabolic processes that produce glucose and free fatty acids (FFAs). In healthy individuals, insulin secretion is suppressed during exercise in order to allow hepatic release of glucose and FFAs, thus providing a constant energy source and preventing profound hypoglycemia. Increased secretion of glucagon and catecholamines also contributes to the increased availability of glucose and FFAs to the muscles (61). Exercise also enhances muscle sensitivity to the effect of insulin, allowing for an increased uptake of glucose without a change in insulin concentration.

The risk of hypoglycemia during exercise is greater for individuals with IDDM than for those with NIDDM. In IDDM, excess insulin, often present in individuals with tightly controlled glucose levels, could potentially lead to enhanced insulin effects and profound hypoglycemia. Insufficient insulin during exercise, which can occur in an individual with poorly controlled blood glucose, can result in rapid hyperglycemia and ketosis (61). The exogenous insulin dose appropriate for an individual who does not participate in a regular exercise regimen is often excessive when physical activity is increased, so the athlete needs to decrease the insulin dose in anticipation of increased physical activity. In addition, exercise of greater duration or greater intensity requires additional lowering of the dose. The modification of the insulin dose must be altered to suit the individual, based on his specific response, the type, length, and intensity of exercise, and the time of day (62). Ingestion of carbohydrate-rich food during prolonged activity is also helpful (63).

The site of the insulin injection may also play a role in hypoglycemia in the physically active diabetic. For the individual at rest, absorption from an abdominal injection is usually faster than from the extremities. With exercise, absorption of insulin from an injection in an extremity may vary, often increasing. Therefore, the abdomen is recommended as the best site for insulin injection before activity because of the more reliable absorption pattern (61).

The risk for hypoglycemia increases during the 6–14 hours following vigorous or prolonged physical activity (64). Increased glucose uptake, glycogen synthesis, and insulin sensitivity, all induced by exercise, persist after exercise is completed. Because muscle tends to replenish glycogen more quickly than does liver tissue, carbohydrate requirements are often increased for up to 24 hours, especially following prolonged activity (63). The post-exercise insulin regimen and caloric intake must take these effects into consideration to avoid the possibility of nocturnal hypoglycemia (61). Exercising earlier in the day may help minimize the risk of exercise indu..d hypoglycemia (65). Careful post-exercise glucose monitoring is critical.

Individuals with poorly controlled IDDM who increase their level of physical activity are at risk for hyperglycemia, ketosis, and acidosis. The lack of insulin during exercise results in an increased hepatic release of glucose and production of ketones (probably due to increased lipolysis), coupled with impaired glucose uptake by muscles (62). The presence of urinary ketones prior to exercise usually suggests the potential for this complication (61).

Non-insulin-dependent diabetes mellitus is characterized by an impaired response to insulin at the level of the receptor. Treatment usually includes alteration in dietary intake, a program of weight loss, and oral hypoglycemic agents. Exogenous insulin is not usually needed unless other management strategies have failed. Exercise has become a highly recommended adjunct to management of NIDDM, since it increases the body's sensitivity to insulin and decreases obesity, resulting in better overall control of serum glucose (61). Hypoglycemia during exercise is infrequent, because endogenous insulin and its effect (glycogen synthesis) can still decrease in NIDDM, although at less effective levels than normal. Regular exercise may also allow the individual to reduce the dose of a hypoglycemic agent. The athlete with NIDDM who uses exogenous insulin for control of serum glucose runs the same type of risks as the athlete with IDDM (61). Occasionally, mildly symptomatic hypoglycemia can occur in individuals with NIDDM who are taking oral hypoglycemics if the exercise activity is prolonged, such as a five-hour round of golf.

For every individual with diabetes mellitus who is starting a new exercise regimen, the physician should take a complete history and perform a physical exam. Because of the high incidence of silent ischemia and heart disease in people with diabetes, a stress test is recommended for all individuals over 35 years and for those of any age who have had diabetes for more than 10 years (66,67). Autonomic neuropathy may result in an impaired cardiovascular response to exercise, which can also be detected in an exercise stress test (61). These individuals tend to have difficulty with aerobic exercise because of an elevated baseline heart rate and an inability to increase their heart rate appropriately upon exertion. Autonomic neuropathy is suggested by heat intolerance, impotence, dependent edema, and inability to recognize hypoglycemia (68); post-exercise hypotension may also occur—all of which place these individuals at a higher risk of cardiac ischemia (69). More specific evidence for autonomic neuropathy includes resting tachycardia, drop in blood pressure by more than 20–30 mm Hg after standing for 2 minutes, and no pupillary dilation in darkness (68).

Evaluation for peripheral neuropathy, as evidenced by decreased deep tendon reflexes, sensation, or proprioception, is important. If this is detected, the individual should be advised to avoid activities involving running or repetitive impact on the lower limbs. Swimming or bicycling may be a better choice for aerobic conditioning. All diabetic athletes should be made aware of the possibility of peripheral neuropathy and should inspect their feet regularly and carefully, especially if they run or walk regularly (61). Shoe wear should be chosen carefully for good cushioning and fit.

Preexisting proliferative retinopathy may lead to either retinal or vitreous hemorrhage with a sudden increase in blood pressure, which may occur during weight lifting or isometric training (62). Affected individuals should avoid heavy resistance training, but they may continue with a muscle-resistance program using a low-resistance weight coupled with a higher-repetition program. Rapid correction of chronic hyperglycemia may result in an abrupt worsening of retinopathy (70). Joint flexibility may be limited, and the incidence of adhesive capsulitis in multiple joints is higher in diabetics, especially those with a long history of poorly controlled blood glucose. Capsulitis may be due to glycosylation of collagen and can be detected by an inability to fully oppose the fingers when hands are placed palm-to-palm in a prayer position (70). These individuals need to include stretching in their exercise regimen, with good warm-up and cooldown.

The extent of change in serum glucose level and insulin requirements during exercise cannot be precisely predicted, so blood glucose monitoring before, during, and after exercise is critical. A log to record these measurements, along with the type and length of exercise, level of exertion, amount of insulin required, as well as any symptoms, can be useful in helping to predict requirements for any type of conditioning. The athlete with diabetes must be willing to comply with a regimen of multiple blood glucose measurements, at least at the initiation of the exercise regimen and periodically, thereafter and self-monitoring of any hypoglycemic symptoms. Because the sympathetic response to hypoglycemia in long-term diabetes may become impaired, the usual warning signs of impending hypoglycemia (i.e., diaphoresis, tremulousness, weakness) may be absent, thus placing the individual at risk of sudden and severe hypoglycemia (61).

A gradual increase in aerobic exercise over a period of several weeks is recommended, thus allowing for gradual adjustment to increased insulin sensitivity. Daily exercise is best, which will help avoid large day-to-day adjustments in the insulin dosage (61). Certain other general strategies may be useful, such as timing the insulin dose so as to avoid peak activity of the insulin during exercise. Short-acting insulin taken in multiple doses during the day allows greater flexibility in altering dosage. In general, the dose of short-acting insulin should be decreased by 30% for exercise activity lasting less than 1 hour, 40% for activity lasting between 1 and 2 hours, and 50% for activity lasting longer than 3 hours. Again, monitoring blood glucose during prolonged activity is advised. For individuals using an insulin pump, a 50% reduction in the basal rate of insulin 1–2 hours before exercise and during exercise is recommended (68). Individuals using a sulfonylurea oral agent may also need to decrease dosage as insulin sensitivity increases with regular exercise. Interestingly, other oral agents are less likely to contribute to exercise-induced hypoglycemia. If the athlete has elevated pre-exercise serum glucose or ketonuria, exercise should be deferred (61). During the initial stages of exercise, checking serum glucose at 1 or 2 A.M. may help prevent post-exercise late-onset hypoglycemia (61). Adequate hydration is critical, since dehydration can affect blood glucose and cardiovascular function. Individuals who become dehydrated while taking metformin risk developing lactic acidosis.

The general exercise program should include a low-intensity warm-up period of 5–10 minutes, followed by proper stretching; athletes should avoid bouncing and holding their breath during this warm-up. The exercise period should last 20–45 minutes. For a maximal cardiovascular benefit, the intensity should be between 50% and 70% of VO_{2max}. This requires specific testing and is not a practical measure for most individuals. Heart-rate monitoring is a more feasible method of determining intensity. For an individual starting a new exercise regimen, 50% of maximal heart rate (HR) is a reasonable intensity and can be calculated by the equation:

$$50\% \text{ max. heart rate} = 0.5(HR_{max} - HR_{rest}) + HR_{rest}$$

As noted earlier, the maximal heart rate can also be roughly estimated as 220 – age (in years), but it is better determined individually using a heart-rate monitor (67). Gradual discontinuation of the exercise and 5–10 minutes of low-intensity cooldown are also recommended to help minimize any post-exercise blood pressure fluctuations and cardiac dysrhythmias (66).

The presence of an autonomic neuropathy places individuals at an increased risk of cardiovascular events during exercise. These patients should undergo an exercise stress test before beginning an exercise program, and their first few workouts should be monitored closely. The physician should instruct patients to report the development of dizziness, weakness, or dyspnea, since these symptoms may be associated with cardiac disease. Because orthostatic hypotension may occur after exercising in the upright position, swimming or bicycling are better forms of physical activity than running or walking for these individuals. Disrupted thermoregulation makes exercising in heat or cold inadvisable (68).

The endurance athlete with diabetes mellitus should maintain adequate hydration and euglycemia by taking fluids and carbohydrate supplements (in the form of complex carbohydrates). Hydration is of particular importance for athletes using NSAIDs, and they should be made aware of this fact. Various types of energy supplements designed for use by athletes are available in fluid, gel, and solid forms, so an athlete can find one that is both appropriate and palatable. It is critical that the athlete experiment with various fluid and energy supplements in a controlled setting before depending on one in a game or race. Glucocorticoids should be used sparingly by the diabetic athlete. If they are required, the physician and athlete should be aware of abnormally elevated serum glucose levels as a critical secondary effect. The serum glucose levels need to be monitored even more closely before, during, and after exercise.

Team sports may make glucose control more difficult; players are often sent into play at varying intervals, rendering predictions of energy expenditure and insulin requirements almost impossible. In such cases, it is critical to have rapidly acting carbohydrates (Gatorade, oranges, or apple juice) available for the player to take either before or during participation, as needed. Parents, coaches, and other players should be knowledgeable about the signs of hypoglycemia and the need for expedient and appropriate management if a team member has symptoms (69).

The initial symptoms of hypoglycemia include dizziness, fatigue, weakness, hunger, and headache, and tend to occur with a serum glucose of 50–70 mg/dL. At this stage, further decrease in glucose level may be avoided with a rapidly absorbable sugar source, such as fruit juice, candy, or glucose tablets. The athlete should then receive further supplementation with food containing complex carbohydrates and protein, in order to allow maintenance of a normal serum glucose level. Fluid intake should also be encouraged. If the diabetic athlete is semiconscious or unconscious, confirmation of a low serum glucose is helpful, but treatment should not be delayed while awaiting this. The preferred treatment is parenteral glucagon, 1 mg subcutaneously, which stimulates the release of glycogen from the liver. Parenteral glucagon should always be available to the team or athlete's trainer or health care provider, and it should be replaced yearly to ensure effectiveness (61). Before deciding to allow the participation of a player who has experienced symptoms but has been treated appropriately with both simple and complex carbohydrates, the coach should keep in mind that both physical performance and judgment may be impaired for a period even after the serum glucose has normalized (69).

ASTHMA: EXERCISE-INDUCED BRONCHOCONSTRICTION

Diagnosis

Exercise induces bronchoconstriction in most people with asthma. Approximately 80% of asthmatics and 40% of individuals with allergic rhinitis experience exercise-induced asthma, or what is more commonly termed exercise-induced bronchoconstriction (EIB) (71). Fifteen percent of the general population suffers from EIB, although 9% of these individuals have no history of asthma or allergies (71,72). EIB is more common in children and young adults (perhaps because of their high levels of physical activity), but it can occur at any age (73).

Exercise-induced bronchoconstriction is characterized by an initial mild bronchodilation followed by bronchoconstriction within 3–8 minutes during an exercise challenge (71). Some disagreement used to exist as to whether the bronchoconstriction occurs after exercise ceases. Most studies (using longer periods of exercise) now indicate that the constriction occurs during exercise (74–76). This reaction subsides spontaneously, with complete remission in 2–4 hours, depending on the severity of the constriction (77). It is also well established that a delayed response (constriction occurring several hours after exercise) does not occur in EIB (71,74,76,77). Interestingly, a "refractory" period occurs within 30 minutes from the initial constriction, which is associated with 50% less reduction in pulmonary function than in the initial response (71,77,78). The characteristic features of EIB—initial bronchodilation followed by bronchoconstriction, a refractory period, and the absence of a delayed response—distinguish it from asthma related to other stimuli, such as allergens (76,77). EIB rarely produces bronchoconstriction significant enough to be life threatening; if it does, this is usually associated with poorly controlled disease or confounding factors, such as environmental allergens (78).

Although the exact mechanism of EIB is not known, the most popular hypothesis attributes bronchoconstriction to vascular engorgement secondary to respiratory heat loss during exercise followed by rapid rewarming (79). Other theories include a mediator release related to a change in the hypertonicity of airway lining fluid and stimulation of neural reflexes, and release of certain neuropeptides (77).

Symptoms of EIB include wheezing, dyspnea, chest tightness, and hypoxemia. Occasionally, a cough is the sole symptom (73). Athletes with EIB may also seem to remain in poor condition throughout the season. The diagnosis of EIB is best performed with serial measurements of peak expiratory flow rates (PEFR) during an exercise challenge on a treadmill or stationary bicycle. The intensity of the exercise is critical: it should be at 85–90% of the maximal heart rate (80). The

PEFR should be measured prior to exercise (the average of three trials is best), during the challenge (every 3–4 minutes), and after completion of the exercise for 15 minutes. The challenge does not need to last longer than 20 minutes. The percentage reduction in PEFR can then be calculated by comparing the resting PEFR with the lowest post-exercise PEFR. Most experts define EIB as a reduction in PEFR of greater than 10–15% (80–82). Of course, the individual should not be allowed to use an inhaler or oral anti-asthmatic agent within 4 hours before the exercise test.

The greatest difficulty faced by persons with EIB and asthma is the limitation or perceived limitation on their activities. Individuals with asthma are capable of any form of exercise, and many are able to compete in sports at elite levels (83). In 1984, 11.2% of the athletes on the U.S. Olympic teams were asthmatic; between them they won 41 medals (84). Nevertheless, one long-held misconception about asthmatic individuals is that they have an inherent decreased ability to perform aerobic activities compared with nonasthmatics. Several studies suggest that asthmatics have a lower fitness level, but no explanation is given (85,86). More recently, studies have demonstrated that no difference exists in the cardiopulmonary response to exercise between asthmatic and nonasthmatic individuals, if the asthmatic individuals are receiving proper treatment (87,88). Indeed, the level of activity tolerated is more likely to be related to the level of inactivity or aerobic conditioning, as in nonasthmatic people (88).

In one study, more than 60% of the asthmatic patients perceived their disease as a major obstacle in their ability to exercise (88). These same individuals felt that the wheezing, coughing, and dyspnea experienced during the first few minutes of exercise precluded their further participation. Most indicated that they had never been instructed in the proper methods to minimize or prevent symptoms during exercise. It is imperative that the physician ask questions about any symptoms that might be related to mild asthma or EIB during the preparticipation exam. These questions should include inquiries as to a history of asthma or environmental allergies, cough after exertion, and use of an inhaler, either prescription or over-the-counter (80). Any individual with possible asthma symptoms should undergo testing in order to receive proper treatment and thus be able to participate fully in any sport.

Treatment

Aerosolized beta-agonists are the most effective agents for the prevention of EIB. Albuterol and terbutaline are the only beta-agonists permitted by the U.S. Olympic Committee (USOC) and the International Olympic Committee (IOC). These medications are more beta-2 selective than metaproterenol (71,89). They are generally effective in preventing symptoms in 80–95% of individuals with EIB when administered 20 minutes before exercise. Their action may last from 2 to 4 hours, and they can also alleviate EIB once it has occurred (71). Interestingly, the bronchodilating capacity of the beta-agonists has proved to be independent of their ability to prevent EIB (90). Although metaproterenol and albuterol have comparable bronchodilatory effects, albuterol seems to protect against EIB longer (91). The duration of the bronchodilatory effect of beta-agonists also seems to be longer than the duration of the protective effect against EIB (74,92,93). Therefore, rather than increasing the dose if a beta-agonist is not completely effective, increasing the frequency of the dosage may be preferable, since this will also reduce the side effects (94). Inhaled beta-agonists are also more effective (95).

If an aerosolized beta-agonist is ineffective or only partially effective, cromolyn sodium or nedocromil sodium (also permitted by the USOC and IOC) may be used as a second-line agent, either alone or in combination with a beta-agonist (71,74,96,97). The cromolyn should be taken 0–20 minutes before exercise. The effectiveness of cromolyn is between 70% and 80% alone and up to 98% in combination with beta-agonists (71). More recent studies have challenged the superior effect of combination therapy and suggest that it is no more effective than beta-agonist treatment alone (98,99). Because cromolyn treatment is not associated with any systemic side effects and long-term use may reduce baseline hyperreactivity in some individuals, it deserves a trial of use (78,97). One disadvantage is that the effect often lasts less than 2 hours, possibly requiring more frequent use.

Nebulized ipratropium bromide (allowed by the USOC and IOC) may also be effective in some individuals with asthma (100). Although it is less effective than beta-agonists and cromolyn (rated only 50% effective in EIB), it may allow better control of baseline pulmonary function in asthmatics with more severe disease who wish to exercise (101–103). It may also allow certain individuals using beta-agonists who are intolerant of their side effects to reduce the dose (100).

Other agents that may be effective either alone or in combination with a beta-agonist or cromolyn include antihistamines (such as astemizole, azelastine, chlorpheniramine, and terfenadine) (104), theophylline (for individuals with baseline asthma) (71), alpha-agonists, and calcium channel blockers (which may prevent mast cell degranulation) (71). For patients with refractory EIB, the physician should carefully review and optimize their baseline asthma regimen, since EIB may indicate poor control (78). An exercise challenge test with the standard premedication regimen can be quite useful to determine other possible causes of poor exercise tolerance such as poor conditioning or muscle weakness (78). A concomitant sinusitis or allergic rhinitis should also be treated. Of note, oral steroids are banned by the USOC and IOC, but inhaled steroids may be allowed, as approved on an individual basis for specific medical situations.

Another, nonpharmacological approach to optimizing exercise capacity for asthmatic athletes is an awareness of the exercise environment. The severity and incidence of EIB are exacerbated by cold dry air (105,106). If possible, athletes should choose sports in environments where the air is warm and humid (such as swimming in a heated pool), or breath slowly through the nose, or use a mask or scarf over their mouth and nose to help warm the air in cold environments. Swimming is considered a "less asthmagenic" exercise than running or cycling (77), which may be related to the environment rather than the exercise itself. EIB is also triggered by a rapid increase in exercise intensity. A less intense or submaximal warm-up period for 20 minutes, with increasing intensity just before the actual exercise program, may protect against severe bronchoconstriction by facilitating catecholamine release (107) and may also allow the individual to take advantage of the "refractory" period (108). Some sports are associated with a higher risk of precipitating or exacerbating asthma (such as soccer, basketball, long-distance running, hockey), and the health care provider can direct athletes toward or away from a particular sport, depending on the degree of their disease.

Reports of improvement in fitness from 10% to 92% in asthmatics in exercise programs have been made (109). Improved aerobic conditioning has been shown to improve exercise tolerance in individuals with

EIB (76,80,83). Regular aerobic training, in addition to increasing the maximal oxygen consumption and work capacity at a given heart rate, also reduces the minute ventilation (MV) (the number of respirations per minute) (71,76). A higher MV results in greater airflow obstruction and exacerbates EIB (77). A lower MV, occurring at the same level of exercise intensity after a period of conditioning, reduces the stimulus for EIB (76). The lessened sense of breathlessness also allows the individual to tolerate a longer duration of the exercise activity. The value of maintaining aerobic fitness during the off-season should be emphasized to athletes with EIB (80).

In order to improve cardiorespiratory fitness, an individual must engage in aerobic exercise—continuous and rhythmic exercise for a minimum of 20 minutes at a time—at least three times a week. The intensity must raise the heart rate to at least 70% of the maximally predicted rate (83); this is the accepted prescription for all individuals. Exercise capacity may be limited in individuals with pulmonary disease, because of their inadequate ventilatory reserve, thus preventing the achievement of the required duration of exercise for maximal benefit. Studies exploring the effects of various exercise programs have demonstrated that many asthmatic individuals do have sufficient ventilatory reserve (83). The exercise program must be individualized to allow an adequate increase in heart rate and to maintain an adequate ventilatory reserve for at least 20 minutes of continuous exercise (78,110). Most individuals do not need formal testing or instruction in an exercise program, although this can be helpful. Individuals should be encouraged to measure their own heart rate to monitor exercise intensity (best done with a heart-rate monitor) while maintaining an awareness of their sense of breathlessness (perhaps inability to maintain light conversation).

Individuals who are unable to sustain exercise of sufficient intensity or duration due to dyspnea may require special assistance to condition peripheral muscles, as well as to monitor their function for safety reasons (83). Those with moderate to severe pulmonary disease can use low-intensity isotonic training of individual muscle groups in order to improve muscle strength and endurance and, eventually, overall physical fitness as Vo_{2max} improves (111). The improvement in quality of life and lifestyle often gives them an enhanced sense of well-being and confidence.

Pulmonary renaviiitatiu.. ¸¸·grams are the best environments for these individuals to begin exercise and strengthening programs, ·viii·!. may also include breathing retraining exercises. The individual should take an exercise stress test before embarking on such a program. Pulse oximetry can detect arterial desaturation during exercise, and ECG monitoring, at least during the initial stages, is also critical (111). The usual mode of aerobic exercise is walking, but other possibilities are swimming or use of a stationary bicycle. The few individuals whose oxygen saturation drops below 88% should undergo special supervised conditioning programs with oxygen supplementation, conducted by trained specialists (83).

EPILEPSY

Because of the long-held concern that exercise may have a deleterious effect on individuals with epilepsy, it has been estimated that only 20% of epileptics participate regularly in sports (112). Information on the effect of exercise on seizure frequency is sparse and controversial.

Among the most common concerns about sports and epilepsy are that any injury in an epileptic could lead to an increased incidence of seizures and that a head injury might trigger the onset of seizures in a previously nonepileptic person. Overall, penetrating head trauma or an injury associated with a prolonged period of unconsciousness does have a higher risk of producing epilepsy. One large study reported a relative risk of development of posttraumatic epilepsy as 4.0 in individuals with a history of "moderate" head trauma, defined as a skull fracture or more than 30 minutes of post-injury amnesia or unconsciousness. With less severe head injuries, associated with less than 30 minutes of post-injury amnesia or unconsciousness, the relative risk of developing epilepsy was 1.5 (113). In addition, in children most seizures occur within 24 hours after injury, but they do not always occur in this period for adults. Head injury–related seizures usually occur within 2 years of the trauma, and 50–65% of patients with head injury experience them within 12 months after injury (114). Of those who do have a seizure after head injury, about 50% experience a single seizure and 25% have two or three.

Clinically, seizures are described as partial (or secondary generalized) or primary generalized, each of which responds differently to medications. Partial seizures can be controlled to some degree with medications in 60% of patients, and generalized seizures in 80% (114–116). A primary concern for epileptics is the possibility of a seizure during exercise—that is, exercise lowering the seizure threshold and precipitating a seizure.

Various secondary effects of exercise, often metabolic, have been associated with a decrease in the seizure threshold. Hyperventilation, which usually occurs to some degree with most exercise, is an established precipitant of seizures (117). Athletes who scuba dive or exercise at high altitudes are at highest risk of hypocapneic hyperventilation (118). Exercise causing a lowered seizure threshold is of most concern to endurance athletes, such as triathletes and marathon runners. Hyperthermia (118), hypoglycemia (119), and hyponatremia (which can occur with excessive sweating and rehydration with isotonic or hypotonic solutions) all can result from extreme exercise (120). Endurance athletes with epilepsy should be aware of these possible complications in order to take precautions to avoid them. Excessive fatigue may also lower the seizure threshold, although disturbances in the sleep rhythm and, more specifically, sleep deprivation seem to have a greater influence on seizure activity (121). Stress, especially psychological, is another established precipitant of seizures and may be an important issue in an epileptic athlete in competitive sports (122).

More recent reports support the concept that exercise may increase the seizure threshold and thus confer a level of protection against seizures (118,123,124). One study found exercise produced a decrease in seizure frequency among a subgroup of individuals with recurrent, frequent seizures despite therapeutic levels of anti-seizure medication (112). In addition, exercise may contribute to better seizure control by helping to control stress and depression (both of which have been correlated with seizure frequency) (125). The release of beta-endorphins during exercise may also influence the incidence of epileptiform discharges found on electroencephalogram (EEG), thus decreasing seizure frequency (126). In addition, the increased focus of attention and awareness that accompany exercise may increase the seizure threshold. Increased mental concentration appears to reduce seizure incidence; the mechanism of this effect is not known (127).

The effect of exercise on the pharmacokinetics of anti-seizure med-

ication remains unclear. One study did not find any statistically significant difference between pre- and post-conditioning serum levels of carbamazepine, phenobarbital, and valproic acid (128). Unfortunately, the
potential side effects of anti-seizure medication include lethargy,
drowsiness, decreased level of concentration or coordination, and prolonged reaction time, all of which may profoundly alter an athlete's performance, even if only subtly. The incidence of the side effects is not pre-
dictable and occurrence is not always dose-related. The side effects may
be an indication to switch to another medication or try combination
therapy. Newer anti-seizure medications have recently become available and may be another alternative. No anti-seizure medication is considered hazardous for use while exercising or participating in sports
(127). Many athletes with epilepsy need to try different medications to
determine both efficacy and effect on performance. Of note, however,
estrogenic and androgenic steroids may alter the hepatic metabolism of
anti-seizure medication and lower serum drug level.

Given the more recent data on exercise and decreased frequency of
seizures, as well as the multiple benefits of exercise, participation in
sports should be evaluated on an individual basis (112,127–129).
Epilepsy is no longer considered a contraindication for participation in
contact sports. The minor head injuries that may occur in some competitive contact sports have not been associated with an increase in
seizures in individuals with epilepsy (121,130). Epileptics do have a
higher risk of drowning, which can be minimized with the appropriate
precautions: never swimming alone, avoiding rough water, and using
safety belts for rough-water sports such as wind surfing and water skiing. These are reasonable precautions that should not impede participation in water sports. Individuals with well-controlled seizures should be
allowed to participate in sports without restriction. On the other hand,
individuals with frequent seizures associated with the risk of a sudden
fall should be advised to avoid certain sports, such as parachuting, hang
gliding, high-altitude climbing, and boxing, until their seizures are under better control (129). The coach, other players, and any trainers or
persons involved in a sport in which an athlete with epilepsy is participating should be aware of the possibility of a seizure and be acquainted
with the appropriate management. If a player does have a seizure on the
field or court, the focus of management is to prevent self-injury. The

athlete should be guided to a safe area where she can sit down (during partial seizure), or the area should be cleared of people and dangerous objects (during a generalized seizure). Never insert any object or fingers into the athlete's mouth or restrain her. It is helpful to remember that most seizures are self-limiting and last less than 5 minutes (131).

ANEMIA

The term *sports anemia* was first used to describe a hemoglobin value less than the accepted norm, as found in a group of elite athletes in a study in 1970 (132). The prevalence of anemia among individuals who participate in regular exercise has been difficult to establish. The existence of a true anemia has also been questioned (133–135). However, a compilation of large studies comparing athletes with non-athletes has revealed a true, often mild anemia in athletes (136,137).

The finding of anemia in a well-conditioned athlete at first seems counterintuitive. Athletic performance should be enhanced with a higher hemoglobin level (for more efficient oxygen delivery to the muscles), which has been demonstrated in studies on the effects of blood doping (138). Various theories have been proposed to explain the existence of anemia in athletes, but none has been completely accepted. These include plasma expansion, intravascular hemolysis, and iron deficiency.

Vigorous activity has been shown to decrease the plasma volume by 10–20% (139–142). This shift is considered to be secondary to an increase in both intravascular hydrostatic pressure and tissue osmotic pressure, which drives plasma into the surrounding tissues (139). A significant volume of plasma may also be lost as sweat. Plasma volume begins to return to baseline within 3 hours after cessation of exercise and is fully corrected after 3–5 days (143). The increase in plasma volume often exceeds the baseline level, resulting in a dilutional decrease in hemoglobin but an overall increase in blood volume by up to 25% (141, 144–146). With regular exercise, this decrease in hemoglobin concentration (although the total hemoglobin may actually be higher than normal) will persist, assuming adequate hydration. The expected negative effect of the anemia on performance seems to be offset and possibly enhanced by the resulting increase in cardiac output and stroke volume

(139,147). The overall increase in blood volume enhances oxygen delivery to active muscle tissue. The dilution may also dilute plasma fibrinogen and lessen the risk of blood clot formation within blood vessels (148).

"March hemoglobinuria" was first described in 1881 (149). Since then, the possibility of anemia as a result of hemolysis in athletes has been studied extensively. The evidence supporting an association of intravascular hemolysis with exercise includes a fall in serum haptoglobin (150–152) and overall increase in plasma hemoglobin (153,154) and reticulocyte counts (151). Overt hemoglobinuria seems to be rare. The amount of change in these factors appears to correlate directly with the degree of exertion and the duration of exercise (143). A drop in serum haptoglobin has been documented not only in sports involving running but also in rowing (155) and swimming (156). Therefore, factors other than trauma or impact must also play a role. Possible mechanisms include a fragility of the red blood cell (RBC) membrane (157), trauma to the RBC resulting from increased body temperature or compression by active muscles (157), and acute acidosis (153). Catecholamines may enhance the osmotic and mechanical fragility of the RBC as well (158, 159). The body can utilize the iron from the destroyed RBCs fairly efficiently, so hemolysis should not result in an iron-deficient state unless the individual has low baseline ferritin stores and poor iron intake or absorption (160). In general, however, hemolysis is not considered a clinically important factor in exercise-related anemia.

Iron deficiency, with or without frank anemia, is prevalent in U.S. athletes. Data on the prevalence are conflicting, most likely because of the use of different parameters. Low serum ferritin levels, with and without associated anemia, have been reported in up to 29% of male and 82% of female athletes (161). This may be a reflection of dilution by plasma rather than decreased iron stores. A gradual decrease in iron stores among endurance athletes over a training period has been documented (162), and studies show the bone marrow of long-distance runners to contain iron stores below normal (163,164). More recent studies suggest that true iron-deficiency anemia is relatively uncommon, occurring in up to 3% of the athletic populations examined (143).

The athlete is at a high risk of becoming iron deficient, however, especially female athletes between 15 and 40 years of age. Female athletes are notorious for poor dietary intake, often because of their attempts to control weight to improve athletic performance. Menstruation also plays a key role. Decreased absorption of iron in endurance athletes may also be a factor (165).

Gastrointestinal (GI) bleeding associated with vigorous training has been observed, especially in marathon runners (166,167). The incidence seems to vary and will peak 24–48 hours after exercise (168,169). Dehydrated and exhausted athletes seem to be at highest risk, perhaps explaining the higher incidence following competitive events (169–172). In male athletes, GI bleeding is the most likely cause of blood loss and secondary iron deficiency. The source of the GI bleeding is often not found. The most frequent lesion is a transient hemorrhagic gastritis, which usually resolves without treatment (173–175). No association with the use of NSAIDs has been found, although the use of NSAIDs certainly enhances the potential blood loss (176). Recurrent and clinically significant episodes respond to H_2-blockers (histamine H_2 antagonists) (177–179). The colon may also be a source of bleeding, possibly related to a decrease in blood flow (20–50%) resulting in ischemia (180–182). The incidence and significance of GI blood loss remain to be determined.

The physician should evaluate any true iron deficiency in an athlete, as evidenced by serum hemoglobin, mean cell volume (MCV), total serum iron, and total iron-binding capacity of transferrin, with the usual diagnostic tests. GI bleeding primarily due to exercise is often a diagnosis of exclusion.

The occurrence of iron deficiency without an associated anemia does seem to be prevalent in athletes. Although even mild anemia may impede maximal exercise performance, the effect of pure iron deficiency remains unclear. The use of iron supplements increases serum ferritin levels and possibly serum hemoglobin levels by a minimal amount, but evidence on the effect on performance is conflicting. Increases in both Vo_{2max} and endurance have been reported with an increase in serum ferritin (183–185). There have also been reports of no change in exercise capacity with similar replacement therapy (76,96,110,139,186, 187).

The distinction between an anemia due to iron deficiency and a dilutional anemia (or the contribution of each to the hemoglobin level) may be difficult. After attempts to increase iron intake from dietary sources, an empiric trial of iron replacement with ferrous iron tablets, up to three a day for 2 months, may be reasonable. A change in the hemoglobin level of at least 1g/dL reflects a component of iron deficiency (139). The prophylactic use of iron supplements is not widely recommended.

SICKLE CELL DISEASE

The athlete with sickle cell disease (sickle cell anemia, SSA) presents a unique situation for the sports physician. No study has shown sufficient evidence warranting the complete exclusion of these individuals from exercise and sports (188). The exercise capacity of the individual with SSA may be limited by mechanisms leading to lower oxygen affinity, such as acidosis, dehydration, and hyperthermia. These effects may be further complicated by the impaired ability of the kidney in these individuals to appropriately concentrate urine (due to multiple microinfarcts and subsequent damage to the medulla) (188). With adequate hydration and avoidance of high-temperature situations, however, individuals with SSA should be able to enjoy the multiple cardiovascular and psychological benefits of regular exercise.

REFERENCES

1. Sherman C: Sudden death during exercise. Physician and Sportsmedicine 21(9):92–102, 1993

2. Maron BJ, Epstein SE, Roberts WC: Causes of sudden death in competitive athletes. J Am Coll Cardiol 7:204–214, 1986

3. American College of Sports Medicine, Preventive and Rehabilitative Exercise Committee: Guidelines for Exercise Testing and Prescription, ed 4. Philadelphia, Lea & Febiger, 1991

4. Spirito P, Maron BJ, Bonow RO, et al: Prevalence and significance of an abnormal S-T segment response to exercise in a young athletic population. Am J Cardiol 51:1663–1666, 1983

5. McHenry PL, O'Donnell J, Morris SN, et al: The abnormal exercise electrocardiogram in apparently healthy men: a predictor of angina pectoris as an initial coronary event during long-term follow-up. Circulation 70:547–551, 1984

6. Weiner DA, Ryan TJ, McCabe CH, et al: Exercise stress testing: correlations among history of angina ST segment response and prevalence of coronary ar-

tery disease in the Coronary Artery Surgery Study (CASS). N Engl J Med 302:230–235, 1979

7. Franklin BA, Haskell WL, Van Camp SP: Exercise and cardiac complications. Physician and Sportsmedicine 22(2):56–68, 1994

8. Moy CS, Songer TJ, LaPorte R, et al: Insulin-dependent diabetes mellitus, physical activity, and death. Am J Epidemiol 137:74–81, 1993

9. 16th Bethesda Conference: Task Force VI: arrhythmias. J Am Coll Cardiol 6:1222–1224, 1985

10. Balady GJ, Cadigan JB, Ryan TJ: Electrocardiogram of the athlete: an analysis of 289 professional football players. Am J Cardiol 53:1339–1343, 1984

11. Balady GJ, Weiner DA, McCabe CH, et al: Value of arm exercise testing in detecting coronary artery disease. Am J Cardiol 55:37–39, 1985

12. Balady GJ, Weiner DA: Exercise testing for sports and the exercise prescription. Cardiol Clin 5:183–196, 1987

13. Kaplan NM, Deveraux RB, Miller HS Jr: 26th Bethesda conference: recommendations for determining eligibility for competition in athletes with cardiovascular abnormalities. Med Sci Sports Exerc 26(10):5268–5270, 1994

14. Rames LK, Clarke WR, Connor WE, Reiter MA, Lauer RM: Normal blood pressures and the evaluation of sustained blood pressure elevation in childhood: the Muscatine study. Pediatrics 61:245–251, 1978

15. National Center for Health Statistics: Blood pressure of adults by age and sex, United States, 1960–1962. Vital Health Stat 11(4), 1964

16. Physical exercise in the management of hypertension: a consensus statement by the World Hypertension League. J Hypertens 9:283–287, 1991

17. MacKnight, JM: Hypertension in athletes and active patients. Physician and Sportsmedicine 27(4):35–44, 1999

18. Lim PO, MacFadyen RJ, Clarkson PBM, MacDonald TM: Impaired exercise tolerance in hypertensive patients. Annals of Internal Medicine 124:41–55, 1996

19. Shapiro LM: Morphologic consequences of systematic training. Cardiol Clin 10:219–226, 1992

20. Effron MB: Effects of resistive training on left ventricular function. Med Sci Sports Exerc 21:694–697, 1989

21. Fleck SJ: Cardiovascular adaptations to resistance training. Med Sci Sports Exerc 20(5 suppl):S146–S151, 1989

22. Fariello R, Boni E, Corda L, Muiesan ML, Agabiti-Rosei E: Exercise-induced modifications in cardiorespiratory parameters of hypertensive patients treated with calcium antagonists. J Hypertens 9:S67–S72, 1991

23. Amery A, Julius S, Whitlock LS, Conway J: Influence of hypertension on the hemodynamic response to exercise. Circulation 36:231–237, 1967

24. Fagard R, Staessen J, Amery A: Maximal aerobic power in essential hypertension. J Hypertens 6:859–865, 1988

25. Goodman JM, McLaughlin PR, Plyley MJ, et al: Impaired cardiopulmonary response to exercise in moderate hypertension. Can J Cardiol 8:364–371, 1992

26. Missault L, Duprez D, Buyzere MD, de Backer GD, Clement D: Decreased exercise capacity in mild essential hypertension: non-invasive indicators of limiting factors. J Hum Hypertens 6:151–155, 1992

27. Siegel WC, Blumenthal JA, Divine GW: Physiological, psychological, and behavioral factors and white coat hypertension. Hypertension 16:140–146, 1990

28. Chick TW, Halperin AK, Gacek EM: The effect of antihypertensive medications on exercise performance: a review. Med Sci Sports Exerc 20:447–454, 1988

29. Goodman JM, McLaughlin PR, Plyley MJ, et al: Impaired cardiopulmonary response to exercise in moderate hypertension. Can J Cardiol 8:363–371, 1992

30. Palatini P: Exercise haemodynamics in the normotensive and hypertensive subject (editorial). Clin Sci (Colch) 87:278–287, 1994

31. Balogun MO, Ajayi AA, Ladipo GO: Spectrum of treadmill exercise responses in Africans with normotension, essential hypertension and hypertensive heart failure. Int J Cardiol 21:293–300, 1988

32. Montain SJ, Jilka SM, Ehsani AA, Hagberg JM: Altered hemodynamics during exercise in older essential hypertensive subjects. Hypertension 12:479–484, 1988

33. Lund-Johansen P, Omvik P: Central hemodynamic changes of calcium antagonists at rest and during exercise in essential hypertension. J Cardiovasc Pharmacol 10:S139–S148, 1987

34. Halperin AK, Icenogle MV, Kapsner CO, Chick TW, Roehnert J, Murata GH: A comparison of the effects of nifedipine and verapamil on exercise performance in patients with mild to moderate hypertension. Am J Hypertens 6:1025–1032, 1993

35. Reid JL, Millar JA, Campbell BC: Enalapril and autonomic reflexes and exercise performance. J Hypertens 1:129–134, 1983

36. van Baak MA, Mooij JMV, Wijnen JAG, Tan FS: Submaximal endurance exercise performance during enalapril treatment in patients with essential hypertension. Clin Pharmacol Ther 50:221–227, 1991

37. Tomten SE, Kjeldsen SE, Nilsson S, Westheim AS: Effect of 1-adrenoreceptor blockade on maximal V_{O_2} and endurance capacity in well-trained athletic hypertensive men. Am J Hypertens 7:603–608, 1994

38. Thompson PD, Cullinane EM, Nugent AM, et al: Effect of atenolol or prazosin on maximal exercise performance in hypertensive joggers. Am J Med 86:104–109, 1989

39. Armstrong LE, Costill DI, Fink WJ: Influence of diuretic-induced dehy-

dration on competitive running performance. Med Sci Sports Exerc 17:456–461, 1985

40. Davies SF, Fraif JL, Husebye DG, et al: Comparative effects of transdermal clonidine and oral atenolol on acute exercise performance and response to aerobic conditioning in subjects with hypertension. Arch Intern Med 149:1551–1556, 1989

41. Gordon NF, Duncan JJ: Effect of beta-blockers on exercise physiology: implications for exercise training. Med Sci Sports Exerc 23:668–676, 1991

42. Nilsson OR, Attenhog JH, Castenfors J, et al: A comparison of 100 mg atenolol and 100 mg metoprolol once a day at rest and during exercise in hypertensives. Acta Med Scand 216:301–307, 1984

43. Kaiser P, Hylander B, Eliasson K, Kaijser L: Effect of beta-1-selective and non-selective beta blockade on blood pressure relative to physical performance in men with systemic hypertension. Am J Cardiol 55:79D–84D, 1985

44. Luurila OJ, Grohn P, Heikkila J, et al: Exercise capacity and hemodynamics in persons aged 20 to 50 years with systemic hypertension treated with diltiazem and atenolol. Am J Cardiol 60:1092–1095, 1987

45. Myburgh DP, Gordon NF: Comparison of diltiazem and atenolol in young physically active men with essential hypertension. Am J Cardiol 59:98A–107A, 1987

46. McLeod AA, Kraus WE, Williams RS: Effects of beta-selective and non-selective beta-adrenoceptor blockade during exercise conditioning in healthy adults. Am J Cardiol 53:1656–1661, 1984

47. Chrysant SG, Miller E: Effects of atenolol and diltiazem-SR on exercise and pressure load in hypertensive patients. Clin Cardiol 17:670–674, 1994

48. Stewart KJ: Weight training in coronary artery disease and hypertension. Prog Cardiovasc Dis 35:159–168, 1992

49. MacDougal JD, Tuxen D, Sale G, Moroz JR, Sutton JR: Arterial blood pressure response to heavy resistance exercise. J Appl Physiol 58:785–790, 1985

50. DeBusk RF, Valdez R, Houston N, et al: Cardiovascular responses to dynamic and static efforts soon after myocardial infarction. Circulation 58:369–375, 1978

51. Logan R, Burridge P: Pre-discharge exercise testing involving weight carrying after myocardial infarction. N Z Med J 93:69–71, 1981

52. Markiewicz W, Houston N, DeBusk RA: A comparison of static and dynamic exercise after myocardial infarction. Isr J Med Sci 11:984–987, 1979

53. Taylor LJ, Copeland RB, Cousin AL, et al: The effect of isometric exercise on the graded exercise test in patients with stable angina. J Cardiol Rehab 1:450–458, 1981

54. Sheldahl LM, Wilke NA, Tristani FE, et al: Responses of patients after myocardial infarction to carrying a graded series of weight loads. Am J Cardiol 52:698–703, 1983

55. Vander LB, Franklin BA, Wrisley D, et al: Acute cardiovascular responses

to Nautilus exercise in cardiac patients: implications for exercise training. Ann Sports Med 2:165–169, 1986

56. Hagberg JM, Ehsani AA, Goldring D, et al: Effect of weight training on blood pressure and hemodynamics in hypertensive adolescents. J Pediatr 104: 147–151, 1984

57. Harris KA, Holly RG: Physiological response to circuit weight training in borderline hypertensive subjects. Med Sci Sports Exerc 19:246–252, 1987

58. Tanji JL: Exercise and the hypertensive athlete. Clin Sports Med 11:291–302, 1992

59. Ebeling P, Tuominen JA, Bourey R, Koranyi L, Koivisto VA: Athletes with IDDM exhibit impaired metabolic control and increased lipid utilization with no increase in insulin sensitivity. Diabetes 44:471–477, 1995

60. Richter EA, Turcotte L, Hespel P, Kiens B: Metabolic responses to exercise. Diabetes Care 15:1767–1776, 1992

61. Landry GL, Allen DB: Diabetes mellitus and exercise. Clin Sports Med 11:403–418, 1992

62. Wasserman DH, Zinman B: Exercise in individuals with IDDM. Diabetes Care 17:924–937, 1994

63. Horton ES: Role and management of exercise in diabetes mellitus. Diabetes Care 11:201, 1988

64. MacDonald MJ: Postexercise late-onset hypoglycemia in insulin-dependent diabetic patients. Diabetes Care 10:584, 1978

65. Kemmer FW: Prevention of hypoglycemia during exercise in type I diabetes. Diabetes Care 15:1732–1735, 1992

66. Morgado A, Schneider SH: Sports medicine for the diabetic athlete. N J Med 88:651–654, 1991

67. Schneider SH, Ruderman NB: Exercise and NIDDM. Diabetes Care 13: 785–789, 1990

68. White RD, Sherman C: Exercise in diabetes management: maximizing benefits, controlling risks. Physician and Sportsmedicine 27(4):63–76, 1999

69. Hough DO: Diabetes mellitus in sports. Med Clin North Am 78:423–437, 1994

70. Rosenbloom AL, Siverstein JH, Lexotte DC, et al: Limited joint mobility in childhood diabetes mellitus indicates increased risk for microvascular disease. N Engl J Med 305:192, 1981

71. Spector SL: Update on exercise-induced asthma. Ann Allergy 71:571–577, 1993

72. McCarthy P: Wheezing and breezing through exercise-induced asthma. Physician and Sportsmedicine 17:125–130, 1989

73. McFadden ER Jr, Gilbert IA: Exercise-induced asthma. N Engl J Med 330:1362–1367, 1994

74. Woolley M, Anderson SD, Quigley BM: Duration of protective effect of

terbutaline sulfate and cromolyn sodium alone and in combination on exercise-induced asthma. Chest 97:39–45, 1990

75. Suman OE, Babcock MA, Peglow DF, Jarjour NN, Reddan WG: Airway obstruction during exercise in asthma. Am J Respir Crit Care Med 152:24–31, 1995

76. Karjalainen J: Exercise response in 404 young men with asthma: no evidence for a late asthmatic reaction. Thorax 46:100–104, 1991

77. Makker HK, Holgate ST: Mechanisms of exercise-induced asthma. Eur J Clin Invest 24:571–585, 1994

78. Cypcar D, Lemanske RF: Asthma and exercise: clinical exercise testing. Clin Chest Med 15:351–368, 1994

79. McFadden ER Jr: Respiratory heat and water exchange: physiological and clinical implications. J Appl Physiol 54:331–336, 1983

80. Kyle JM, Walker RB, Hanshaw SL, Leaman JR, Frobase JK: Exercise-induced bronchospasm in the young athlete: guidelines for routine screening and initial management. Med Sci Sports Exerc 24:856–859, 1992

81. Shephard RJ: Exercise-induced bronchospasm—a review. Med Sci Sports 9:1, 1977

82. Anderson SD: Issues in exercise-induced asthma. J Allergy Clin Immunol 76:763–772, 1985

83. Freeman W, Williams C, Nute MG: Endurance running performance in athletes with asthma. J Sports Sci 8:103–17, 1990

84. Voy RO: The US Olympic Committee experience with exercise-induced bronchospasm. Med Sci Sports Exerc 18:328–330, 1986

85. Clark CJ, Cochrane LM: Assessment of work performance in asthma for determination of cardiorespiratory fitness and training capacity. Thorax 43: 745–749, 1988

86. Chryssanthopoulos C, Maksud MG, Fundhashi A, Hoffman RG, Barboriak JJ. An assessment of cardiorespiratory adjustments of asthmatic adults to exercise. J Allergy Clin Immunol 63:321–327, 1979

87. Ingemann-Hansen T, Bundgaard A, Halkjaer-Kristensen J, Siggaard-Anersen J, Weeke B: Maximal oxygen consumption rate in patients with bronchial asthma: the effect of 2-adrenoreceptor stimulation. Scand J Clin Lab Invest 40:99–104, 1980

88. Garfinkel SK, Kesten S, Chapman KR, Rebuck AS: Physiologic and non-physiologic determinants of aerobic fitness in mild to moderate asthma. Am Rev Respir Dis 145:741–745, 1992

89. Afrasiabi R, Spector SL: Exercise induced asthma: it needn't sideline your patients. Physician and Sportsmedicine 19(5):49–62, 1991

90. Sly RM: Beta-adrenergic drugs in the management of asthma in athletes. J Allergy Clin Immunol 73:680, 1984

91. Lemanske RF Jr, Henke KG: Exercise-induced asthma. In Gisolfi CV, Lamb RD (eds): Perspectives in Exercise Science and Sports Medicine, vol 2: Youth, Exercise and Sport. Indianapolis, IN, Benchmark Press, 1989, 465

92. Eggleston PA, Beasley PP: Bronchodilatation and inhibition of induced asthma by adrenergic agonists. Am Rev Respir Dis 20:505, 510, 1981

93. Ahrens RC, Bonhan AC, Maxwell GA, Weinberger MM: A method of comparing the peak intensity and duration of action of aerosolized bronchodilators using broncho-provocation with methacholine. Am Rev Respir Dis 129: 903–906, 1984

94. Smith CM, Anderson SD, Seale JP: The duration of action of the combination of fenoterol hydrobromide and ipratropium bromide in protecting against asthma provoked by hypernea. Chest 94:709–717, 1988

95. Newnham DM, Ingram CG, Earnshaw J, Palmer JBD, Dhillon DP: Salmeterol provides prolonged protection against exercise-induced bronchoconstriction in a majority of subjects with mild, stable asthma. Respir Med 87:439–444, 1993

96. Todaro A, Faina M, Alippi B, Dal Monte A, Ruggieri F: Nedocromil sodium in the prevention of exercise-induced bronchospasm in athletes with asthma. J Sports Med Phys Fitness 33:137–145, 1993

97. Kleiner SM: The role of meat in an athlete's diet: its effect on key macro- and micronutrients. Sports Science Exchange 8:1–6, 1995

98. Clark PS, Ratowsky DA: Effect of fenoterol hydrobromide and sodium cromoglycate individually and in combination on postexercise asthma. Ann Allergy 64:187, 1990

99. Woolley M, Anderson SD, Quigley BM: Duration of protective effect of terbutaline sulfate and cromolyn sodium alone and in combination on exercise-induced asthma. Chest 97:39, 1990

100. Freeman W, Javaid A, Cayton RM: The effect of ipratropium bromide on maximal exercise capacity in asthmatic and non-asthmatic men. Respir Med 86:151–155, 1992

101. Borut TC, Tashkin DP, Fischer TJ, et al: Comparison of aerosolized atropine sulfate and SCH 1000 on exercise-induced bronchospasm in children. J Allergy Clin Immunol 60:127–133, 1977

102. Wolkove N, Kreisman H, Frank H, Gent M: The effect of ipratropium on exercise-induced bronchoconstriction. Ann Allergy 47:311–315, 1981

103. Pasterkamp H, Tal A, Leahy F, Fenton R, Chernick V: The effect of anticholinergic treatment on postexertional wheezing in asthma studied by phono-pneumography and spirometry. Am Rev Respir Dis 132:16–21, 1985

104. Virant FS: Exercise-induced bronchospasm: epidemiology, pathophysiology, and therapy. Med Sci Sports Exerc 24:851–855, 1992

105. Weinstein RE, Anderson JA, Kvale P, Sweet LC: Effects of humidification on exercise-induced asthma (EIA). J Allergy Clin Immunol 57:250–251, 1976

106. Chen WY, Horton DJ: Heat and water loss from the airways and exercise-induced asthma. Respiration 34:305–313, 1977

107. Reiff DB, Choudry NB, Pride NB, et al: The effect of prolonged submaximal warm-up exercise on exercise-induced asthma. Am Rev Respir Dis 139: 479–484, 1989

108. Mckenzie DC, Mcluckie SL, Stirling DR: The protective effects of continuous and interval exercise in athletes with exercise-induced asthma. Med Sci Sports Exerc 26:951–956, 1994

109. Clark CJ: Exercise and asthma. *In* Casaburi R, Petty T (eds): The Principles and Practice of Pulmonary Rehabilitation. Philadelphia, WB Saunders, 1992

110. Clark CJ: The role of physical training in asthma. Chest 101:293S–298S, 1992

111. Mink BD: Pulmonary concerns and the exercise prescription. Clin Sports Med 10:105–116, 1991

112. Erikson HR, Ellertsen B, Grønningsæter H, Nakken KO, Løyning Y, Ursin H: Physical exercise in women with intractable epilepsy. Epilepsia 35: 1256–1264, 1994

113. Annegers JE, Grabow JD, Groover RV, et al: Seizures after head trauma: a population study. Neurology 30(7, pt 1):683–689, 1980

114. Wyllie E: The Treatment of Epilepsy: Principles and Practice, ed 2. Baltimore, Williams & Wilkins, 1997

115. Mattson RH, Cramer JA, Collins JE, et al: Comparison of carbamazepine, phenobarbital, phenytoin, and primidone in partial and secondarily generalized tonic-clonic seizures. N Engl J Med 313:145–151, 1985

116. Mattson RH, Cramer JA, Collins JF: A comparison of valproate with carbamazepine for the treatment of complex partial seizures and secondarily generalized tonic-clonic seizures in adults: The Department of Veterans Affairs Epilepsy Cooperative Study No. 264. N Engl J Med 327:765–771, 1992

117. Gotze W, Kubicki ST, Munter M, et al: Effect of physical exercise on seizure threshold investigated by electroencephalographic telemetry. Dis Nerv Syst 28:664–667, 1967

118. Millington JT: Should epileptics scuba dive? (correspondence). JAMA 254:3182–3183, 1985

119. French JK: Hypoglycaemia-induced seizures following a marathon. N Z Med J 96:407, 1983

120. Noakes ID, Goodwin N, Raymer BL, Branken T, Taylor RKN: Water intoxication: a possible complication during endurance exercise. Med Sci Sports Exerc 17:371–375, 1984

121. O'Donohoe NV: Epilepsies of Childhood, ed 2. Butterworth, London, 1985

122. Temkin NR, Davis GR: Stress as risk factors for seizures among adults with epilepsy. Epilepsia 25:450–456, 1984

123. Livingston S: Epilepsy and sports. JAMA 224:239, 1978

124. Denio LS, Drake ME Jr, Pakalnis A: The effect of exercise on seizure frequency. J Med 20:171–176, 1989

125. Roth DL, Goode KT, Williams VL, Faught E: Physical exercise, stressful life experience, and depression in adults with epilepsy. Epilepsia 35:1248–1255, 1994

126. Albrecht H: Endorphins, sport and epilepsy: getting fit or having one? (letter). N Z Med J 99:915, 1986

127. van Linschoten R, Backx FJG, Mulder OGM, Meinardi H: Epilepsy and sports. Sports Med 10:9–19, 1990

128. Nakken KO, Bjørholt PG, Johannessen SI, Løyning T, Lind E: Effect of physical training on aerobic capacity, seizure occurrence, and serum level of antiepileptic drugs in adults with epilepsy. Epilepsia 31:88–94, 1990

129. Gates JR: Epilepsy and sports participation. Physician and Sportsmedicine 19(3):98–104, 1991

130. Livingston S, Berman W: Participation of epileptic patient in sports. JAMA 224:236–238, 1973

131. Sirven JI, Varrato J: Physical activity and epilepsy: what are the rules? Physician and Sportsmedicine 27(3):63–70, 1999

132. Yoshimura H: Anemia during physical training (sports anemia). Nutr Rev 28:251, 1970

133. De Wijn JF, de Jongste JL, Mosterd W, et al: Haemoglobin, packed cell volume, serum iron and iron binding capacity of selected athletes during training. J Sports Med 11:42, 1971

134. Balaban EP, Cox JV, Snell P, et al: The frequency of anemia and iron deficiency in the runner. Med Sci Sports Exerc 21:643, 1989

135. Brune M, Magnusson B, Persson H, et al: Iron losses in sweat. Am J Clin Nutr 43:438, 1986

136. Clement DB, Asmundson RC, Medhurst CW: Hemoglobin values: comparative survey of the 1976 Canadian Olympic team. Can Med Assoc J 117:614, 1977

137. Stewart GA, Steel JE, Toyne AH: Observations on the haemotology and the iron and protein intake of Australian Olympic athletes. Med J Aust 2:1339, 1972

138. Gledhill N: Blood doping and related issues: a brief review. Med Sci Sports Exerc 14:183, 1982

139. Eichner ER: Sports anemia, iron supplements, and blood doping. Med Sci Sports Exerc 24:S315–S318, 1992

140. Costill DL, Fink WJ: Plasma volume changes following exercise and thermal dehydration. J Appl Physiol 37:521, 1974

141. Davidson RJL, Robertson JD, Galea G, et al: Hematological changes associated with marathon running. Int J Sports Med 8:19, 1987

142. Wells CL, Stern JR, Hecht LH: Hematological changes following a marathon race in male and female runners. Eur J Appl Physiol 48:41, 1982

143. Balaban EP: Sports anemia. Clin Sports Med 11:313–325, 1992

144. Brotherhood J, Brozovic B, Pugh LGC: Haematological status of middle- and long-distance runners. Clin Sci 48:139, 1975

145. Dill DB, Braithwaite K, Adams WC, et al: Blood volume of middle-

distance runners: effect of 2,300-m altitude and comparison with non-athletes. Med Sci Sports Exerc 6:1, 1974

146. Richieri GV, Mel HC: Temperature effects on osmotic fragility, and the erythrocyte membrane. Biochim Biophys Acta 813:41, 1985

147. Pate R: Sports anemia: a review of the current research literature. Physician and Sportsmedicine 11:115, 1983

148. Bunch TW: Blood test abnormalities in runner. Mayo Clin Proc 55:113, 1980

149. Fleischer R: Uber eine neue Form van Hamoglobinurie beim Menschen. Berlin Klin Wochenschr 18:691, 1881

150. Hunding A, Jordal R, Paulev P-E: Runner's anemia and iron deficiency. Acta Med Scand 209:315, 1981

151. Schmidt W, Maassen N, Tegtbur U, et al: Changes in plasma volume and red cell formation after a marathon competition. Eur J Appl Physiol 58:453, 1989

152. Selby GB, Eichner ER: Endurance swimming, intravascular hemolysis, anemia, and iron depletion. Am J Med 81:791, 1986

153. Weight LM, Byrne MJ, Jacobs P: Haemolytic effects of exercise. Clin Sci 81:147–152, 1991

154. Gilligan DR, Altschule MD, Katersky EM: Physiological intravascular hemolysis of exercise: hemoglobinemia and hemoglobinuria following cross-country runs. J Clin Invest 22:859, 1943

155. Eichner ER, Strauss RH, Sherman WM, et al: Intravascular hemolysis in elite college rowers. Med Sci Sports Exerc 21:S78, 1989

156. Probart CK, Bird PJ, Parker KA: Diet and athletic performance. Clin Nutr 77:757–772, 1993

157. Banga JP, Pinder JC, Gratzer WB, Linch DC, Huehns ER: An erythrocyte membrane-protein anomaly in march haemoglobinuria. Lancet 2:1043–1044, 1979

158. Davidson RJ: Exertional haemoglobinuria: a case report on three cases with studies on the haemolytic mechanism. J Clin Pathol 17:536–540, 1964

159. Shiraki K, Yamada T, Yoshimura T: Relation of protein nutrition to the reduction of red blood cells induced by physical training. Jpn J Physiol 27:413–421, 1977

160. Eichner ER: Runners macrocytosis: a clue to footstrike haemolysis; runner's anaemia as a benefit vs runner's haemolysis as a detriment. Am J Med 78:321–325, 1985

161. Clement DB, Asmundson RC: Nutritional intake and hematological parameters in endurance runners. Physician and Sportsmedicine 10:37, 1982

162. Rowland TW, Black SA, Kelleher JF: Iron deficiency in adolescent endurance athletes. J Adolesc Health Care 8:322, 1987

163. Ehn L, Carlmark B, Hoglund S: Iron status in athletes involved in intense physical activity. Med Sci Sports Exerc 12:61, 1980

164. Wishnitzer R, Vorst E, Berichi A: Bone marrow depression in competitive distance runners. Int J Sports Med 4:27, 1983

165. Ehn L, Carlmark B, Holgund S: Iron status in athletes involving intense physical activity. Med Sci Sports Exerc 12:61–64, 1980

166. McCabe ME, Peura DA, Kadakia SC, Bocek Z, Johnson LF: Gastrointestinal blood loss associated with running a marathon. Dig Dis Sci 31:1229–1232, 1986

167. McMahon LF, Ryan MJ, Larson D, Fisher RL: Occult gastrointestinal blood loss in marathon runners. Ann Intern Med 100:846–847, 1984

168. Stewart JG, Ahlquist DA, McGill DB, Ilstrup DM, Schwartz S, Owen RA: Gastrointestinal blood loss and anemia in runners. Ann Intern Med 100:843–845, 1984

169. Baska RS, Moses FM, Deuster PA: Cimetidine reduces running-associated gastrointestinal bleeding: a prospective observation. Dig Dis Sci 35:956–960, 1990

170. Selby G, Fram D, Eichner ER: Effort-related gastrointestinal blood loss in distance runners during a competitive season. Med Sci Sports Exerc 20:S79, 1988

171. Dobbs TW, Akins M, Ratliff R, et al: Gastrointestinal bleeding in competitive cyclists. Am Coll Sports Med 20:S78, 1988

172. Viala JJ, Ville D: Anémie des coureurs de fond liée à des hémorragies digestives. Presse Med 20:386, 1991

173. Hilpert G, Gaudin B, Devars Du Mayne JF, et al: Gastrite ulcereusse chez un coureur de fond. Gastroenterol Clin Biol 8:983, 1984

174. Papaioannides D, Giotis CH, Karaginnis N, et al: Acute upper gastrointestinal hemorrhage in long distance runners. Ann Intern Med 101:719, 1984

175. Scobie BA: Recurrent gut bleeding in five long distance runners. N Z Med J 98:966, 1985

176. Moses FM: Gastrointestinal bleeding and the athlete. Am J Gastroenterol 88:1157–1159, 1993

177. Cooper DT, Douglas SA, Firth LA, et al: Erosive gastritis and gastrointestinal bleeding in a female runner: prevention of bleeding and healing of the gastritis with H2-receptor antagonist. Gastroenterology 92:2019–2023, 1987

178. Gaudin C, Zerath E, Guezennec CY: Gastric lesions secondary to long-distance running. Dig Dis Sci 35:1239–1243, 1990

179. Mack D, Sherman P: Iron deficiency anemia in an athlete associated with campylobacter pylori-negative chronic gastritis. J Clin Gastroenterol 11:445–447, 1989

180. Schaub N, Spichtin HP, Stadler GA: Ischamische kolitis als ursache einer darmblutung bei marathonlauf? Schweiz Med Wochenschr 115:454–457, 1985

181. Merlin P, Roche JF, Aubet JP, et al: Colite ischemique lors d'un effort inhabituel. Gastroenterol Clin Biol 13:108–109, 1989

182. Beaumont AC, Teare JP: Subtotal colectomy following marathon running in a female patient. J R Soc Med 84:4339–4440, 1991

183. Hunding A, Jordal R, Paulev PE: Runner's anemia and iron deficiency. Acta Med Scand 209:315–318, 1981

184. Gardner GW, Edgerton VR, Barnard RJ, Bernauer EM: Cardiorespiratory, hematological and physical performance responses of anemic subjects to iron treatment. Am J Clin Nutr 28:982–988, 1975

185. Plowman SA, McSwegin PC: The effect of iron supplementation on female cross country runners. J Sports Med 21:407–416, 1981

186. Matter M, Stittfall T, Graves J, et al: The effect of iron and folate therapy on maximal exercise performance in female marathon runners with iron and folate deficiency. Clin Sci 72:415–422, 1987

187. Clark N: The power of protein. Physician and Sportsmedicine 24(4):11–12, 1996

188. Kark JA, Ward FT: Exercise and hemoglobin S. Semin Hematol 31:181–225, 1994

Chapter 3

INFECTIOUS DISEASES

The influence of exercise on both the probability of contracting an infection and its ensuing severity and duration has long been debated. The effect of exercise seems to depend upon multiple factors, including the type of infection (viral, bacterial, or fungal) and the type, duration, and intensity of the particular exercise. Moderate exercise may provide increased resistance to infection, whereas prolonged and intense exertion may increase susceptibility and prolong the duration of the infection (1). The issue of exercise during an infection is also still under debate, but intense and prolonged exercise may not be as detrimental as was once thought.

UPPER RESPIRATORY INFECTION AND INFLUENZA

Upper respiratory infections (URI) cause far more disabilities among athletes of all levels than do any other types of infection (2). One report comparing the occurrence of infections in athletes in the Summer and Winter Olympics found a considerably higher incidence of respiratory infections than of GI and skin infections in both groups (3). Prolonged and exhaustive exertion, poor air quality, and inadequate recovery time, with or without the mental stress of competition, appear to increase the risk of contracting a URI (4–6).

This effect seems to be related to the direct influence of exercise on immune function (7,8). Suppression of lymphocyte function was demonstrated in runners who ran 42 km (26 miles); lymphocyte function then returned to baseline after 24 hours (9). The function of the mucosal immune system is also suppressed with exercise, which may further increase the susceptibility to URIs (10). Simple psychological stress increases adrenaline levels and may result in inhibition of humoral and cell-mediated immunity (11).

Compared with the average, more sedentary individual, the athlete participating in moderate exercise training has a lower risk of contracting a URI. However, this risk appears to increase and eventually exceed that of the sedentary individual as training intensity increases (12,13). Athletes who run more than 60 miles per week have been shown to experience URI symptoms twice as often as those running less than 20 miles per week (14,15). In addition, one bout of exhaustive exercise may also influence the susceptibility to URI. The incidence of URI symptoms in runners who competed in the Los Angeles marathon in 1987 was found to be six times greater than that among athletes of similar experience who registered but then withdrew for reasons other than illness (14).

A URI impairs physical performance and endurance via alteration in respiratory, cardiac, and musculoskeletal functions (16). Athletes are more sensitive to any alteration in physical functions and may therefore notice the effect of what would be a subclinical infection in an average individual. Controversy also exists regarding the effect of exercise on a viral infection versus a bacterial infection. Exercise during active viral or parasitic infections may increase both morbidity and mortality, even at levels thought to confer resistance. Exercise may increase an athlete's risk of developing viral myocarditis, which has rarely been associated with sudden death but could result in some level of permanent cardiac impairment (17,18). Bacterial infections seem to be less affected by exercise (1).

Advice on training during a URI is a common request from a physician caring for athletes. It is generally accepted that athletes with a URI without any constitutional symptoms may be allowed to participate in exercise activity as tolerated (19,20). A simple method for the athlete to determine the extent of a URI is to do a "neck check" (21). If symptoms originate above the neck, such as rhinorrhea, sneezing, or scratchy throat, and are not associated with any other systemic symptoms such as a fever, the athlete may exercise at a moderate intensity or as tolerated. If the symptoms appear to worsen or spread, exercise should be reduced or avoided (if possible) for a few days until the symptoms resolve. Any symptoms originating below the neck, such as myalgias or coughing, should be treated with rest: 10–14 days is the optimal rest period, but this is not feasible for most competitive athletes. Rest for at least a few days (or until fever resolves) and gradual return to full training help minimize the risk of more serious (although rare) complications such as myocarditis (22). Performance during a URI will also be affected, which should be taken into consideration before placing the athlete in a competitive situation. Of course, athletes with any history of asthma should reduce exercise during the acute stage of a URI (which will probably occur anyway) and optimize their anti-asthma treatment (23).

Prevention is always preferred. The athlete should try to minimize exposure to any possible infection, especially during an intense period of training such as prior to an important event. Athletes should be encouraged to maintain a healthy diet and closely monitor their individual response to increased or heavier training schedules. Team members who have an active infection should try to avoid direct contact with other members. A closed air space, such as on an airplane, is a prime situation for exposing others to an infection. Depending on the situation, the coach should consider not allowing a team member with an infection to travel. Individuals need to be reminded that viruses are primarily transmitted by hand contact, so hands should be washed frequently (24). Requiring a hepatitis vaccination and yearly flu shots for all team members is another means of optimizing performance.

A URI in a competitive athlete will usually receive aggressive treatment. Instead of waiting to determine whether the infection is bacterial, physicians prescribe antibiotics sooner and more often for athletes than for the general population. Early antibiotic treatment may also prevent a viral URI from deteriorating into a secondary bacterial infection. The risk to the athlete is small and therefore acceptable. Minimizing down time and optimizing performance are critical at high levels of competition.

INFECTIOUS MONONUCLEOSIS

Infectious mononucleosis (IM), which is caused by the Epstein-Barr virus (EBV), is another common infection encountered by the sports physician. EBV is transmitted by the exchange of oral secretions. Contrary to popular belief, it cannot be transmitted to teammates or roommates unless direct exchange of saliva occurs. As long as the saliva contains EBV, which can be for several months after the acute infection, it can be a source of infection (25). The incubation period is approximately 30–45 days. Up to 50% of infected individuals experience the classic symptoms, which begin with malaise, myalgias, excessive fatigue, and anorexia, followed after 1 week by a moderate to high fever, often with chills, sore throat with enlarged tonsils, and cervical and possibly generalized lymphadenopathy. By the second week, 50–70% of infected individuals have an enlarged spleen. A macular rash may also occur, but this is less common (22).

Laboratory tests reveal a leukocytosis, up to 20,000/mm^2, associated with more than 50% lymphocytes, many of which will be described as atypical. A mild or transient leukopenia or thrombocytopenia may be seen, but severe cytopenias are rare. During the second week of symptoms, 80% of individuals have elevated liver enzymes consistent with a mild hepatitis. Most of the laboratory tests return to normal by the fifth week of symptoms (22).

Diagnosis can be made on the basis of symptoms and laboratory tests. Many physicians rely on the "Monospot test," which reflects the presence of the heterophil antibody IM-related immunoglobulin IgM (25). Interpretation of this test needs to be made with caution, since other viral infections such as cytomegalovirus (CMV), hepatitis A, adenovirus, and toxoplasmosis may cross-react and give a false-positive result (25). In addition, the heterophil IgM is not produced in 15% of cases of IM, thus giving a false-negative result. More specific laboratory tests for EBV-related IgM and IgG levels can be performed in suspicious cases. Tests for IgM for CMV and hepatitis A are also available (25).

Complications from IM are relatively rare. The most serious are splenic rupture and airway obstruction due to enlarged tonsils. Although splenomegaly is present in 50% of cases, frank rupture occurs in less than 0.2% (22). Most cases of documented rupture do not result from direct trauma in athletic activities but rather occur during common activities associated with increased intra-abdominal pressure, such as lifting or defecating (22). Splenic rupture can be associated with sudden onset of left upper quadrant pain. An ultrasound or computed tomography (CT) scan can document splenomegaly and possible rupture. Treatment often requires splenectomy.

Tonsillar enlargement may be associated with airway compromise and possible obstruction. Intubation is rarely necessary if the condition is recognized early enough and treated with steroids, which can shrink the tonsils within hours (22). Severe hepatitis is also rare, and even fewer cases of Guillain-Barré encephalitis have been documented. Myocarditis and severe thrombocytopenia, neutropenia, and anemia have also been described.

Treatment for general IM is primarily supportive, with adequate rest and Tylenol for fevers, myalgias, and headaches. The use of steroids in uncomplicated cases of IM has not been demonstrated to alter the course of recovery and is indicated only for complications such as severe tonsillar enlargement or cytopenias (26). Recovery from IM-associated hepatitis may be hindered by the use of steroids (27). Strict or prolonged bed rest is not necessary, although the physician should remind infected individuals that recovery will be gradual and overexertion too soon may prolong recovery. Most individuals recover within 4–6 weeks, but competitive and elite athletes may not regain their high level of conditioning and performance for 3 months (25).

During the initial few weeks of symptoms, most athletes are incapable of exercising strenuously. Once the symptoms begin to resolve, the issue of resumption of training arises. The possibility of splenic rupture is the most important consideration in evaluating the athlete for return to participation. Splenomegaly usually resolves after the third week of symptoms. The clinical examination is often sufficient to ensure that the spleen has returned to normal size within the area protected by the lower rib cage. For large athletes, for whom palpation of the spleen can be less than optimal, an ultrasound to document splenic size is recommended (28,29). Once the spleen has returned to normal size and fevers have resolved, the athlete may gradually return to training, starting at 50% of maximal effort. Both the athlete and the trainer or physician should evaluate tolerance to the activities daily. Return to contact sports is allowed once spleen size returns to normal.

HUMAN IMMUNODEFICIENCY VIRUS

The issue of human immunodeficiency virus (HIV) infection and exercise has been controversial in the past, primarily regarding both the effect of exercise on the HIV-positive individual and the possible risk of transmission of infection through physical contact. HIV-positive individuals participating in exercise conditioning programs exhibit levels of improved fitness similar to those of matched controls who are HIV-negative (30). Infection with HIV does not seem to prevent or diminish the ability to improve cardiovascular fitness with exercise (30–32). Similar improvements in strength and body mass can also be achieved by HIV-positive individuals participating in strength-training programs (30,33). Increasing and maintaining body mass is particularly important in HIV disease, since general wasting and loss of lean body mass are among the most common effects of HIV infection. Strength training may help delay, if not reverse, the loss of muscle tissue (34).

Exercise can also help improve the HIV-positive individual's sense of well-being and quality of life (31). Infection with HIV leads to a progressively worsening immunosuppressed state, reflected by decreasing numbers of CD4 and T-helper cells, which are also dysfunctional. Moderate aerobic exercise has been shown to increase the absolute CD4 cell counts in HIV-positive individuals (35–39). This increase has also been demonstrated in individuals with symptoms of HIV infection (without superimposed opportunistic infection) (40,41).

Asymptomatic HIV-positive individuals who are otherwise healthy should be allowed to participate in sports without restrictions and encouraged to adopt a regular exercise program. Recommendations on participation in sports and exercise activities may vary, depending upon the extent of HIV infection. Exercise can allow HIV-positive individuals to actively participate in the management of their disease, as well as improving quality of life and reducing stress (42). Some of the medications used to treat HIV disease can affect the individual's response to exercise. For example, zidovudine (AZT) can be associated with a myopathy characterized by muscle weakness, myalgias, diminished physical endurance, and possibly an elevated serum creatinine kinase (CK). The myopathy is reversible with discontinuation of AZT (43). The effect of protease inhibitors on exercise has yet to be documented; however, the associated improvement in overall symptoms and increased CD4 levels will most likely allow individuals to tolerate exercise and improve cardiovascular fitness.

Concern about the potential for transmission of HIV during a sporting activity or event is certainly understandable, especially given the increasing incidence of HIV infection among young people. The Centers for Disease Control and Prevention estimates that 1 in 200 college-aged individuals is infected with HIV (44). A survey of NCAA members found that of 548 member institutions, 12 knew of at least one HIV-positive team member (45). HIV can be transmitted through sexual contact and blood inoculation, and from mother to fetus (46). It cannot be transmitted by sweat or by saliva (47). The American Academy of Pediatrics has issued a statement that no documentation of transmission of HIV from one athlete to another during participation in a sporting event exists (48). The World Health Organization consensus statement supports this view (49). One report described the possible transmission of HIV infection from one athlete to another after each incurred scalp wounds after collision (50). A careful examination of the history of the athlete thought to have been previously uninfected revealed other possible exposures to HIV. The possibility that the minimal exchange of blood following the collision resulted in transmission of HIV was dismissed (51).

The American Medical Society for Sports Medicine and the American Academy of Sports Medicine have issued position statements on HIV and sports. Both support the participation of HIV-infected athletes in sports activities. Both state that the risk of transmission of HIV during a sports event is "too low to quantify." The presence of HIV infection in an individual is not sufficient reason to deny participation in athletic activity. Neither society supports the use of mandatory testing for HIV as a criterion for clearance for participation in a sport (52). Exclusion of an infected athlete is reasonable if he cannot meet the physical demands of the sport, but it is inappropriate to assume that his physical capabilities are reduced (44).

Despite the view that the risk of HIV transmission during a sporting event is minimal, the principle of "universal precautions" should be implemented. This has already been established at NCAA, U.S. Olympic, and most professional sporting events. Athletes, coaches, trainers, and physicians should treat every injury associated with blood as a potential source of HIV infection (and hepatitis B infection; see below). Most athletic leagues stop play if an athlete is bleeding and allow him to return to play only after the bleeding is controlled and the wound properly covered. All wounds should be bandaged and all playing surfaces and clothes exposed to blood should be properly disinfected or changed before the athlete returns to play (45,51,53).

HEPATITIS B

Though not often discussed, the hepatitis B virus (HBV), another blood-borne pathogen, has a much greater chance of transmission than HIV and is spread by the same routes (52). Estimates suggest that the United States alone has more than 1 million carriers of HBV (54). An athlete with an acute HBV infection should be treated symptomatically, as for any other viral infection. Considerations about return to play are similar to those for IM, since hepatosplenomegaly can be present. For the previously infected individual, no evidence of any adverse effects from high-level, intense, competitive training has been found (52). No athletic association has issued a requirement for HBV vaccination, but several other groups highly recommend immunization for the general public as infants (as part of the required childhood immunizations) and for college-aged students (55,56). Immunization should also be strongly considered for any competitive team, in order to avoid a catastrophic loss in the number of healthy players if one player becomes infected and subsequently infects other team members.

Only one case of HBV transmission during a sports activity has been documented (57). It involved an outbreak of HBV in sumo wrestlers in Japan, all of whom had contact with an asymptomatic wrestler who was found to have significant serum levels of hepatitis B surface antigen and hepatitis B_e antigen (which is associated with high levels of virus and therefore a higher degree of contagion). This wrestler had multiple scars all over his body and was known to bleed frequently from lesions incurred while wrestling. Universal precautions during sporting events will minimize exposure and possible transmission of HBV.

DERMATOLOGICAL INFECTIONS

Bacterial, viral, and fungal infections are prevalent among athletes, especially in contact sports. The ease of transmission is probably related to the weakening of the outermost layers of skin secondary to excessive sweating and skin friction, as well as direct trauma (58,59). Certain infections are more common with particular sports or types of exercise, such as herpes simplex type 1 and impetigo in wrestling.

Miliaria is a common form of dermatitis in athletes wearing heavy, hot clothing, such as football or baseball players (60). Although the small, clear, and often pruritic blisters seem to suggest an infectious process, they are secondary to sweat duct occlusion in the lower epidermis (61). Treatment is not necessary, since the lesions usually resolve with cooling and airing out of the affected areas.

Minor lacerations or abrasions in the skin, resulting from direct trauma or irritation from pads or tape, occur in every sport and may allow penetration by bacteria. Impetigo is a common superficial skin infection often seen in wrestlers, swimmers, and gymnasts (22). Caused by beta-hemolytic streptococci or *Staphylococcus aureus* bacteria, it is highly contagious and can be transmitted through contact with contaminated mats, towels, or equipment or by direct contact with an infected person. Clinically, it is characterized by multiple vesicles filled with clear, yellow fluid, which then forms a crust. Diagnosis can be confirmed with direct culture. If impetigo is suspected, a urinalysis should also be performed because of a small risk of post-streptococcal glomerulonephritis. Treatment with a 7- to 10-day course of oral antibiotics such as erythromycin or a penicillinase-resistant penicillin is most effective, with topical cleansing of weeping lesions with hydrogen peroxide (62). Infected athletes should not be allowed to participate in any water or contact sport until the lesions have resolved (63,64).

Superficial folliculitis (acne mechanica) may occur with pressure or friction and occlusion caused by athletic clothing or equipment (65). It is most common in football and hockey players, who wear heavy equipment over the areas of the body with high concentrations of sebaceous glands. It may also be seen on the backs of weight lifters, resulting from lying on vinyl-covered weight benches (66). Characteristic lesions are small pustules with a protruding hair in the center; the pustules can be pruritic or tender. Treatment is not always simple. Athletes should be encouraged to wear clean T-shirts under their protective equipment and to change into fresh clothing as soon as possible after working out. Immediate showering is useful, as are topical drying lotions. In severe cases, anti-acne medication, such as retinoin, may be required; however, it needs to be used with caution since side effects include myalgias and fatigue (66). Antibiotics are usually not needed but may be used in recurrent or persistent cases. Although the risk of transmission is minimal, athletes should not share towels and should wear equipment over a clean T-shirt or underwear.

Furuncles occur when the sebaceous glands associated with a hair follicle become infected, usually with *S. aureus;* they appear as warm, tender, enlarged nodules or abscesses. Treatment with oral antibiotics (penicillinase-resistant penicillin or erythromycin) and drainage of any abscesses is required. Risk of transmission is low, but reports of outbreaks involving several members of some teams (particularly football) do exist (67,68). Contact sports and water sports should be avoided until the lesions clear.

Certain dermatological conditions are associated with the use of anabolic steroids, which seems to be reaching epidemic proportions worldwide. It is important for the sports physician to be aware of these conditions, since cutaneous lesions may be the first indication of steroid use. The most common are acne, folliculitis, and furunculosis.

HERPES SIMPLEX VIRUS

Herpes simplex virus (HSV), type 1 (usually affecting lips and areas above the waist) and, less often, type 2 (genital area and below the waist), is a highly contagious skin infection, which can easily be transmitted among athletes, especially those in contact sports, such as wrestling and rugby (62). Termed herpes gladiatorum, the incidence in wrestlers has been estimated to be as high as 20% overall (69). Multiple cases of rapid transmission between several team members or competitors have been documented (70–72). The most commonly affected sites are the head and neck, due to direct contact with the opponent's face and neck, such as in the rugby scrum or the "lock-up" position in wrestling (62).

The typical herpes lesion is a painful blister with a red inflamed base. The lesions often occur in clusters and may coalesce with the rapid ulceration that follows. The infected individual may experience a tingling or burning at the site of the blisters before they appear. During the primary infection, fever, malaise, and lymphadenopathy may accompany the lesions; systemic symptoms are not usually as severe during a recurrence (73,74). The physician should obtain a swab of the base of a blister for a viral culture in order to make an accurate diagnosis, since it is vital for an individual with HSV to make certain lifestyle changes to avoid transmission to others.

The lesions usually resolve spontaneously in 10–14 days, but may recur at the same site in the future. A variety of factors, such as sunlight, illness, stress, or menses, may trigger a recurrence (75). The current treatment for a recurrence is oral acyclovir, 200–400 mg five times a day for 10–14 days, which helps decrease the viral shedding and accelerate healing. Acyclovir may also help to prevent secondary keratitis, meningitis, arthritis, and disseminated disease (76). Topical antiviral treatments are not considered effective (77). Prophylactic acyclovir, 200 mg three times a day, may reduce recurrent outbreaks; however, it should not be used for more than 6 months at a time. Newer antiviral agents, valacyclovir and famciclovir, are also useful and are preferred because of the decreased frequency of dosing (500 mg of valacyclovir or 125 mg famciclovir twice a day for 10 days for an acute attack and twice a day for 5 days for a recurrent attack). Topical drying solutions such as 5% benzoyl peroxide gel applied two or three times a day may help (62). Given the highly contagious nature of HSV, an athlete with active lesions should not be allowed to participate in any water or contact sports for at least 7 days (75) or until the lesions are completely healed (78). Pain medication may be needed for management, but the choice of analgesic should always be made within the restrictions of the USOC, NCAA, or professional league, if appropriate.

HUMAN PAPILLOMA VIRUS (WARTS)

Warts are due to infection with one of the multiple types of human papilloma virus and can be quite disabling to the affected athlete. Plantar warts, found on the sole of the foot, can be transmitted from pool decks, shower rooms, and exercise equipment. For this reason, the use of sandals is highly encouraged in common sports areas. Treatment can be quite frustrating: plantar warts should generally not be removed by curettage, electrodesiccation, or laser. The risk of a painful scar and possible recurrence is high with these treatments, and liquid nitrogen is not always successful unless given deeply, requiring local anesthesia. Slow removal using a keratolytic agent applied constantly under an occlusive dressing, with weekly paring of excess tissue (which can be performed by the athlete), is quite successful. A corn pad over the wart and under the dressing allows the athlete to continue exercising (79).

Hand warts may be transmitted by use of equipment or apparatus in gyms. Treatment is somewhat easier. Cryotherapy produces a blister under the wart, which subsequently heals and sloughs off the wart. The only drawback is that the individual must avoid heavy pressure to the area for 1 week in order to ensure proper healing (80).

FUNGAL INFECTIONS

Fungal infections of the skin are well known to athletes ("athlete's foot" and "jock itch"), because of, among other factors, the constant moist environment from sweat, occlusive footwear and clothes, contaminated locker room floors, and direct and close contact with other, possibly infected individuals.

Tinea pedis (athlete's foot) is a superficial fungal infection of the skin of the foot. The infected area may be an asymptomatic reddish patch with scaling and central clearing or may have painful itchy blisters. A good diagnostic clue is involvement of the web of skin between the 4th and 5th toes, which is almost always present in fungal infections (63). Topical antifungals such as clotrimazole are not always successful, since relapse is not uncommon. Terbinafine (Lamisil) is a topical cream with both antifungal and anti-inflammatory properties that can eradicate fungal infection in 1–2 weeks (79). The excessive scaling of the skin may allow secondary infection with bacteria, often gram-negative or diphtheroids. Macerated and malodorous lesions in the toe webs suggest secondary infection, and in these cases oral antibiotics have successfully eradicated what had previously been a chronic fungal infection (79). Prophylactic use of powder to keep the skin dry and frequent changing of socks should always be encouraged.

Tinea cruris (jock itch) is a similar fungal infection, affecting the groin and upper thighs. The scrotum is not usually affected. The lesions are similar to those of tinea pedis—red, scaly, and itchy—and often occur secondary to infection of the feet. The treatment is the same as for tinea pedis. Good hygiene can prevent these fungal infections, as can toweling the feet dry last after a shower and putting on socks before under-wear (82).

Tinea corporus (ringworm) involves the trunk and is caused by the same fungi as tinea pedis and cruris; however, the lesions in tinea cor-porus are annular with an erythematous border and central clearing. Epidemic outbreaks among wrestlers have been reported (83). Treat-ment is similar to those outlined above. Oral fluconazole may be used for resistant or recurrent lesions.

Candida albicans infection, less common than tinea, is another type of fungal skin infection seen in athletes, especially those in running sports and swimming (84). Warm and moist areas, such as the groin, per-ineum, vagina, and interdigital web spaces, are the usual sites of in-volvement. Transmission is similar to that for other fungal infections of the skin. The typical lesion is a slightly raised, inflamed plaque in the typical site, sometimes associated with smaller satellite papules (62). Topical antifungal agents are usually effective; however, oral flucona-zole works more quickly.

For all fungal infections, athletes should keep affected areas covered and avoid sharing towels and walking barefoot. At all times, all mats and apparatus should be disinfected regularly, especially if an athlete is found to have an infection. Athletes with a fungal infection can be al-lowed to participate only if affected areas are adequately covered.

REFERENCES

1. Brenner I, Shek PN, Shephard RJ: Infection in athletes. Sports Med 17:86–107, 1994

2. Ryan AJ, Dalrymple W, Dull B, et al: Round Table: upper respiratory in-fections in sports medicine. Physician and Sportsmedicine 3:29, 1975

3. Hanley DF: Medical care of the US Olympic team. JAMA 236:147, 1976

4. Cohen S, Tyrrell DA, Smith AP: Psychological stress and susceptibility to the common cold. N Engl J Med 325:606, 1991

5. Graham NMH, Douglas RM, Ryan P: Stress and acute respiratory infection. Am J Epidemiol 124:389, 1986

6. Heath WG, Ford ES, Craven TE: Exercise and the incidence of upper res-piratory tract infections. Med Sci Sports Exerc 23:152, 1991

7. Berk LS, Nieman DC, Youngberg WS, et al: The effect of long endurance running on natural killer cells in marathoners. Med Sci Sports Exerc 22:207, 1990

8. Mackinnon LT, Chick TW, van As A, et al: The effect of exercise on secretory and natural immunity. Adv Exp Med Biol 216A:869, 1987

9. Eskola J, Ruuskanen O, Soppi E, et al: Effect of sport stress on lymphocyte transformation and antibody formation. Clin Exp Immunol 32:339–345, 1978

10. Ahlborg A, Ahlborg G: Exercise leukocytosis with and without beta-adrenergic blockade. Acta Med Scand 187:241–246, 1970

11. Jeammott JB, Borysenko JZ, Borysenko M, et al: Academic stress, power motivation and decrease in secretion rate of salivary secretory IgA. Lancet 1:1400–1402, 1983

12. Nieman DC, Johanssen LM, Lee JW, et al: Infectious episodes in runners before and after a roadrace. J Sports Med Phys Fitness 29:289, 1989

13. Nieman DC, Nehlsen-Cannarella SL: The effects of acute and chronic exercise on immunoglobulins. Sports Med 11:183, 1991

14. Nieman DC, Johanssen LM, Lee JW, Arabatzis K: Infectious episodes in runners before and after the Los Angeles marathon. J Sports Med Phys Fitness 30:316–328, 1990

15. Stewart KJ: Weight training in coronary artery disease and hypertension. Prog Cardiovasc Dis 3:159–168, 1992

16. Daniels WL, Sharp DS, Wright JE, et al: Effects of virus infection on physical performance in man. Mil Med 150:8, 1985

17. Phillips MM, Robinowitz M, Higgins JRM, et al: Sudden cardiac death in airforce recruits: a twenty year review. JAMA 256:2696–2699, 1986

18. Drory Y, Kramer MR, Lev B: Exertional sudden death in soldiers. Med Sci Sports Exerc 23:147–151, 1991

19. Robers JA: Viral illnesses and sports performance. Sports Med 3:296, 1986

20. Simon HB: Exercise and infection. Physician and Sportsmedicine 15:135, 1987

21. Eichner ER: Neck check. Runner's World 27:16, 1992

22. Sevier TL: Infectious disease in athletes. Med Clin North Am 78:389–412, 1994

23. Roberts JA: Viral illnesses and sports performance. Sports Med 3:296–303, 1986

24. Shephard RJ, Shek PN: Athletic competition and susceptibility to infection. Clin J Sport Med 3:75–77, 1993

25. Eichner ER: Infectious mononucleosis: recognizing the condition, "reactivating" the patient. Physician and Sportsmedicine 24(4):49–54, 1996

26. Eichner ER: Infectious mononucleosis: recognition and management in athletes. Physician and Sportsmedicine 15(12):61–72, 1987

27. Chetham MM, Roberts KB: Infectious mononucleosis in adolescents. Pediatr Ann 20:206–213, 1991

28. Ali J: Spontaneous rupture of the spleen in patients with infectious mononucleosis. Can J Surg 36:49–52, 1993

29. Oski FA: Management of a football player with infectious mononucleosis. Pediatr Infect Dis J 13:938–939, 1994

30. Rigsby LW, Dishman RK, Jackson AW, MacLean GS, Raven PB: Effects of exercise training on men seropositive for the human immunodeficiency virus-1. Med Sci Sports Exerc 24:6–12, 1992

31. Macarthur RD, Levine SD, Birk TJ: Supervised exercise training improves cardiopulmonary fitness in HIV infected persons. Med Sci Sports Exerc 25:S45, 1993

32. Spence DW, Galantino MLA, Mossberg KA, Zimmerman SO: Progressive resistance exercise: effect on muscle function and anthropometry of a select AIDS population. Arch Phys Med Rehabil 71:644–648, 1990

33. Soppi E, Varjo P, Eskola J, et al: Effect of strenuous physical stress on circulating lymphocyte number and function before and after training. J Clin Lab Immunol 8:43–46, 1982

34. Eichner ER, Calabrese LH: Immunology and exercise: physiology, pathophysiology, and implications for HIV infection. Med Clin North Am 78:377–388, 1994

35. LaPerriere A, Fletcher MA, Antoni MH, Klimas NG, Ironson G, Schneiderman N: Aerobic exercise training in an AIDS risk group. Int J Sports Med 12:S53–S57, 1991

36. LePerriere A, O'Hearn P, Ironson G, et al: Exercise and immune function in healthy HIV antibody negative and positive gay males. In Proceedings of the Ninth Annual Scientific Sessions of Society of Behavioral Medicine, Boston, 1988, 28

37. LaPerriere AR, Antoni MH, Schneiderman N, et al: Exercise intervention attenuates emotional distress and natural killer cell decrements following notification of positive serologic status for HIV-1. Biofeedback and Self-regulation 15:229–241, 1990

38. LaPerriere AR, Fletcher MA, Antoni MH, Klimas NG, Schneiderman N: Aerobic exercise training in an AIDS risk group. Int J Sports Med 12:S53–S57, 1991

39. Nefzger MD, Chalmers TC: The treatment of acute infectious hepatitis: ten-year follow-up study of the effects of diet and rest. Am J Med 35:299–309, 1963

40. Schlenzig C, Jager H, Rieder H, et al: Supervised physical exercise leads to psychological and immunological improvement in pre-AIDS patients. In Proceedings of the Fifth International Conference on AIDS, Montreal, 1989, 337

41. Keyes C, Rodgers P, Wolert J, et al: Effect of cardiovascular conditioning in HIV infection. In Proceedings of the Fifth International Conference on AIDS, Montreal, 1989, 363

42. Calabrese LH, LaPerriere A: Human immunodeficiency virus infection, exercise and athletics. Sports Med 15:6–13, 1993

43. Cupler EJ, Danon MJ, Jay C, Hench K, Ropka M, Dalakas MC: Early fea-

tures of zidovudine-associated myopathy: histopathological findings and clinical correlations. Acta Neuropathol 90:1–6, 1995

44. Mitten MJ: Athletic participation with a contagious blood-borne disease. Clin J Sport Med 5:153–154, 1995

45. McGrew CA, Dick RW, Schniedwind K, Gikas P: Survey of NCAA institutions concerning HIV/AIDS policies and universal precautions. Med Sci Sports Exerc 25:917–921, 1993

46. Friedland GH, Klein RS: Transmission of the human immunodeficiency virus. N Engl J Med 317:1125–1134, 1987

47. Wormser GP, Bittker S, Forseter G, et al: Absence of infectious human immunodeficiency virus type 1 in "natural" eccrine sweat. J Infect Dis 165:155–158, 1992

48. American Academy of Pediatrics Committee on Sports Medicine and Fitness: Human immunodeficiency virus (AIDS) in the athletic setting. Pediatrics 88:640–641, 1991

49. World Health Organization consensus statement: consultation on AIDS and sports. JAMA 267:1312, 1992

50. Torre D, Sampietro C, Ferraro G, et al: Transmission of HIV-1 infection via sports injuries (letter). Lancet 335:1105, 1990

51. Goldsmith ME: When sports and HIV share the bill, smart money goes on common sense. JAMA 267:1311–1314, 1992

52. American Medical Society for Sports Medicine and American Academy of Sports Medicine: Human immunodeficiency virus (HIV) and other blood-borne pathogens in sports. Am J Sports Med 23(4):510–514, 1995

53. Mitten MJ: AIDS and athletics. Seton Hall Journal of Sport Law 3:5–40, 1993

54. Centers for Disease Control: Guidelines for prevention of transmission of human immunodeficiency virus and hepatitis B virus to health care and public safety workers. Morb Mortal Wkly Rep 38(suppl 6):1–37, 1989

55. Committee on Infectious Diseases (American Academy of Pediatrics): Universal hepatitis B immunization. Pediatrics 89:795–800, 1992

56. Hepatitis B virus: a comprehensive strategy for eliminating transmission in the United States through universal childhood vaccination. Recommendations of the Immunization Practices Advisory Committee (ACIP). Morb Mortal Wkly Rep 40:1–25, 1991

57. Kashiwagi S, Hayshi J, Ikematsu H, Nishigori S, Ishihara K, Kaji M: An outbreak of hepatitis B in members of a high school sumo wrestling club. JAMA 248:213–214, 1982

58. Conklin RJ: Common cutaneous disorders in athletes. Sports Med 9:100–119, 1990

59. Sharp JCM, Girdwood RWA, Watt B, et al: Infections in sport. Br J Sports Med 22:117–121, 1988

60. Freeman MJ, Bergfeld WF: Skin diseases of football and wrestling participants. Cutis 20:333–341, 1977

61. Lever WF, Schaumberg-Lever G: Noninfectious vesicular and bullous diseases. In Histopathology of the Skin. Philadelphia, JB Lippincott, 1983, 92–135

62. Kantor GR, Bergfeld WF: Common and uncommon dermatologic diseases related to sports activities. Exerc Sport Sci Rev 16:215, 1988

63. Basler RS: Skin lesions related to sports activity. Prim Care 10:479–494, 1983

64. Robinson AM: Skin problems in athletes. Md Med J 18:81–82, 1969

65. Conklin RJ: Acne vulgaris in the athlete. Physician and Sportsmedicine 16(10):57–68, 1988

66. Reichel M, Laub D: From acne to black heel: common skin injuries in sports. Physician and Sportsmedicine 20(2):111–118, 1992

67. Bartlett PC, Martin RJ, Cahill BR: Furunculosis in a high school football team. Am J Sports Med 10:371–374, 1982

68. Muller SA: Dermatologic disorders in athletes. J Ky Med Assoc 74:225–228, 1976

69. Becker T, Kodsi R, Bailey P, et al: Grappling with herpes: herpes gladiatorum. Am J Sports Med 16:665–669, 1988

70. Dyke LM, Merikangas UR, Bruton OC, Trask SG, Hetrick FM: Skin infection in wrestlers due to herpes simplex virus. JAMA 194:1001–1002, 1965

71. Porter PS, Baughman RD: Epidemiology of herpes simplex among wrestlers. JAMA 194:150–152, 1965

72. Wheeler CE, Cabaniss WH: Epidemic cutaneous herpes simplex in wrestlers (herpes gladiatorum). JAMA 194:145–149, 1965

73. Corey L: Genital herpes. In Holmes KK, Mardh PA, Sparling PF, et al (eds): Sexually Transmitted Diseases. New York, McGraw-Hill, 1984, 449–473

74. Nahmias AJ, Dannenbarger J, Wickliffe C, et al: Clinical aspects of infection with herpes simplex viruses 1 and 2. In Nahmias AJ, Dowdle WR, Schinazi RF (eds): The Human Herpesviruses. New York, Elsevier, 1981, 3–9

75. Stauffer LW: Skin disorders in athletes: identification and management. Physician and Sportsmedicine 11:101–121, 1983

76. Shelley WB: Herpetic arthritis associated with disseminated herpes simplex in a wrestler. Br J Dermatol 103:209–212, 1980

77. Corey L, Nahmias A, Guinan M: A trial of topical acyclovir in genital herpes simplex infections. N Engl J Med 306:1313–1319, 1982

78. Houston SD, Knox JM: Skin problems related to sports and recreational activities. Cutis 19:487–491, 1977

79. Omura EF, Rye B: Dermatologic disorders of the foot. Clin Sports Med 13:825–841, 1994

80. Conklin RJ: Common cutaneous disorders in athletes. Sports Med 9:100–119, 1990

81. Reyes MP, Lerner AM: Interferon and neutralizing antibody in sera of exercised mice with Coxsackie virus B-3 myocarditis. Proc Soc Exp Biol Med 151:333, 1976

82. Bart B: Skin problems in athletics. Minn Med 66:239–241, 1983

83. Frisk A, Heilborn H, Melen B: Epidemic occurrence of trichophytosis among wrestlers. Acta Derm Venereol 46:453–456, 1966

84. Resnik SS, Lewis LA, Cohen BH: The athlete's foot. Cutis 20:351–353, 355, 1977

Chapter 4

ERGOGENIC AGENTS

The popularity of competitive sports and the prevailing attitude in society that "winning is everything" have led to an intense, almost fervent quest for anything to give the athlete a competitive edge. Some athletes choose unique training programs, exercise protocols, or dietary changes. Unfortunately, an increasing number of athletes are choosing to enhance their performance with pharmacological agents that include various hormones, stimulants, minerals, vitamins, and proteins.

ANABOLIC STEROIDS

The strength-enhancing effects of testosterone were first demonstrated in the 1950s, and by 1960 the first synthetic anabolic, androgenic steroid was produced. Since that time, numerous anabolic and adrenergic steroids have been synthesized, but technology has not successfully produced one agent with only anabolic or only adrenergic properties (1). A wide variety of steroids that maximize anabolic effects and minimize adrenergic effects are available today. The anabolic effects of a steroid include induction of protein synthesis in muscle cells and enhanced utilization of ingested protein (2,3). Anabolic steroids also reverse the catabolic state induced by the release of glucocorticoids during exercise (4). Many weight lifters live in a chronic negative nitrogen balance resulting from the breakdown of proteins for energy within the muscle cells, due, in part, to an inability to keep up with the substantial amount of protein needed to maintain their physical state. Anabolic steroids allow the athlete to maintain a balance of nitrogen through an efficient use of ingested protein and further protein synthesis. These effects may explain why weight lifters who are already training (and probably in a state of negative nitrogen balance) seem to experience the most benefit and increase in strength from anabolic and adrenergic steroids (4).

Resistance exercise stimulates protein synthesis by way of endogenous hormones, most notably growth hormone, insulin, insulin-like growth factor, and testosterone (5,6). Ingested anabolic steroids have also been demonstrated to further stimulate the release of growth hormone. Insulin, one of the most potent anabolic hormones, is generally not significantly affected by resistance exercise; ingestion of carbohydrates stimulates the release of insulin within 30 minutes. Studies have shown that the use of both protein and carbohydrate supplements after resistance training provides the maximal benefit (enhanced muscle mass and strength), resulting from the anabolic effect of the ingested anabolic steroid combined with effects of insulin and other endogenous hormones (7,8). Overall, anabolic steroids increase muscle mass and strength, often at an enhanced rate, and combined with the appropriate dietary restrictions cause significant reductions in body fat, producing the characteristic "body builder's body."

The effect of anabolic steroids on aerobic exercise performance and endurance has also been examined. Anabolic steroids do not affect aerobic performance, endurance, or maximal oxygen uptake (4,9). They can improve performance in sports requiring short bursts of anaerobic exercise. The cardiovascular effects are unclear. Anabolic steroids have been shown to increase left ventricular mass and left ventricular internal diameter (9). Some evidence suggests that anabolic steroids impair left ventricular diastolic filling and result in a cardiomyopathy (10). The effects on ventricular mass, similar to the effects on skeletal muscle, reverse with discontinuation of steroid use. Although most users of anabolic steroids do try to "cycle" the use and spend a period of time off the steroids, this time off is relatively short and steroid use remains, in effect, chronic.

Both the strength- and muscle-enhancing effects of anabolic steroids are quite attractive not only to athletes but to non-athletes seeking a muscular appearance. A multitude of negative side effects have been demonstrated, some of which can be life threatening (table 4.1). Research has associated anabolic steroid use with myocardial ischemia and infarction (11,12,18), ischemic cerebral vascular accident (CVA) (13–16), deep vein thrombosis (DVT), and superior sagittal thrombosis (17)

Table 4.1. Effects of Anabolic Steroids

Positive effects
    Temporary increase in muscular size and weight
Adverse effects
    Cardiovascular
        Hypertension
        Increase in LDL/HDL ratio
        Possible stroke or myocardial infarction (reported cases)
    Hepatic (with oral agents)
        Elevated enzymes
        Peliosis hepatitis
        Tumors (benign and malignant)
    Genitourinary
        Males
            Decreased production of testosterone
            Suppression of spermatogenesis
            Testicular atrophy
            Gynecomastia
        Females
            Altered menstruation
            Clitoral enlargement
            Increased facial and body hair
    Endocrine
        Suppression of thyroid function
        Deepened voice (female)
    Immunological
        Decreased levels of immunoglobulins
    Musculoskeletal
        Premature closure of epiphysis and bone growth centers
        Tendon degeneration and increased risk of rupture
    Dermatological
        Acne, facial and body
        Male-pattern baldness
        Coarsening of skin
    Psychological
        Mood swings (can be severe)
        Enhanced aggression
        Psychotic episodes
        Depression
        Dependency on drug or risk of habitual use
        Suicide attempts (some cases reported)

in young individuals. Anabolic steroids may be thrombogenic, possibly due to an increase in platelet adhesiveness or alterations in prostaglandin synthesis (12). They also increase serum levels of low-density lipoprotein cholesterol (LDL-C) and decrease serum levels of high-density lipoprotein cholesterol (HDL-C). Thus, even though exercise generally decreases the LDL/HDL ratio, athletes taking anabolic steroids tend to experience an overall increase in LDL/HDL ratios (19). The possible acceleration of atherosclerosis that may occur with the use of anabolic steroids, even over the short term, may further increase the risk of an ischemic event.

Oral anabolic steroids may increase liver function tests (LFTs): SGOT (aspartate aminotransferase), SGPT (alanine aminotransferase), alkaline phosphatase, and LDH (lactate dehydrogenase). Weight lifting alone may result in elevated LFTs (with normal alkaline phosphatase), but this effect is enhanced by anabolic steroid use. The elevated LFTs return to normal with discontinuation. Continued use, however, may result in peliosis hepatitis, a rare cystic degeneration of the liver. Liver tumors, benign and malignant, have also been reported with use for longer than 24 months, some of which were reversible with elimination of steroid use (20).

Anabolic steroids are supposedly associated with an enhanced libido, but this is not always the case. Exogenous anabolic steroids can inhibit feedback from the pituitary gland, resulting in decreased levels of follicle-stimulating hormone (FSH) and luteinizing hormone (LH) (21–23). The serum testosterone levels subsequently decrease, and since most anabolic steroids cannot interact with testicular function in the same way as testosterone, hypogonadotropic hypogonadism with possible azoospermia can occur. These effects are usually reversible, but persistent azoospermia and/or hypogonadism have been reported (24).

Few studies have examined the effect of anabolic steroids on women, even though the use in female athletes is rising. Reported effects include hirsutism, deepening of the voice, alopecia, abnormal menses, and acne (25). Clitoral enlargement may also occur and is often not reversible (26,27). Serum testosterone levels seem to be higher in females who use anabolic steroids than in normal males (25).

Anabolic steroids can have adverse effects on the musculoskeletal system as well. Several cases have been reported of tendon ruptures, possibly due to collagen dysplasia and subsequent weakening of the musculotendinous junction (28–30). Adolescents who use anabolic steroids prior to epiphyseal closure may accelerate the closure, resulting in a shorter stature (26).

Perhaps the most worrisome side effect of anabolic steroids is their influence on behavior and personality. The overwhelming majority of steroid users experience some degree of personality change, from increased irritability and aggressiveness to frank psychosis (31,32). The resulting intense personality, aggressiveness, and tendency toward violence may be attractive to some athletes who believe their training and performance is thus enhanced. These same changes, however, often render the individual incapable of maintaining appropriate composure during competition and normal relationships outside athletic events.

These personality changes are reversible, but they are compounded by the strong tendency toward both psychological and physiological addiction (33). Individuals who are attracted to steroid use are often seeking an "edge" or advantage over other athletes (highly competitive or professional athletes), or they may feel that steroid use is imperative to compete on the same level as other athletes, who are assumed to be using steroids as well. These substances may also function to appease a psychological insecurity about performance or appearance (34).

Anabolic steroids can be taken in oral or parenteral form. The doses used exceed the recommended therapeutic doses by up to 100-fold. It is not uncommon for an individual to take an oral and a parenteral steroid simultaneously, in a method known as "stacking." The use of parenteral steroids suggests an increased level of commitment and perhaps of dependence, not unlike the effects seen in recreational drug use. Parenteral steroids cannot be administered using an insulin needle, which often forces the individual to resort to the black market to obtain larger-gage needles. This places the individual at additional risk for contracting HIV or hepatitis through the use of shared needles (35)

Discontinuation of anabolic steroids often results in severe depression, which may have a physiological component (35). The individual experiences a loss of muscle bulk and strength, in addition to a diminished intensity and desire to exercise. These losses are even more significant to the competitive and insecure athlete who is attracted to steroid use. Unfortunately, a significant number of individuals are unable to cope with these losses and return to steroid use, becoming long-term users, and some have even attempted suicide (36,37). The effects of long-term use have not been clearly defined as yet, but the potential for severe and irreversible consequences is undeniable.

Steroid users are almost a unique category of substance abusers. They often consider themselves the epitome of good health, diligently regulating their diet and social activities, avoiding alcohol and nicotine in the name of a maximally "pure" physique. Most serious steroid users are well versed in the potentially deleterious side effects of the steroids. Their rationale for use—to give them a competitive edge—often allows them, in their own minds, to minimize the potential risks. This attitude is also encouraged, not only by other serious users who exhibit their own enhanced physique but also by underground publications, such as the *Underground Steroid Handbook*. This popular text circulates through many gyms and is regularly edited and revised. It emphasizes the complete reversibility of all side effects and discredits the concept of "too much." It also lists the available agents and methods of obtaining them, and gives stepwise instructions on "how to give yourself a shot."

The use of anabolic steroids has escalated to almost epidemic proportions. Initially, use seemed to be predominantly among elite athletes. Reports of use in the Soviet Union and possibly other Soviet-bloc countries have surfaced, perhaps accounting for the premature deaths of a number of Olympic athletes, including 26 gold medalists (38). Lately, the popularity of anabolic steroids has spread to younger and recreational athletes. Surveys of high school students have revealed that between 7% and 11% of high school males (39,40) and 2.5% of females have tried anabolic steroids at one time (41). One-third of these students were not participating in interscholastic sports. Attempts to control the spread of anabolic steroid use led to Congress's passage of the Anti-Drug Abuse Act in 1988, which prohibited the use of anabolic steroids except for the treatment of disease (42). In 1990, anabolic steroids were included as a class III substance under the Controlled Substances Act of 1970 (43). Organized sports, including the NCAA, IOC, and National Football League (NFL), have instituted elaborate drug-testing protocols to discourage the further use of anabolic steroids. However, as different types of steroids become available—especially those produced specifically to hinder detection by present testing methods—detection becomes more difficult. Physicians involved in the care of athletes, as well as adolescents, should actively participate in education programs to discourage and prevent the possible abuse of anabolic steroids. Suspicion of possible use should always remain high.

TESTOSTERONE

Most recently, testosterone has become popular as an anabolic steroid with the advantage of being undetectable. Some have speculated that female Olympians in 1996 used testosterone patches, which deliver a small amount of testosterone but enough to increase strength and speed in women (44).

Some male athletes most likely use testosterone as well, but detection is difficult since synthetic testosterone cannot be differentiated from natural testosterone in the serum (45). In addition, testosterone levels in males seem to vary, making interpretation of a high serum level difficult. Presently, the ratio of serum levels of testosterone to a direct metabolite, epitestosterone—the T/E ratio—is the best means of determining an abnormally high level of testosterone. In most males, the T/E ratio is 1, although recent ingestion of alcohol may increase it to 2 or 3; but it is rarely above 6. The official "abnormal" level, used by the USOC, is 6. Athletes have now begun taking epitestosterone in addition to testosterone, effectively decreasing their serum T/E ratio. It is important for testers to bear in mind that some men (approximately 1 in 2,000) lack the enzyme that converts testosterone to epitestosterone, a deficiency that could increase the T/E ratio. Hopefully, tests will soon be available to allow differentiation between synthetic and natural testosterone, making detection of testosterone use by these athletes easier (44).

HUMAN GROWTH HORMONE

Human growth hormone (hGH) is an endogenous hormone produced by the pituitary gland. Although the primary function is to maintain normal linear growth from birth to adulthood, it also has some anabolic effects. It stimulates the transport of amino acids into muscle tissue, enhancing the synthesis of protein (46); it also increases the release of lipids from adipose tissue and stimulates the preferential use of lipids for energy, thus preserving muscle glycogen (47,48). The potential anabolic effects of exogenous hGH are attractive to athletes interested in enhancing strength and muscle mass without the risk of detection by presently available drug tests. The current popular belief is that hGH produces the same effects as anabolic steroids, and although its use is banned by the NCAA and USOC, it is undetectable in urine (the most commonly used means of drug testing in athletes). Some adolescents have been led to believe that hGH will increase their physical stature, whereas it actually can stunt growth by stimulating early closure of epiphyses.

The anabolic and lipolytic effects of hGH are well documented, but no well-controlled studies exist to support the belief that it improves strength and endurance (49,50). Increases in muscle mass have been demonstrated with the administration of exogenous hGH, but a concurrent increase in strength was not found (51,52). In fact, muscles in patients with acromegaly (overproduction of endogenous hGH) are myopathic (53).

The extent of exogenous hGH use is limited by the high cost, which can range from $1,000 to $1,500 for the 8-week supply needed for an ergogenic effect (54). Because it is available only in parenteral form, needles and syringe are required as well. Certain amino acids, most commonly arginine, ornithine, and lysine, have been shown to stimulate the release of endogenous hGH (55). Many athletes are turning to amino acid supplements as an alternative means of increasing the serum level of hGH. No well-controlled studies exist to support this possible effect.

CLENBUTEROL AND BETA-2 AGONISTS

Clenbuterol, terbutaline, albuterol, and salmeterol are beta-2 agonists and have multiple sympathomimetic effects on muscle, metabolic, and endocrine activities. They are not anabolic steroids, but they all have potential anabolic effects and as such are banned by the NCAA and USOC (44).

Clenbuterol is also classified as a stimulant and has been demonstrated to increase muscle mass and decrease body fat in experimental animals. It also decreases the oxidative potential of the same muscles, although this effect can be eliminated via an exercise regimen (56). No studies of the ergogenic effect of clenbuterol in humans are presently available. Certain athletes—usually weight lifters and body builders, who are always seeking a possible new ergogenic agent—have been using it in combination with anabolic steroids. The safety of long-term use of clenbuterol has not been established, but the sudden death of two European body builders who were using it suggests that this needs to be investigated soon (57).

Other long-acting beta-2 agonists are also banned by the NCAA and USOC, because of the possible ergogenic effect, especially in resistance-exercise sports (58,59). Although this effect has not been proven conclusively, the use of beta-2 agonists is restricted to an inhaled form specifically for treatment of exercise-induced asthma (60,61).

CAFFEINE

Caffeine is one of many drugs in the methylxanthine group, which also includes theophylline and theobromine (62). Available in a multitude of popular drinks (tea, colas), as well as in over-the-counter medications (Midol, Excedrin, No Doz) and chocolate, caffeine is the most commonly used drug worldwide. For years athletes have used it as an ergogenic aid.

Caffeine stimulates lipolysis and enhances the mobilization of FFAs, preserving glycogen stores and thus delaying the onset of glycogen depletion and exhaustion (63,64). It also increases the serum level of catecholamines during and after exercise (34). Skeletal muscle strength may also be enhanced and perhaps less susceptible to exhaustion (47, 65). These effects may be potentiated by a direct influence on the central nervous system to stimulate the release of endorphins, thus modifying the perception of pain and discomfort during exercise (66).

The effect of caffeine on exercise performance is dose-related. Moderate to high levels of caffeine (2–9 mg/kg) have been shown to improve endurance exercise such as running or cycling over prolonged periods (longer than 1 hour) at moderate intensity (75–80% of Vo_{2max}) (67,68).

Sprint performance (defined as the intensity of exercise needed to reach exhaustion in 90 seconds) does not seem to be affected by caffeine ingestion, in either elite or recreational athletes (69). The absorption of 85–250 mg of caffeine is required before improvement in reaction time and dexterity or coordination can be elicited (70). These effects, however, can be strongly attenuated in habitual consumers of caffeine (coffee) (71). The athlete who wants to use caffeine as an ergogenic aid can maximize its effect by avoiding caffeine for a prolonged period (4–5 days), then ingesting it 3–4 hours before the endurance event; this allows the plasma concentration of FFAs to peak and thus maximizes the ergogenic effect (rather than allowing just the plasma concentration of caffeine to peak, which occurs within 1 hour after ingestion) (72).

Side effects of caffeine include dizziness, headaches, insomnia, and GI upset, with palpitations and arrhythmias occurring in some individuals (usually premature ventricular contractions [PVCs] and tachycardia). The occurrence is often dose related and varies with the individual. The probability of side effects increases dramatically with doses greater than 6 mg/kg (73). These side effects can significantly negate the ergogenic effect of the ingested caffeine.

The USOC bans caffeine only if the urinary concentration is greater than 12 µg/mL (74). The NCAA's limit is somewhat higher at 15 µg/mL (75). These concentrations would require the ingestion of 6–10 cups of coffee at one sitting approximately 2–3 hours before the test (74). Ingestion of such large amounts of caffeine at one time most likely reflects the ingestion of caffeine in a form other than the usual coffee or cola, such as caffeine tablets or suppositories (reportedly used by the U.S. cycling team in the 1984 Olympics, although illegal levels were not reported) (76). It is important for the athlete to realize that the rate of elimination of caffeine can vary among individuals, such that even a moderate amount of ingested caffeine may produce a higher than expected level of caffeine in the urine.

AMINO ACID SUPPLEMENTATION

The increased need for protein and amino acids in endurance athletes is primarily to minimize or replace protein broken down during prolonged exercise (73,77). Amino acid supplementation has become popular among many athletes trying to increase their muscle mass and strength. The benefits are considered, at least by the athletes, to be multifold. The rationale is that the mere excess of amino acids will promote protein synthesis and increase muscle mass, rather than just replace what has been lost.

Certain amino acids do have an anabolic effect. Amino acids have been demonstrated to promote insulin secretion, which in turn enhances the uptake of amino acids and further decreases the catabolic degradation of protein (78,79). Branch-chain amino acids (BCAAs)—leucine, arginine, isoleucine—can also stimulate further release of hGH, another anabolic hormone (as discussed above). But a chronically elevated level of hGH may actually be detrimental, since it can result in chronically elevated serum glucose levels, hyperinsulinemia, hyperglucagonemia, and a possible diabetogenic state resulting from the diminished sensitivity of the target cells (80,81). BCAAs may also prevent clearance of testosterone in exercising muscles—another indirect anabolic influence (82).

The possibility that a combination of ornithine and arginine can stimulate the synthesis of creatine and creatine phosphate (another endogenous anabolic chemical; see below) has been suggested. This effect in turn may lead to an increase in muscle mass, although it has not been demonstrated (83). The importance of BCAAs in muscle physiology has been supported primarily by the finding that during prolonged and intense exercise, degradation of BCAAs in muscle tissue increases significantly, while plasma concentration of BCAAs decreases to a lesser degree (84,85). The direct implication of these changes is unclear, but an adverse effect on strength, muscle mass, and endurance has not been shown.

Although BCAAs may stimulate the release of hGH, insulin, and possibly creatine, the ergogenic effect has recently been challenged (86). The concentrations of BCAAs needed to raise the serum levels of hGH to a physiologically significant concentration may require a dose too large to be ingested orally without severe side effects, such as GI cramping and nausea (87). The large doses needed may cause a significant increase in serum ammonia level, which would adversely affect muscle metabolism (88,89). The small doses of BCAAs usually present in popular energy supplements such as fluid replacement drinks are certainly not enough to affect performance or endurance.

ERYTHROPOIETIN AND BLOOD DOPING

The concept that increasing the total number of red blood cells will enhance physical performance, especially endurance exercise, through an increase in oxygen delivery to active muscles has interested athletes for several years. Athletes initially tried training at high altitudes in an attempt to physiologically stimulate the production of RBCs (90). A 10–20% increase in the serum hemoglobin is known to enhance oxygen consumption and delivery, resulting in a significant improvement in endurance exercise performance (43).

These findings have led to attempts to increase serum hemoglobin by other means, most notably by "blood doping." Blood doping is the intravenous infusion of autologous blood for the sole purpose of temporarily raising the serum hemoglobin to enhance athletic performance. The most popular method involves removing two units of blood, separating the RBCs, and freezing them for 4–8 weeks while the athlete's bone marrow regenerates sufficient numbers of RBCs to return hemoglobin to its baseline level. The athlete continues to train at the usual level in the interim, and the RBCs are re-infused within 1 week prior to the competitive event. The dramatic effect of blood doping has been demonstrated, for example, by an improvement of up to 35% in running time to exhaustion (91,92) or by a 45-second improvement in a 5-mile run (93).

In 1985, synthetic erythropoietin (epo) became widely available. Epo is an endogenous glycoprotein responsible for the stimulation of RBC formation in the bone marrow. Intravenously administered epo has a half-life of only 4–5 hours, but increased RBC production following a subcutaneous dose continues for up to 2 weeks (94). Studies have shown the similar effect of epo and blood doping on elevation of hemoglobin and enhanced performance (95,96). The availability of epo and its ease of administration make it particularly attractive to athletes as a shortcut to blood doping and an increase in hemoglobin.

Blood doping, either indirectly through epo or by direct infusion of autologous blood, poses a serious health threat. Hypertension is associated with administration of epo (97). The viscosity of the serum increases with the concentration of RBCs, and this is often compounded by the dehydration commonly present in endurance athletes during an event. The resulting increase in hematocrit can be as high as 60%. This self-induced "erythrocythemia" places the athlete at substantial risk for coronary and cerebral arterial occlusion, a risk that rises exponentially as the hematocrit increases above 55%. In fact, the 19 unexplained deaths in competitive Belgian and Dutch cyclists between 1987 and 1990 are most likely related to blood doping and epo use (43).

Blood doping is banned by the IOC and USOC, but detecting its use is close to impossible at present. Epo is excreted in the urine in such a small amount that measurement is of little use. Measurement of epo levels in the blood is not helpful either, since epo is metabolized so quickly. Serum hemoglobin levels could be an indirect means of detecting blood doping. Use of this test would require a general agreement between athletic governing bodies (the IOC and others) as to what hemoglobin level is acceptable for an endurance athlete and what suggests the use of an endogenous agent. This has yet to be done.

CREATINE

Creatine is another ergogenic agent that has recently become popular among athletes. The primary source of creatine is animal proteins in the diet, but some is produced endogenously. It is present in the body in both free and phosphorylated forms. Skeletal muscle contains more than 95% of the body's store of creatine, of which more than two-thirds is phosphorylated (98).

Creatine phosphate is degraded into creatine and phosphate with intense exercise and high energy demand. The phosphate is then added to adenosine diphosphate (ADP) to produce adenosine triphosphate (ATP), the primary energy source for skeletal muscle contraction. Free creatine accumulates during activity, then is converted back to creatine phosphate during rest. It has been suggested that the limiting factor for the maintenance of muscle force may be the concentration of creatine phosphate in type II muscle fibers (99).

Athletes can take creatine as an oral supplement in a water-soluble form such as creatine monohydrate (98). The goal is to increase the level of creatine phosphate, which will then supposedly increase the supply of ATP to allow a higher energy output, delay fatigue, and improve overall performance. The concentration of creatine in muscle fibers has been shown to increase with supplementation, but once the maximal concentration is reached, any excess creatine is excreted in the urine (100,101). Data suggest that creatine supplements may improve performance in short intermittent periods of high-intensity exercise (less than 10 seconds) (102–104). The overall higher concentration of creatine in muscles achieved with supplementation may allow less dependence on anaerobic glycolysis, leading to a smaller decrease in muscle pH and a higher rate of resynthesis of creatine phosphate during recovery (98).

Creatine may be a useful ergogenic aid for athletes in sports that require intermittent short sprints or all-out efforts, such as football, hockey, or tennis (98,102,103,105). It has not been demonstrated to have any effect on performance in endurance exercise (103,106). The IOC does not presently include creatine on the list of banned substances, probably because of the difficulty in detecting the use of oral supplementation. No data presently exist on the effects of long-term supplementation.

BICARBONATE

High-intensity exercise quickly leads to the accumulation of lactic acid in muscle. The relative acidemia can interfere with continued ATP production in the muscle fibers by slowing glycolysis (107,108). Lactic acidosis may also impair the release of calcium from the endoplasmic reticulum of the muscle, thus interfering with contraction (109,110). The possibility that lactic acidosis contributes to muscle exhaustion has led to the use of bicarbonate as a buffer to reduce the level of acidosis in muscle and in the bloodstream and thus delay the onset of complete exhaustion.

Data on the use of oral bicarbonate and its effect on exercise performance are contradictory and seem to depend on the amount of bicarbonate ingested, the form (calcium carbonate, sodium citrate, or sodium chloride), and duration of exercise (111). Higher doses of bicarbonate (300 mg/kg vs. 200 mg/kg) tend to improve performance to some extent, although not always significantly (112–114). In addition, calcium carbonate and sodium chloride seem to be more beneficial than sodium citrate (115). Bicarbonate also improves performance in repeated exercise periods of short duration to exhaustion (112,115–117). Short-term anaerobic exercise or endurance exercise has not shown any benefit from bicarbonate supplementation (115,118).

CHROMIUM PICOLINATE

Chromium is classified as an essential trace mineral. It is present in various foods, including nuts, grains, and cereals. The average American diet provides only 50% of the recommended daily allowance (119).

Chromium supplementation seemed to gain popularity after studies associated increased chromium loss with regular exercise (120). Chromium is a cofactor that enhances the action of insulin. The results of studies showing its ergogenic potential have not been impressive. Early studies suggested an increase in lean body mass and resistance strength with chromium supplementation (121–123). More recently, vigorous studies have not demonstrated any ergogenic potential with supplementation (124,125). The safety of chromium supplementation is also questionable. Supplements are usually in the form of chromium picolinate, which helps to increase absorption. Adverse effects, some serious, have been reported; these include anemia (126), cognitive impairment (127), and interstitial nephritis (128).

DEHYDROEPIANDROSTERONE

Dehydroepiandrosterone (DHEA) is an endogenous androgen produced in the adrenal glands. It is a precursor to androgenic steroids and thus has gained popularity among athletes. Athletes using DHEA consider it an indirect means of increasing serum testosterone levels, producing the same ergogenic effect as testosterone supplementation (129). No studies demonstrate any ergogenic effect of DHEA.

AMPHETAMINES

Amphetamines are indirect sympathomimetic amines that stimulate the release of catecholamines (34). Amphetamines improve strength, speed, and endurance and increase alertness, all of which enhances athletic performance (130,131). They may also be used as appetite suppressants by athletes involved in sports that focus on body weight, such as wrestling and gymnastics (132,133). Amphetamine use places the athlete at a higher risk for hyperthermia and may impair performance through insomnia, anxiety, and nervousness. The potential for both tolerance and abuse are well established. Amphetamines are banned by both the NCAA and USOC.

COCAINE

More than 25% of American adults between the ages of 20 and 40 years and more than 15% of high school seniors have tried cocaine at least once (134,135). It stimulates the release of norepinephrine and blocks its reuptake. The use of cocaine before a sports event may give the athlete an overall feeling of euphoria and a perception of fantastic performance; however, it actually impairs reflexes and coordination and impairs performance (34). Cocaine is a dangerous drug for an athlete; it can cause a severe hyperthermia resulting from peripheral vasoconstriction and cardiac or cerebral vasoconstriction, and may result in a myocardial infarction, possibly fatal, or a stroke (136,137). Ventricular arrhythmias and seizures have also been associated with its use. Cocaine may be detected in the urine 18–36 hours after ingestion. It is banned by the USOC and NCAA.

TESTING FOR BANNED ERGOGENIC AGENTS

With increasing pressure to improve performance, the popularity of ergogenic agents has grown astronomically. Both the NCAA and USOC have had to produce a list of banned ergogenic agents, as well as legally sound rules and regulations for testing. (Table 4.2 presents the NCAA's list of all banned drugs.)

Athletes participating in sports sanctioned by the NCAA must sign a consent to be tested in order to be eligible to play. Unfortunately, only some of the banned drugs can be detected in a urine-screening test (presently the most commonly used test). Testing occurs at all individual and team championship events and at some football games. The testing is random and based on athletes' position and finish at the particular event, player position, or suspicion of drug use (34). The testing protocol is quite rigid. It allows athletes to perform as much of the procedure themselves as is possible in order to minimize the potential for tampering and thus ensure both the athletes and the NCAA of the validity of the results. During testing the athlete is observed closely at all times (including while voiding) by a member of the NCAA. Each athlete first selects two containers from a given batch and then gives two samples of urine, which must have a specific gravity greater than 1.010 for optimal testing sensitivity. The athlete makes up his own identification number, places the number on each container, and then places the containers in plastic bags. He is the only person who seals them. The samples are screened individually, and any sample that gives a positive result is further tested by more sensitive and specific methods, usually immunoassay or gas chromatography (presently the only tests allowed for the basis of legal action) (75,138,139). Both samples are retested within a 24-hour period; the athlete is allowed to be present for the second test.

The team physician plays a critical role in the testing process. Certain medications may be allowed by the NCAA, such as specific asthma medications or steroids, only if the physician informs the NCAA of this prior to testing of the athlete and confirms the need for the medication. Athletes must also inform the NCAA of their use of any over-the-counter sympathomimetic medications or diet drugs before testing. The NCAA then makes a decision on the athlete's eligibility based on the levels of the medication or by-products detected in the urine as consistent with the athlete's statement. If an athlete has a positive test result on one occasion, she is automatically tested at the next event. Participation in any competition is prohibited for the following 90 days after a positive result and the athlete is retested for restoration of eligibility. If she is found to

Table 4.2. NCAA Banned Drugs and Restricted Procedures (2000)

Stimulants

amiphenazole
amphetamine
bemigride
benzphetamine
bromantan
caffeine*
chlorphentermine
cocaine
cropropamide
crothetamide
diethylpropion
dimethylamphetamine
doxapram
ephedrine
ethamivan
ethylamphetamine
fencamfamine

meclofenoxate
methamphetamine
methylene-dioxymethamphetamine
   (MDMA) (Ecstasy)
methylphenidate
nikethamide
pemoline
pentetrazol
phendimetrazine
phenmetrazine
phentermine
picrotoxine
pipradol
prolintane
strychnine
and related compounds†

Anabolic agents

anabolic steroids
androstenediol
androstenedione
boldenone
clostebol
dehydrochlormethyl-testosterone
dehydroepiandrosterone (DHEA)
dehydrotestosterone (DHT)
dromostanolone
fluoxymesterone
mesterolone
methandienone
methenolone
methyltestosterone

nandrolone
norandrostenediol
norandrostenedione
norethandrolone
oxandrolone
oxymesterone
oxymetholon
stanozolol
testosterone‡
and related compounds†

Other anabolic agents
   clenbuterol

Substances banned for specific sports

Rifle

alcohol
atenolol
metoprolol
nadolol

pindolol
propranolol
timolol
and related compounds†

Diuretics

acetazolamide
bendroflumethiazide
benzthiazide
bumetanide
chlorothiazide
chlorthalidone
ethacrynic acid
flumethiazide
furosemide
hydrochlorothiazide

hydroflumethiazide
methyclothiazide
metolazone
polythiazide
quinethazone
spironolactone
triamterene
trichlormethiazide
and related compounds[†]

Street drugs

heroin
marijuana[§]
THC (tetrahydrocannabinol)[§]

Peptide hormones and analogues

chorionic gonadotrophin (hCG, human chorionic gonadotrophin)
corticotrophin (ACTH)
growth hormone (hGH, somatotrophin)

All the respective releasing factors of the above-mentioned substances also are banned.

erythropoietin (epo)
sermorelin

Supplements

Nutritional supplements are not strictly regulated and may contain substances banned by the NCAA. For questions regarding nutritional supplements, contact the National Center for Drug Free Sport Resource Exchange Center (REC) at 877-202-0769.

Blood doping

The practice of blood doping (the intravenous injection of whole blood, packed red blood cells, or blood substitutes) is prohibited and any evidence confirming use will be cause for action consistent with that taken for a positive drug test.

Local anesthetics

The Executive Committee will permit the use of local anesthetics under the following conditions:

1. That procaine, xylocaine, carbocaine, or any other local anesthetic may be used—but not cocaine.

(continued)

Table 4.2 *(continued)*

2. That only local or topical injections can be used—not intravenous injections.

3. That use is medically justified only when permitting the athlete to continue competition without potential risk to his or her health.

Manipulation of urine samples

The Executive Committee bans the use of substances and methods that alter the integrity and/or validity of urine samples provided during NCAA drug testing. Examples of banned methods are catheterization, urine substitution, and/or tampering or modification of renal excretion by the use of diuretics, probenicid, bromantan, or related compounds, and epitestosterone administration.

Beta-2 agonists

The use of beta-2 agonists is permitted by inhalation only.

Additional analysis

Drug screening for select nonbanned substances may be conducted for nonpunitive purposes.

Source: Adapted from NCAA Banned Drug Classes, www.ncaa.org/sports (September 7, 2001).

*For caffeine—if the concentration in urine exceeds 15 µg/mL.

†The term *related compounds* comprises substances that are included in the class by their pharmacological action and/or chemical structure. No substance belonging to the prohibited class may be used, regardless of whether it is specifically listed as an example.

‡For testosterone—if the administration of testosterone or the use of any other manipulation has the result of increasing the ratio of the total concentration of testosterone to that of epitestosterone in the urine to greater than 6:1, unless there is evidence that this ratio is due to a physiological or pathological condition.

§For marijuana and THC—if the concentration in the urine of THC metabolite exceeds 15 ng/mL.

have a second positive test result after eligibility has been approved, she is prohibited from all competition for the reminder of the season and for the following academic year (75).

In addition to many other substances, the USOC also bans blood doping—although no test exists to detect it. As with the NCAA rules, certain drugs such as asthma medications and oral steroids are allowed if medically indicated. The period of eligibility loss depends upon the setting and the type of agent detected. For the Olympic Games, the use of anabolic steroids, amphetamines or related substances, caffeine, beta-blockers, diuretics, narcotics, or designer drugs leads to 2 years of ineligibility for the first offense and a lifelong ban for the second offense. For ephedrine, phenylpropanolamine, and codeine, the period of ineligibility is 3 months for the first offense, 2 years for the second offense, and lifelong for the third (34). At any Olympic trial events, detection of banned substances results in disqualification and loss of eligibility for 6 months for the first offense, 4 years for the second offense.

REFERENCES

1. Cowart V: Steroids in sports after four decades: time to return these genies to the bottle? JAMA 257:421–427, 1987

2. Alen M, Hakkinen K, Komi P: Changes in neuromuscular performance and muscle fiber characteristics of elite power athletes self-administering androgenic and anabolic steroids. Acta Physiol Scand 122:535–544, 1984

3. Kopera H: The history of anabolic steroids and a review of clinical experience with anabolic steroids. Acta Endocrinol Suppl 271:11–18, 1985

4. Haupt HA, Rovere GD: Anabolic steroids: a review of the literature. Am J Sports Med 12(6):469–484, 1984

5. Kraemer WJ, Gordon SE, Fleck SJ, et al: Endogenous anabolic hormonal and growth factor responses to heavy resistance exercise in males and females. Int J Sports Med 12:228–235, 1991

6. Kraemer WJ, Marchitelli LJ, Gordon SE, et al: Hormonal and growth factor responses to heavy resistance exercise protocols. J Appl Physiol 69:1442–1450, 1990

7. Rabinowitz D, Merimee TJ, Maffezzoli R, Burgess JA: Patterns of hormonal release after glucose, protein, and glucose plus protein. Lancet 2:454–457, 1966

8. Reed MJ, Brozinick JT, Lee MC, Ivy JL: Muscle glycogen storage postexercise: effect of mode of carbohydrate administration. J Appl Physiol 66:720–726, 1989

9. Sachtleben TR, Berg KE, Elias BA, Cheatham JP, Felix GL, Hofschire PJ: The effects of anabolic steroids on myocardial structure and cardiovascular fitness. Med Sci Sports Exerc 25:1240–1245, 1993

10. Mochizuki RM, Richter KJ: Cardiomyopathy and cerebrovascular accident associated with anabolic-androgenic steroid use. Physician and Sportsmedicine 16(11):109–114, 1988

11. McNutt RA, Ferenchick GS, Kirlin PC, Hamlin NJ: Acute myocardial infarction in a 22-year-old world class weight lifter using anabolic steroids. Am J Cardiol 62:164, 1988

12. Ferenchick GS: Are androgenic steroids thrombogenic? N Engl J Med 322:476, 1990

13. Nagelberg SB, Lane L, Loriaux DL, Liu L, Sherins RJ: Cerebrovascular accident associated with testosterone therapy in a 21-year-old hypogonadal man. N Engl J Med 314:649–650, 1986

14. Mochizuki RM, Richter KJ: Cardiomyopathy and cerebrovascular accident associated with anabolic-androgenic steroid use. Physician and Sportsmedicine 16:109–114, 1988

15. Frankle MA, Eichberg R, Zachariah SB: Anabolic androgenic steroids and a stroke in an athlete: case report. Arch Phys Med Rehabil 69:632–633, 1988

16. Laroche GP: Steroid anabolic drugs and arterial complications in an athlete: a case history. Angiology 41:946–969, 1990

17. Shiozawa Z, Yamada H, Mabuchi C, et al: Superior sagittal sinus thrombosis associated with androgen therapy for hypoplastic anemia. Ann Neurol 12:578–580, 1982

18. Huie MJ: An acute myocardial infarction occurring in an anabolic steroid user. Med Sci Sports Exerc 26:408–413, 1994

19. Hurley BF, Seals DR, Hagberg JM, et al: High-density-lipoprotein cholesterol in bodybuilders vs powerlifters: negative effects of androgen use. JAMA 252:507–513, 1982

20. Haupt HA, Rovere GD: Anabolic steroids: a review of the literature. Am J Sports Med 12:469–484, 1984

21. Alen M, Reinila M, Vihko R: Response of serum hormones to androgen administration in power athletes. Med Sci Sports Exerc 17:354–359, 1985

22. Clerico A, Ferdeghini M, Palombo C, et al: Effect of anabolic treatment on the serum levels of gonadotropins, testosterone, prolactin, thyroid hormones and myoglobin of male athletes under physical training. J Nucl Med Allied Sci 25:79–88, 1981

23. Holma P, Adlercreutz H: Effect of an anabolic steroid (metandienon) on plasma LH, FSH, and testosterone and on the response to intravenous administration of LRH. Acta Endocrinol 83:856–864, 1976

24. Jarow JP, Lipshultz LI: Anabolic steroid-induced hypogonadotropic hypogonadism. Am J Sports Med 18(4):429–431, 1990

25. Malarkey WB, Strauss RH, Leizman DJ, et al: Endocrine effects in female weight lifters who self-administer testosterone and anabolic steroids. Am J Obstet Gynecol 165:1385–1390, 1991

26. Lamb DR: Anabolic steroids in athletics: how well do they work and how dangerous are they? Am J Sports Med 12:31–38, 1984

27. Wilson JD, Griffin JE: The use and misuse of androgens. Metabolism 29:1278–1295, 1980

28. Bach BR, Warren RF, Wickiewicz TL: Triceps rupture: a case report and literature review. Am J Sports Med 15:285–289, 1987

29. Herrick RT, Herrick S: Ruptured triceps in a powerlifter presenting as cubital tunnel syndrome: a case report. Am J Sports Med 15:514–516, 1987

30. Hill JA, Suker JR, Sacks K, Brigham C: The athletic polydrug abuse phenomenon. Am J Sports Med 11:269–271, 1983

31. Pope HG Jr, Katz DL: Affective and psychotic symptoms associated with anabolic steroid use. Am J Psychiatry 145:487–490, 1988

32. Pope HG, Katz DL: Bodybuilder's psychosis. Lancet 1:863, 1987

33. Tennant FS Jr, Black DL, Voy RO: Anabolic steroid dependence with opioid type features. N Engl J Med 319:578, 1988

34. Haupt HA: Drugs in athletics. Clin Sports Med 8:561–582, 1989

35. DuRant RH, Rickert VI, Ashworth CS, Newman C, Slavens G: Use of multiple drugs among adolescents who use anabolic steroids. N Engl J Med 328: 922–926, 1993

36. Brower M, Aziaian C: Trouble: steroids built Mike Keys up; then they tore him down. People Magazine, March 20, 107–108, 1989

37. Brower KJ, Blow FC, Eliopulos GA, et al: Anabolic androgenic steroids and suicide (letters to the editor). Am J Psychiatry 146:1075, 1989

38. Harries M: Deaths of athletes. BMJ 290:656, 1985

39. Johson MD: Anabolic steroid use in adolescent athletes. Pediatr Clin North Am 37:1111, 1990

40. Johson M, Jay M, Shoup B, et al: Adolescent steroid use in adolescent males. Pediatrics 83:921, 1989

41. Cowart VS: Blunting "steroid epidemic" requires alternatives, innovative education. JAMA 264:1641, 1990

42. Council on Scientific Affairs: Medical and nonmedical uses of anabolic-androgenic steroids. JAMA 264:2923, 1990

43. Wadler GI: Drug use update. Med Clin North Am 78:439–455, 1994

44. Eichner ER: Ergogenic aids. Physician and Sportsmedicine 25(4):70, 1997

45. Catlin DH, Murray TH: Performance-enhancing drugs, fair competition, and Olympic sport. JAMA 276:231–237, 1996

46. Frankle MA, Eichberg R, Zachariah SB: Anabolic androgenic steroids and a stroke in an athlete: case report. Arch Phys Med Rehabil 69:632–633, 1988

47. Goodman LS, Gilman A: The Pharmacologic Basis of Therapeutics, ed 5. New York, Macmillan, 1975, 1376–1382

48. Macintyre JG: Growth hormone and athletes. Sports Med 4:129–142, 1987

49. DiPasquale MG (ed): Clenbuterol: a new anabolic drug. Drugs in Sports (Hamilton, Ont., Decker Periodicals) 1(Feb.):8–10, 1992

50. DiPasquale MG (ed): Use and side effects of growth hormone. Drugs in Sports (Hamilton, Ont., Decker Periodicals) 1(Feb.):5, 1992

51. Rogol A: Growth hormone: physiology, therapeutic use, and potential for abuse. Exerc Sports Sci Rev 17:353, 1989

52. Smith DA, Perry PJ: The efficacy of ergogenic agents in athletic competition. Part I: anabolic-androgenic steroids. Ann Pharmacother 26:653, 1992

53. Nagulesparen M, Trickey R, Davies MJ, et al: Muscle changes in acromegaly. BMJ 2:914, 1976

54. Cowart VS: Human growth hormone: the latest ergogenic aid? Physician and Sportsmedicine 3:175–185, 1988

55. Lemon PWR, Chaney MM: Physiologic effects of amino-acid supplementation. *In* Garrett WE Jr, Malone TR (eds): Muscle Development: Nutritional Alternatives to Anabolic Steroids, Report of the Ross Symposium. Columbus, OH, Ross Laboratories, 1988, 62–67

56. Ingalls CP, Barnes WS, Smith SB: Interaction between clenbuterol and run training effects on exercise performance and MLC isoform content. J Appl Physiol 80:795–801, 1996

57. Prather ID, Brown DE, North P, et al: Clenbuterol: a substitute for anabolic steroids? Med Sci Sports Exerc 27:1118–1121, 1995

58. Martineau L, Horan MA, Rothwell NH, et al: Salbutamol, a beta-2-adrenoceptor agonist, increases skeletal muscle strength in young men. Clin Sci 83:615–621, 1992

59. Caruso JF, Signorile JF, Perry AC, et al: The effects of albuterol and isokinetic exercise on the quadriceps muscle group. Med Sci Sports Exerc 27:1471–1476, 1995

60. Robertson W, Simkins J, O'Hickey SP, et al: Does single dose salmeterol affect exercise capacity in asthmatic men? Eur Respir J 7:1978–1984, 1994

61. Morton AR, Joyce K, Paplia SM, et al: Is salmeterol ergogenic? Clin J Sports Med 6:220–225, 1996

62. Conlee RK: Amphetamine, caffeine, and cocaine. *In* Lamb DR, Williams MH (eds): Ergogenics: Enhancement of Performance in Exercise and Sport. Dubuque, IA, Brown & Benchmark, 1991, 285–325

63. Spriet LL, MacLean DA, Dyck DJ, Hultman E, Cederblad G, Graham TE: Caffeine ingestion and muscle metabolism during prolonged exercise in humans. Am J Physiol 262:E891–E898, 1992

64. Costill JD, Dalsky GP, Fink WJ: Effects of caffeine ingestion on metabolism and exercise performance. Med Sci Sports 10:155–158, 1978

65. Goodman LS, Gilman A: The Pharmacologic Basis of Therapeutics, ed 5. New York, Macmillan, 1975, 367–378

66. Rossier J, French ED, Rivier C, Ling N, Guillemin R, Bloom FE: Footshock induced stress increases beta-endorphin levels in blood but not brain. Nature 270:618–620, 1977

67. Graham TE, Spriet LL: Performance and metabolic responses to a high caffeine dose during prolonged exercise. J Appl Physiol 71:2292–2298, 1991

68. Sasaki H, Maeda J, Usui S, Ishiko T: Effect of sucrose and caffeine ingestion on performance of prolonged strenuous running. Int J Sports Med 8:261–265, 1987

69. Spriet LL: Caffeine and performance. Int J Sport Nutr 5:S84–S99, 1995

70. Wadler GI, Hainline B: Drugs and the Athlete. Philadelphia, FA Davis, 1989, 107–111

71. Nehlig A, Daval JL, Debry G: Caffeine and the central nervous system: mechanisms of action, biochemical, metabolic and psychostimulant effects. Brain Res Rev 17:139–170, 1992

72. Flinn S, Gregory J, McNaughton LR, Tristan S, Davies P: Caffeine ingestion prior to incremental cycling to exhaustion in recreational cyclists. Int J Sports Med 11:188–193, 1990

73. Graham TE, Spriet LL: Caffeine and exercise performance. Sports Science Exchange (Gatorade Sports Science Institute) 9:1–6, 1996

74. Guide to banned medications. Sportsmediscope 7:1–5, 1988

75. National Collegiate Athletic Association. The 1988–89 NCAA Drug-Testing Program. September 1988

76. Rogers CC: Cyclists try caffeine suppositories. Physician and Sportsmedicine 13(3):38–40, 1985

77. Graham TE, Spriet LL: Performance and metabolic responses to a high caffeine dose during prolonged exercise. J Appl Physiol 71:2292–2298, 1991

78. Castellino P, Luzi L, Simonson DC, Haymond M, DeFronzo RA: Effect of insulin and plasma amino acid concentrations of leucine metabolism in man. J Clin Invest 80:1784–1793, 1987

79. Garkick PJ, Grant I: Amino acid infusion increases the sensitivity of muscle protein synthesis in vivo to insulin. Biochem J 254:579–584, 1988

80. Nakagawa K, Horiuchi Y, Mashimo K: Responses of plasma growth hormone and corticosteroids to insulin and arginine with or without prior administration of dexamethasone. J Clin Endocrinol Metab 29:35–40, 1969

81. Ohneda A, Parada E, Eisentraut AM, Unger RH: Characterization of response of circulating glucagon to intraduodenal and intravenous administration of amino acids. J Clin Invest 47:2305–2322, 1968

82. Blomstrand E, Hassmen P, Ekblom B, Newsholme EA: Administration of branched-chain amino acids during sustained exercise—effects on performance and on plasma concentration of some amino acids. Eur J Appl Physiol 63:83–88, 1991

83. Meduski JW: Promoters of the Anabolic State. Nutritional Consultants Group, 1985

84. Blomstrand E, Celsing F, Newsholme EA: Changes in plasma concentrations of aromatic and branched-chain amino acids during sustained exercise in men and their possible role in fatigue. Acta Physiol Scand 133:115–121, 1988

85. Conlay LA, Wurtman RJ, Lopez I, et al: Effect of running the Boston marathon on plasma concentration of large neutral aminoacids. J Neural Transm 76:65–71, 1989

86. Varnier M, Sarto P, Martines D, et al: Effect of infusing branched-chain

amino acid during incremental exercise with reduced muscle glycogen content. Eur J Appl Physiol 69:26–31, 1994

87. Gater DR, Gater DA, Uribe JR, Bunt JC: Effects of arginine/lysine supplementation and resistance training on glucose tolerance. Am J Physiol 72(4):1279–1284, 1992

88. Banister WW, Cameron BJC: Exercise-induced hyperammonemia: peripheral and central effects. Int J Sports Med 11(suppl 2):S129–S142, 1990

89. Wagenmakers AJM, Bechers EJ, Brouns F, et al: Carbohydrate supplementation, glycogen depletion, and amino acid metabolism during exercise. Am J Physiol 260:E883–E890, 1991

90. Spriet LL: Blood doping and oxygen transport. In Lamb DR, Williams MH (eds): Perspective in Sports Medicine. Vol 4: Ergogenics-Enhancement of Performance in Exercise and Sport. Indianapolis, Brown & Benchmark, 1991, 213

91. Buick FJ, Gledhill N, Froese AB, Spriet L, Meyers EC: Effect of induced erythrocythemia on aerobic work capacity. J Appl Physiol 48:636–642, 1980

92. Ekblom B, Goldbarg AN, Gullbring B: Response to exercise after blood loss and reinfusion. J Appl Physiol 40:175–180, 1972

93. Eichner ER: Sports anemia, iron supplements, and blood doping. Med Sci Sports Exerc 24(9):S315–S318, 1992

94. McMahon F, Vargas R, Ryan M, et al: Pharmacokinetics and effects of recombinant human erythropoietin following intravenous and subcutaneous injections in healthy volunteers. Blood 76:1718–1722, 1990

95. Ekblom B, Berglund B: Effect of erythropoietin administration on maximal aerobic power. Scand J Med Sci Sports 1:88–93, 1991

96. Spence M: Doctors concerned about side effects of chemical erythropoietin. The Olympian 1990, 61

97. Berglund B, Ekblom B: Effect of recombinant human erythropoietin treatment on blood pressure and some hematological parameters in healthy males. J Intern Med 229:125–130, 1991

98. Balsom PD, Soderlund K, Ekblom B: Creatine in humans with special reference to creatine supplementation. Sports Med 18:268–280, 1994

99. Bogdanis GC, Nevill ME, Boobis LH, et al: Recovery of power output and muscle metabolites following 30 s of maximal sprint cycling. J Physiol 482(pt 2):467–480, 1995

100. Hunter A: Monographs on Biochemistry: Creatine and Creatinine. London, Longmans, Green, 1928

101. Harris R, Soderlund K, Hultman E: Elevation of creatine in resting and exercise muscles of normal subjects by creatine supplementation. Clin Sci 83:367–374, 1992

102. Greenhaff PL, Casey A, Short AH, et al: Influence of oral creatine supplementation on muscle torque during repeated bouts of maximal voluntary exercise in man. Clin Sci 84:565–571, 1993

103. Balsom PD, Ekblom B, Soderlund K, et al: Creatine supplementation

and dynamic high-intensity intermittent exercise. Scand J Med Sci Sports 3:143–149, 1993

104. Soderlund K, Balsom PD, Ekblom B: Creatine supplementation and high-intensity exercise: influence on performance and muscle metabolism. Clin Sci 87(suppl):120, 1994

105. Birch R, Noble D, Greenhaff PL: The influence of dietary creatine supplementation on performance during repeated bouts of maximal isokinetic cycling in man. Eur J Appl Physiol 69:268–270, 1994

106. Balsom PD, Harridge SDR, Soderlund K, et al: Creatine supplementation per se does not enhance endurance exercise performance. Acta Physiol Scand 149:521–523, 1993

107. Kirkendall D: Mechanisms of peripheral fatigue. Med Sci Sports Exerc 22:444–449, 1990

108. Sutton JR, Jones NL, Toews CJ: Effect of pH on muscle glycolysis during exercise. Clin Sci 61:331–338, 1981

109. Fabiato A, Fabiato F: Effects of pH on the myofilaments and the sarcoplasmic reticulum of skinned cells from cardiac and skeletal muscles. J Physiol 276:233–235, 1978

110. Heigenhauser G, Jones N: Bicarbonate loading. In Lamb D, Williams M (eds): Ergogenics: Enhancement of Performance in Exercise and Sport. Dubuque, IA, Brown & Benchmark, 1991, 183–212

111. Kozak-Collins K, Burke ER, Schoene RB: Sodium bicarbonate ingestion does not improve performance in women cyclists. Med Sci Sports Exerc 26: 1510–1515, 1994

112. Gao J, Costill DL, Horswill CA, Park SH: Sodium bicarbonate ingestion improves performance in interval swimming. Eur J Appl Physiol 58:171–174, 1988

113. Lavender G, Bird SR: Effects of sodium bicarbonate ingestion upon repeated sprints. Br J Sports Med 23:41–45, 1989

114. Parry-Billings M, Maclaren DPM: The effect of sodium bicarbonate and sodium citrate ingestion on anaerobic power during intermittent exercise. Eur J Appl Physiol 55:524–529, 1986

115. Linderman J, Fahey TD: Sodium bicarbonate ingestion and exercise performance: an update. Sports Med 11:71–77, 1991

116. Costill DL, Verstappen F, Kuipers H, Janssen E, Fink W: Acid-base balance during repeated bouts of exercise: influences of HCO_3. Int J Sports Med 5:228–231, 1984

117. Wilkes D, Gledhill N, Smyth R: Effect of acute induced metabolic alkalosis on 800-m racing time. Med Sci Sports Exerc 15:277–280, 1983

118. Goldfinch J, McNaughton L, Davies P: Induced metabolic alkalosis and its effects on 400-m racing time. Eur J Appl Physiol 57:45–48, 1988

119. Clarkson PM: Do athletes require mineral supplements? Sports Med Digest 16(4):1–3, 1994

120. Campbell WW, Anderson RA: Effects of aerobic exercise and training on trace mineral chromium, zinc, and copper. Sports Med 4:9–18, 1987

121. Evans GW: The role of picoline acid in metal metabolism. Life Chem Rep 1:57–67, 1982

122. Evans GW: The effect of chromium picolinate on insulin controlled parameters in humans. Int J Biosoc Med 11:163–180, 1989

123. Hasten DL, Rome EP, Franks ED, et al: Effects of chromium picolinate on beginning weight training students. Int J Sport Nutr 2:343–350, 1994

124. Clancy SP, Clarkson PM, DeCheke ME, et al: Effects of chromium picolinate supplementation on body composition, strength, and urinary chromium loss in football players. Int J Sport Nutr 4:142–153, 1994

125. Hallmark MA, Reynolds TH, DeSouza CA, et al: Effects of chromium and resistive training on muscle strength and body composition. Med Sci Sports Exerc 28:139–144, 1996

126. Lefavi RG: Sizing up a few supplements. Physician and Sportsmedicine 20(3):190–191, 1992

127. Huszonek J: Over-the-counter chromium picolinate (letter). Am J Psychiatry 150:1560–1561, 1993

128. Wasser WG, Felman NS: Chronic renal failure after ingestion of over-the-counter chromium picolinate (letter). Ann Intern Med 126:410, 1997

129. Armsey TD, Green GA: Nutrition supplements. Physician and Sportsmedicine 25(6):77–92, 1997

130. Ivy JL: Amphetamines in sports: are they worth the risk? Sports Med Dig 6:1–3, 1984

131. Smith GM, Beecher HK: Amphetamine sulfate and athletic performance. I. Objective effects. JAMA 170:542–557, 1959

132. Goodman LS, Gilman A: The Pharmacologic Basis of Therapeutics, ed 5. New York, Macmillan, 1975, 496–500

133. Lombardo JA: Stimulants and athletic performance. I. Amphetamines and caffeine. Physician and Sportsmedicine 11:128–142, 1986

134. Lombardo JA: Stimulants and athletic performance. II. Cocaine and nicotine. Physician and Sportsmedicine 12:85–89, 1986

135. Tennant FS Jr: Dealing with cocaine use by athletes. Sports Med Dig 6:1–3, 1984

136. Cantwell JD, Rose FD: Cocaine and cardiovascular events. Physician and Sportsmedicine 11:77–82, 1986

137. Crack. Med Lett Drugs Ther 28:69–72, 1986

138. A round table: drug testing in sports. Physician and Sportsmedicine 12:69–82, 1985

139. Rovere GD, Haupt HA, Yates CS: Drug testing in a university athletic program: protocol and implementation. Physician and Sportsmedicine 14:69–76, 1986

Chapter 5

INJURIES TO THE HEAD AND SPINE

DENTAL INJURIES

Many competitive sports can place an athlete at risk for dental injury. Some sports are higher risk than others, but only football, ice hockey, lacrosse, and women's field hockey require mouth guards for play at the NCAA level. In sports such as soccer and basketball, not traditionally considered contact sports, almost 10% of injuries are dental or oral injuries (1,2). Therefore it is vital that the physician caring for athletes in any sport at any level be aware of important initial management protocols to minimize any long-term adverse effects from an injury.

Dental trauma can be divided into three types: fracture, dislocation, and avulsion (3). On initial evaluation, the physician should note any lost teeth or asymmetry and should evaluate the athlete's ability to open her mouth, since dislocation of the mandible is not uncommon. Teeth and gums should be closely examined for stability and local damage; this may require local or topical anesthesia (3).

A fractured tooth is not always painful. If the fracture is only to the enamel, pain may occur only on exposure to air or water. If the fracture exposes the dentin, a yellow hue is usually visible and the tooth will be extremely sensitive to water and breathing. A follow-up x-ray is recommended. A fracture through to the pulp of the tooth causes excruciating pain and requires immediate treatment. Hemorrhage in the center of the tooth will be visible and should be controlled with sterile gauze. Application of a local anesthetic such as lidocaine 1% (with or without epinephrine) by insertion of a small-gage needle (30-gage if possible) into the canal, slowly and without force, controls the bleeding and relieves the pain (3). Immediate referral to a dentist for a probable root canal should follow. Infection is also a risk with this level of fracture. A fracture below the gum line may be difficult to diagnose, but mobility in the socket is a clue (3). Again, immediate referral to a dentist is critical for stabilization. Whether the athlete will suffer permanent loss of the tooth depends on the level of the fracture.

Any impact directly on a tooth can result in displacement. Only a dentist should reposition the tooth. The tooth may be abnormally mobile, out of position, or displaced into the bone. The physician should evaluate surrounding structures promptly and refer the athlete to a dentist. Again, early treatment will significantly improve the prognosis.

With complete avulsion of a tooth, immediate action is critical: the tooth should be rinsed with milk or saline and gently placed back into the socket, after removing the blood clot; the surface of the root should not be scraped or touched, since this may kill reparative cells (3). If the tooth cannot easily be placed back into the socket, it should be stored in whole milk, sterile saline (not tap water or drinking water), or saliva until the athlete can receive emergency dental attention. If the tooth is replaced intraorally within 30 minutes, the chance of successful reimplantation is 90% (4,5). After 2 hours, the failure rate is 95%.

The importance of having an emergency dental consultant available cannot be overemphasized. Prevention of dental injury is also important. Athletes should be encouraged to wear mouth guards at an early age, so they can get used to playing with the guard in place. Custom-made mouth guards can be expensive, but plastic "boil and bite" guards are affordable and easier to obtain. Mouth guards not only protect teeth and surrounding soft tissues but also absorb the force transmitted between the mandible and maxilla during a forceful blow, thus reducing the risk of concussion and mandibular fracture (3).

EYE INJURIES

Eye injuries can occur in any sport. The physician should have appropriate equipment available to evaluate eye injuries, even though most athletes will need to be referred to an ophthalmologist for follow-up care. The sports physician should have access to a vision card, fluorescent penlight and fluorescein strips, sterile eye pads and sterile irrigating solution, and an ophthalmoscope.

Lid lacerations are common. Bleeding can be heavy and should be controlled with direct pressure if possible. The eye itself should be evaluated for injury before any attempt at suturing is made in order to detect a possible emergency situation. Most simple lacerations can be sutured by the physician, if she is comfortable with the procedure. Certain lacerations should be repaired only by an ophthalmologist or eye surgeon: these include any complicated laceration; lacerations through the lid margin, especially those on the medial side of the lid, since the lacrimal drainage system may be involved; and any puncture lacerations of the lids (6).

Foreign bodies in the eye are not uncommon. A simple way to examine under the upper eyelid, where many foreign bodies can migrate, is to use a cotton swab to help evert the eyelid; the object can often be removed with a sterile cotton swab. The eye may first be anesthetized using Pontocaine or Ophthetic if available. If the object cannot be removed easily, the athlete should be promptly referred to an ophthalmologist.

Corneal injuries often cause the sensation of "something in the eye." They are also associated with excessive tearing, photophobia, and blepharospasm. Simple corneal abrasions can be detected with fluorescein and an ultraviolet light, used in a dark area. The fluorescein pools and outlines the abrasion. An ophthalmic antibiotic should be applied and the eye covered with a sterile eyepad for 24 hours. The patient should have a follow-up examination by an ophthalmologist on the following day. Sulfa-based ophthalmic antibiotics should be avoided, since allergic reaction and further irritation to the eye are not uncommon (6). A corneal laceration is associated with severe pain, lacrimation, and photophobia. If the eye can be opened (doing so in a darkened area is helpful), the pupil may appear irregular and the anterior chamber shallow. The eyelid should never be forced open, since this can lead to further injury. A corneal laceration should be evaluated by an ophthalmologist immediately.

The lens may be damaged with any blunt trauma to the eye. In milder cases, the iris is forced against the anterior lens capsule, which leaves a circular mark against the lens capsule, visible as the pupil dilates. In more serious cases, the lens capsule itself may rupture, allowing aqueous fluid from the anterior chamber to enter. A cataract may later form over the lens as a further complication.

Blunt trauma can also result in a hyphema, or collection of blood in the anterior chamber of the eye. In this case, the athlete's vision will be blurred, and examination will reveal an irregular pupil, slow to react to light. A faint haze in the iris may also be evident. A hyphema is an emergency. Long-term complications include glaucoma and blood staining of the cornea.

More severe intraocular complications resulting from blunt trauma are less frequent, but again need to be promptly recognized to minimize complications. These injuries include choroidal rupture or hemorrhage, macular edema, and retinal hemorrhage or detachment. They are usually associated with some form of visual impairment or loss. Some level of permanent visual loss is common.

Repeated eye trauma can also be associated with permanent visual impairment. Up to 19% of boxers have subcapsular cataracts. They also have a high incidence of retinal tears, known to correlate directly with the total number of bouts and knockouts (6). Most likely the result of contusive blows to the eye, the tears can be small and asymptomatic initially, but they slowly accumulate and result in significant visual impairment. The physician must always have a high level of suspicion of serious eye injury in examining athletes in such high-risk sports, in order to allow early treatment and prevention of permanent disability.

Fractures of the orbital rim are the result of high-velocity blunt trauma to the eye. When the eye is forced posteriorly into the orbit, the weak orbital floor can blow out under the increase in pressure. Enophthalmos is usually present as the eye itself herniates into the maxillary sinus. Limitation of eye movement and diplopia, especially with upward gaze, are also common, as the extraocular muscles can become entrapped in the fracture. Diagnosis can be made with CT scan or x-rays.

Direct palpation of the anterior orbital rim can be helpful in diagnosing an anterior orbital rim fracture. An irregularity is highly suggestive of a fracture. A suspected fracture of the roof of the orbital rim should be evaluated by a neurosurgeon. Air in the orbital cavity can produce crepitus on palpation; this is seen in patients with a fracture involving the maxillary sinus. All should be evaluated promptly (6).

EAR INJURIES

The most common injury to the inner ear structures is rupture of the tympanic membrane resulting from a pressure change of greater than 30 mm Hg/cm^2 within the outer ear canal, which can occur with a slap or blow to the ear (7). The injury is usually quite painful, with otorrhea and conductive hearing loss. Bleeding may also occur. In order to visualize the tympanic membrane with an otoscope, the physician may need to remove blood clots and cerumen: warm water should be used for irrigation, since cold water may cause caloric stimulation. Blood may also enter the eustachian tube and appear in the nose or oral cavity (8). Rupture of the tympanic membrane can be a special risk for scuba divers. An influx of cold water into the middle ear may result in unilateral coldwater labyrinthine stimulation. The consequent vertigo, disorientation, and vomiting place the diver at a high risk for drowning (8).

Treatment is conservative. The majority of ruptured tympanic membranes heal spontaneously, usually by 8 weeks (9). All patients should still be referred to an otolaryngologist for monitoring until the injury heals. It is important to prevent contamination in order to avoid infection of the middle ear. If seawater could have entered the ear canal, the patient should be given antibiotics, either local or oral. Divers should not be allowed to resume diving until the tympanic membrane has healed. The only other concern following this type of injury may be airplane travel. In order to avoid a severe headache or ear pain, an individual with compromised function of the eustachian tube can take a decongestant approximately 2 hours before landing (8).

Lacerations of the auricle are often difficult to repair and can be deforming even under the best of circumstances. Lacerations involving cartilage should be repaired within 12–24 hours. Prior to suturing, the entire area should be meticulously cleansed. Either a through-and-through cartilage suture or suture of only the perichondrium can be used. Both techniques are effective (8). The patient should take oral antibiotics to cover possible staphylococcal or streptococcal contamination (8).

Auricular hematomas result from tangential or shearing trauma or blunt trauma to the ear, which tears the perichondrium from the cartilage. Auricular hematomas are most commonly seen in wrestlers but are not uncommon in rugby players and boxers. The perichondrium is the only source of blood supply to the cartilage. If a hematoma or seroma forms, it will separate the cartilage from the perichondrium, resulting in excessive fibrosis and deformation, commonly referred to as a "cauliflower ear" (10). Separation of the cartilage from the perichondrium may also predispose the athlete to infection with necrosis of the cartilage (11). Both treatment and prevention are of primary concern to the treating physician.

Management of an auricular hematoma depends upon the timing of presentation. Because it is a painful condition, most individuals consult a physician soon after the injury. The hematoma should be drained within 24 hours of injury, using sterile technique. A syringe with an 18-gage needle is usually sufficient. Local anesthesia with 1% lidocaine with epinephrine is helpful to minimize further bleeding. Some physicians advocate observation for 1 hour after aspiration; if the hematoma does not recur, a pressure dressing is not considered necessary. Close observation for recurrence and avoidance of NSAIDs are usually recommended. Many physicians prefer to apply a pressure dressing after drainage as a precaution, because of the high frequency of reaccumulation. Repeat drainage may be performed if the hematoma recurs (8). If aspiration and pressure are not sufficient to control the hematoma, an incision of 4 or 5 mm may be necessary, with a local drain left in place for a few days; the incision should be made as close to the crevice of the ear as possible to minimize any deformation. The patient should take oral antibiotics for 10 days (8).

A more aggressive technique for management of an auricular hematoma has become popular recently. It involves the use of dental rolls, one on either side of the ear, held in place by a through-and-through mattress suture for local pressure after drainage (12). Antibacterial ointment should then be applied locally over the dental rolls with a local gauze dressing. The dressing can be removed after 24 hours, and the athlete may return to play with appropriate ear protection. The athlete should apply a generous amount of antibacterial ointment frequently, especially before showering. The dental rolls may be removed after 10–14 days (12). This technique is suitable either for primary management or after initial drainage and pressure dressing have failed.

Since it is an invasive procedure, the patient should take oral antibiotics for 1 week. The NCAA requires the use of headgear for wrestling competition, but use during practices is up to the individual athletic departments.

HEAD INJURY

Approximately 6,000 children and adults die each year as a direct result of sports-related traumatic injuries (13). A significant proportion of these deaths result from closed head traumatic injuries. Football, ice hockey, and boxing have the highest incidence of serious closed head injuries, at both the amateur and professional levels, despite the use of helmets. Careful documentation of neurological status and history of previous head injuries are an important part of the preparticipation exam.

Initial on-field evaluation of the injured athlete should include observation of facial expression, symmetry of the pupils, orientation to place, person, and time, and ability to recall play leading up to and after injury, and a quick assessment of motor function. The immediate post-injury state does not always reflect the severity of the injury, and frequent, repeated evaluations of the athlete are important to detect any deterioration of neurological status.

The term *concussion* generally refers to a transient change in neural function. Management of head injury in athletes poses a particular problem, since the physician must make the clinical decision as to when the athlete can return to play (and to a similar situation and risk of injury). In order to simplify the decision and minimize the risk of further injury, grading of concussions is useful. At one time grading was based primarily on duration of unconsciousness: mild concussion, no loss of consciousness; moderate concussion, a loss of consciousness associated with retrograde amnesia; and severe concussion, loss of consciousness lasting longer than 5 minutes (14). More recently, however, the grading of concussions has changed, since it has become evident that even a mild concussion, without loss of consciousness, can vary in severity and affect both the individual's ability to return to the usual level of play and the likelihood of long-term complications. A more useful grading of concussions includes four grades (15).

Grade 1 concussion is associated with only mild confusion that clears within 5–15 minutes. Posttraumatic and retrograde amnesia are not prominent. If the athlete is asymptomatic and has a normal level of concentration, normal neurological findings, and ability to run and maneuver at the same level as prior to injury (and remain asymptomatic), she can return to play (15). She should first be monitored for at least 20–30 minutes. If she has nausea, vomiting, headache, unsteady gait, photophobia, or labile emotions, return to play should be prohibited. If the athlete does return to play, the physician should reevaluate her condition, even if quickly, after the competition and a few hours later, depending on her symptoms. Some symptoms, such as a headache, may begin a few hours after the injury. The athlete should be made aware of this possibility.

Grade 2 concussion is associated with posttraumatic amnesia and possibly a mild unsteady gait, but no loss of consciousness (15). The athlete should not be allowed to return to play and should be observed closely for at least 24 hours or until symptoms clear. If any deterioration in mental status occurs, immediate referral to an emergency room is essential. The athlete is at risk of developing a "post-concussion syndrome," characterized by a persistent headache, labyrinthine disturbance, lethargy, irritability, or inability to concentrate. Persistence of these symptoms is an indication for an MRI of the head and neurological testing (16). Participation in sports activities should be prohibited until symptoms completely resolve and normal dexterity and concentration return. The athlete should also demonstrate the ability to perform at the same level as before the injury without the precipitation of any symptoms before being cleared to play without restriction. If he incurs a second concussion in the same season, participation should be deferred for 2 weeks after symptoms resolve. After the third concussion in one season, contact sports should be prohibited for the remainder of the season.

Grade 3 concussion is similar to a grade 2 concussion, with the addition of retrograde amnesia. The symptoms may also be associated with an epidural or subdural hemorrhage, and the athlete should therefore be closely observed in case of sudden deterioration or collapse. If he has disorientation or difficulty with ambulation and rising, prompt referral to an emergency facility for further evaluation is advisable. Requirements for return to activities are similar to those for a grade 2 concussion.

Grade 4 concussion is a head injury associated with any loss of consciousness, even if only for a few seconds. A spinal injury may also be associated with a loss of consciousness. The decision to move the athlete without protection of the spine with a cervical collar and board should be made cautiously, with a high level of suspicion for associated injury. The athlete should be evaluated at an emergency facility immediately.

More serious head injuries are not common, but the physician needs to be aware of the signs and symptoms of expanding intracranial masses in order to minimize permanent sequelae. An epidural hematoma is the most rapidly progressive intracranial hemorrhage (17). It is usually associated with an initial period of consciousness followed by rapid loss of consciousness, and it can be in fatal within 30 minutes if not diagnosed and treated immediately. Subdural and subarachnoid hematomas may also be associated with moderate head trauma. The patient usually has symptoms of altered level of consciousness or severe headache (18).

No universally accepted criteria are available for decisions about return to contact sports for athletes with a history of documented brain injury, but certain recommendations can be made (19–21). Any history of a severe brain injury requiring surgical intervention precludes participation in all contact sports. Noncontact sports are generally allowed, but only after clearance from a neurosurgeon. An athlete with a history of a closed head injury that required hospitalization but no surgical intervention can usually participate in contact sports, but only after several months without symptoms and with normal neurological examination. An athlete with a history of any abnormality revealed by an MRI of the head should return to contact sports only after clearance by a neurosurgeon (18). Individuals with hydrocephalus should not be allowed to participate in contact sports (22).

The "second impact syndrome" (SIS) gained recognition as a sequela of head injury in 1973 (23). SIS can occur when an athlete who has already sustained a head injury receives a second head injury before the symptoms of the first injury, such as headache, concentration impairment, or visual or motor symptoms, have completely resolved. The second injury can be quite minor, even trauma to the chest or ribs that forces the head to snap back or forward (which can subject the brain to acceleration forces) (17). The etiology is considered to be related to sudden loss of autoregulation of the blood supply to the brain (23–25). The subsequent vascular engorgement leads to a rapid increase in intracranial pressure and herniation of the brain through the foramen magnum (24,26). Herniation occurs rapidly, usually within 2–5 minutes after impact, followed by coma and respiratory failure. Initially the athlete may seem somewhat stunned and may be capable of completing the play or walking unaided (26). Within a minute, he collapses and respiratory failure ensues. Death occurs much sooner than with a subdural or epidural hematoma.

Data suggest that SIS may occur more often than previously reported (27–29). Between 1980 and 1993, the National Center for Catastrophic Sports Injury Research described 35 probable cases among football players in the United States. Eighteen other probable cases were also identified (17). Football is not the only high-risk sport; ice hockey, soccer (goalie), skiing, and equestrian sports also have a higher rate of head injury and thus of SIS. Given a mortality rate of close to 100%, prevention is critical. An athlete with any suggestion of symptoms after a head injury should be prohibited from contact sports until symptoms subside, and preferably for the following week (17).

Repeated head trauma, even mild concussions, may eventually result in a decline in mental function. This effect has been recognized for over 50 years and is often referred to as the "punch drunk syndrome" (30). Some data even suggest that intellectual function can deteriorate following a second severe concussion (21,31,32). Boxing is the only sport in which the primary goal is to inflict a concussion on an opponent. Reviews of CT scans have shown a direct relationship between the cumulative number of bouts fought and the presence and severity of a chronic encephalopathy (33).

NECK INJURIES

The neck can be particularly vulnerable to catastrophic injury. Although only a small number of sports-related injuries to the cervical spine result in permanent neurological deficits, improper management of an unstable injury without neurological deficit can incur permanent injury. The National Center for Catastrophic Sports Injury Research found that all cases of quadriplegia were the result of a fracture or dislocation of the cervical spine (17). Multiple injuries to the neck are possible in sports.

Initial on-field management is critical. The physician in charge needs to be well acquainted with techniques proven to minimize permanent damage. A spine board and rigid cervical collar should always be available—as well as a telephone. The cervical spine should be stabilized manually while the basic ABCs are assessed. If the athlete is face down, he should be shifted to a spine board by log rolling the body while manually stabilizing the cervical spine; this should be performed by individuals familiar with the procedure. If the athlete is not breathing, respiratory resuscitation should be performed using a jaw thrust technique rather than the head tilt. If he is wearing a helmet with a face mask, the mask should be removed using bolt cutters—never remove the helmet on site.

Once the cervical spine is stabilized, a quick neurological assessment of the level of consciousness, pupil reaction, response to pain, and muscle strength is the next step. Any suggestion of a neurological deficit, persistent pain, or inability to achieve full range of motion requires immediate evaluation at an emergency facility. Increasing neck pain with flexion or extension or upon palpation of the spinous processes is suggestive of a spinal injury. Exacerbation of pain on rising from a lying position is more suggestive of a muscular injury (34).

The position of the neck during direct impact to the top of the head is critical. In a normal head-up position, the natural lordotic curve allows the force of the impact to be dissipated by the cervical muscles. If the neck is flexed, the vertebral bodies line up and the force of the direct impact is transmitted directly to the vertebrae, which may result in a compression fracture if the force exceeds the strength of the bone (17). This explains the decreased incidence of serious cervical injuries in football since prohibition of the "spear" tackle (head-first drive into the opponent). Injury to the neck can also occur with hyperflexion or extension ("whiplash") secondary to sudden acceleration or deceleration. Flexion is limited by the sternum, but forceful flexion may result in injury to the posterior elements of the cervical spine—that is, rupture of the longitudinal, interspinal, or supraspinal ligaments. The posterior half of an intervertebral disc may also rupture. Forceful hyperextension can result in a more serious injury. The anterior elements of the cervical spine, such as the anterior longitudinal ligament or intervertebral disc, may rupture or injury may occur to posterior bones, facets, spinous processes, or neural arch (17).

Less serious and more common injuries to the neck include cervical strains and sprains. A cervical sprain—injury to ligamentous or capsular structures along the cervical spine—occurs most commonly in contact sports. The associated pain is localized to the neck and interscapular region and is nonradicular and without neurological symptoms. Management involves brief immobilization and administration of NSAIDs. Rehabilitation with isometric exercises, as tolerated, should follow. When pain resolves and muscle strength is normal, the athlete may return to contact sports (34). A cervical strain is a tear in one of the musculotendinous units. The most commonly involved muscles include the erector spinae, scalenes, levator scapulae, sternocleidomastoid, and trapezius. The tear occurs when a force overloads the extensor mechanism of the neck (34). Initially the athlete experiences only mild localized pain. Over the following several hours, muscle soreness and local swelling increase, limiting the range of motion. Swelling and pain usually maximize 24–48 hours after injury. Recovery may be slow; rehabilitation is the same as for cervical strain (34).

Injuries to a cervical intervertebral disc can occur through the same mechanisms as other cervical injuries in sports, most often by axial compression of the cervical spine (35). Repeated microtrauma may also result in disc protrusion. Sports-related cervical disc injuries can be secondary to premature cervical spondylosis (slippage of one vertebral body on an adjacent vertebral body) (36). The ligamentous stability of the cervical spine depends upon the anterior and posterior longitudinal ligaments and the annulus fibrosus of each intervertebral disc (37). Weakening of these structures due to degeneration usually occurs at the 4th or 5th intervertebral disc space, which can result in protrusion of the disc under excessive axial load (35). Athletes with neurological symptoms due to cervical disc injury generally need longer periods of rehabilitation and may have residual symptoms.

A brachial plexopathy, a "burner" or "stinger," occurs when the head and neck are forced suddenly toward the shoulder, resulting in a transient unilateral neurapraxia (15). Most often it is the result of a direct blow to the head, but it can also occur if the head and shoulder are forced in opposite directions while either the head or shoulder remains in a fixed position. Symptoms are primarily sensory and most often consist of a burning pain and tingling that radiates down one arm, lasting seconds to minutes, rarely longer than a day (17). Occasionally the individual has focal weakness, but pain-free range of motion of the arm and transient sensory symptoms are strongly suggestive of a brachial plexopathy. The symptoms are always unilateral and in the upper extremities (figure 5.1).

The exact mechanism of injury is still a matter of controversy. If the head and neck are forced laterally toward one shoulder while the opposite shoulder is simultaneously depressed or fixed, the brachial plexus or nerve roots on the depressed or fixed side may be stretched, resulting in symptoms on that same side (38,39). A direct impact in the supraclavicular region may also compress the brachial plexus and cause similar symptoms (38). If one shoulder is forcefully depressed while the neck is forced into hyperextension and lateral flexion to the opposite side, the nerve roots on the side of lateral flexion may be compressed by the cervical foramina, producing symptoms on the side opposite to the depressed shoulder (38,40,41). With either mechanism, the nerve roots involved are C5-C6, producing sensory changes along these dermatomes. Any associated weakness tends to involve the deltoid, biceps, infraspinatus, or supraspinatus muscles (17). The "pinch," or compression, mechanism has been gaining recognition recently. Multiple minor compression strains of the cervical spine may result in an accumulation of edematous and scar tissue, thus narrowing the foraminal space and increasing the possibility of compression of the exiting nerve root (34). Data have shown that athletes with demonstrable narrowing of the cervical foramina have a higher incidence of stingers (burners) (42,43). In addition, 45% of athletes who have suffered one stinger will have repeat episodes (42).

The athlete may resume full activity once the symptoms completely resolve. If no associated neck pain is present and the range of motion is normal, she can return to contact sports. Any residual neck pain or sensory or motor symptoms (lasting longer than several minutes) should be evaluated further for possible cervical-spine bone or nerve pathology (17).

Due to the popularity of the Special Olympics, as well as the recognition of the vital role of exercise in maintenance of good health, the

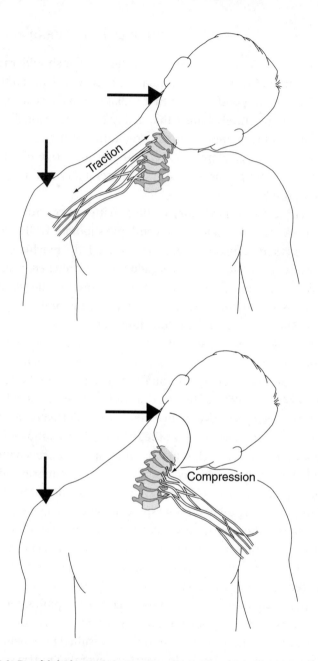

Figure 5.1. Brachial Plexus Injuries. *Top:* Acute brachial plexus injuries ("burners" or "stingers") with shoulder depression and lateral neck flexion and symptoms on the same side as the blow as nerves are stretched. *Bottom:* Lateral neck flexion resulting in symptoms on the opposite side from the blow as nerve roots are compressed.

number of athletes with Down's syndrome is quickly increasing (44). Structural abnormalities of the upper cervical spine are not uncommon in Down's syndrome. Many of these individuals have an increased space between the odontoid and anterior arch of the atlas (45,46); 15–30% have an atlanto-dens interval greater than 5 mm, which places them at an increased risk of cervical spinal cord compression (47).

The natural history of the increased atlanto-dens interval in these athletes is unknown. Usually, individuals with Down's syndrome who develop a cervical myelopathy experience symptoms before the age of 10 years. They also tend to be female and have a generalized ligamentous laxity. Detectable signs and symptoms of spinal cord compression develop for weeks before any catastrophic dislocation occurs (48). Acute dislocation and cord compression are considered exceedingly rare (44). The effect of exercise and certain sports on this type of structural abnormality is not known, but given the overall benefit—both cardiovascular and psychosocial—of exercise and participation in sports activities, complete exclusion from sports participation is not justified.

The guidelines of the Special Olympics Committee on participation in sporting events are ambiguous and refer only to the presence of the C1-C2 instability as revealed by x-ray, without reference to any corresponding neurological symptoms evident on physical examination (44). The sports physician can use the following guidelines for assessing athletes with Down's syndrome in order to allow them to obtain the benefits of exercise and sports with minimal risk of neurological injury:

–All individuals with Down's syndrome should have a cervical spine x-ray at the age of 4 or 5 years (once ossification of the spine is sufficient).
–Any abnormalities evident on x-ray should be followed every 2–3 years, as long as the neurological examination is normal.
–If the x-ray is normal, it does not need to be repeated unless symptoms develop.
–A neurological examination should be performed yearly and x-rays repeated if any changes are noted.

Regular screenings are not justified by the present medical literature (44). It is also recommended that athletes with an increased atlanto-dens interval should avoid sports that can produce any stressful weight bearing to the head or neck, such as tumbling, gymnastics, and diving (44). Present data seem to suggest that, if they avoid the latter activities, individuals with this structural abnormality will not have any difficulty (49,50). Other cervical spine abnormalities present in Down's syndrome include a malformation of the odontoid (51), spondylolysis or spondylolisthesis of the midcervical vertebrae (49), and arthrosis of C4-C6 (49).

BACK INJURIES

Although spine-related injuries are not uncommon among athletes, especially those in physically demanding sports, serious and disabling sports-related injuries are relatively rare (52). Most injuries are minor and tend to be self-limited. Intense and long-term training in sports that place excessive stress on the vertebral column (e.g., gymnastics) has been demonstrated to lead to various spinal disorders (53–56). All types of lumbosacral spine abnormalities occur with higher frequency in athletes than in non-athletes (54). One report found spinal abnormalities on MRI in 63% of Olympic-level gymnasts and 15% of nationally ranked divers (53). Even noncontact sports such as running have been related to a higher incidence of spinal abnormalities, although the incidence of low-back pain in athletes is lower than in non-athletes (57).

The two most common causes of acute low-back pain in athletes are sprains and strains, which can be caused by a sudden twisting motion or flexion, with or without contact. The most common site of a back sprain is in the interspinal ligaments, often in the mid to lower back (58). The athlete experiences acute pain in the midback, which is exacerbated with flexion of the spine. Palpation between the spinous processes at the affected levels also elicits increased pain. Compensatory spasm of the paraspinal muscles may also occur. With a muscle strain in the back, the athlete may feel the sensation of a "tear" in the lower back, with pain that increases in intensity over the following 24–48 hours.

Treatment for both injuries is similar and should include the intermittent use of local ice for reduction of swelling and inflammation for the first 24–48 hours. NSAIDs are useful both for pain relief and to minimize inflammation. If any muscle trigger points develop, local injection can also be useful. Mild stretching can begin once pain is under better control, and the athlete can increase activity as tolerated. He should not return to full activity until he regains full range of motion of the spine and pain has resolved. Continued stretching and strengthening of muscles supporting the spine, including abdominals, is advisable to minimize the risk of recurrent or chronic injury (58).

Acute low-back pain secondary to intervertebral disc disease or herniated nucleus pulposus (HNP) is uncommon in young athletes. Older athletes (over 30 years of age) may be at higher risk, since degenerative changes may already be present, but some athletes who are involved in activities that subject the spine to significant and repetitive axial loads develop degenerative disc disease at an earlier age (59). Younger athletes with HNP may not experience any motor or sensory deficits (60). Radiographs should always be performed to rule out any possible fracture or vertebral abnormality, and further evaluation with either MRI or CT scan is advisable if the pain persists or is associated with any neurological deficits. Lumbar facet arthropathy, which may also be associated with degenerative changes, is increasingly recognized as a cause of back pain and occasional radiculopathy similar to HNP (61,62).

Scheuermann's disease is another uncommon cause of back pain in young athletes, related to the intervertebral disc and generally occurs in the lower thoracic or upper lumbar spine. The disease involves three or more consecutive vertebrae each with anterior wedging of greater than 5 degrees and one or more of the following: irregular endplates, marginal sclerosis, anterior Schmorl's nodules, and narrowed disc spaces (63). In the lumbar spine, only two vertebrae may be involved. Schmorl's nodules occur when disc material is forced into the spongiosa of the vertebrae. They are usually considered secondary to injury or trauma, but sometimes are not detected on radiographs for several months after the inciting injury (64). Anterior Schmorl's nodules are more common in athletes and seem to be associated with vigorous activity (64–66). These are considered characteristic of Scheuermann's disease (66).

Scheuermann's disease in the lower thoracic spine may be associated with dorsal kyphosis. "Swimmers back" is thoracic Scheuermann's disease seen in athletes with a history of excessive and intense training in the butterfly stroke (58). Lumbar Scheuermann's disease is seen more frequently in adolescent males with well-developed musculature. With either type, midline pain is the primary complaint. Chronic overuse or repetitive microtrauma of the lower thoracic and upper lumbar spine can also result in Scheuermann's disease (66,67). Symptoms tend to be less intense and can be treated with rest, pain management, extension exercises, and close monitoring. Scheuermann's associated with a single event, either from forced flexion or compression, needs to be treated as an acute fracture of the vertebral endplate. The associated pain is more intense and often requires a brace for support and pain relief (68).

Spondylolysis and Spondylolisthesis

Spondylolysis and spondylolisthesis are closely associated and common causes of back pain in athletes. Spondylolisthesis is a forward displacement of one vertebral body over an adjacent one. It can occur with either a bilateral elongation or fracture of each pars interarticularis (69). Spondylolysis is specifically a defect in the pars interarticularis, such as an elongation or fracture, which is not necessarily associated with any displacement. The defect may be unilateral or multilevel, but most often occurs at L5 (70,71) (figure 5.2).

The incidence of spondylolisthesis is higher in athletes than in non-exercising individuals, especially athletes in gymnastics (72,73), football (74), and wrestling (75,76). Sports-associated spondylolysis and spondylolisthesis are usually painful. Spondylolysis can occur with repetitive microtrauma or stress resulting in elongation and stress reaction or stress fracture of one or both of the pars interarticularis at a particular level. Initially, pain in the middle of the lower back is associated only with particular activities. Eventually, the pain becomes chronic and may radiate to the buttocks and thighs. The physical examination reveals no abnormalities, but extension of the spine tends to exacerbate the pain. Acute fractures secondary to a single traumatic event can also occur; in this case, pain is usually immediate and focal, without associated neurological deficits.

A stress fracture of the pars interarticularis should always be considered a possibility in an athlete with persistent back pain, especially one involved in intense training in high-risk sports, such as gymnastics and wrestling. Initial evaluation should include x-rays of the lower back in

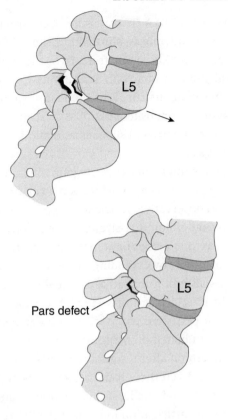

Figure 5.2. Spondylolisthesis and Spondylolysis

anteroposterior, lateral, and oblique views. Any evidence of sclerosis of a pars interarticularis, lamina, or pedicle or an asymmetry of a vertebral body is suggestive of spondylolysis (77). Flexion-extension views of the spine may also help demonstrate any instability. The percentage of slippage (if present at all) is maximized when the person is standing, allowing an easier diagnosis. It is important to remember that spondylolysis may be asymptomatic and present for years prior to detection and therefore can be considered the etiology of an individual's back pain only if previous films are normal.

Both bone scans and CT scans can be used to identify acute spondylolysis before any radiographic changes are evident. The bone scan helps identify a stress reaction in the bone before any elongation and possible spondylolisthesis occur (78). A CT scan is more consistent and accurate for the diagnosis of spondylolysis, since elongation of the pars interarticularis may be due not to an acute fracture or the site of active stress but to a congenital anomaly or an old, healed fracture (neither of which is detected on a bone scan but can allow slippage or spondylolisthesis or asymmetric stress on the opposite pars). The CT scan may also help detect minimal degrees of vertebral slippage and allow evaluation of the apophyseal joints (79).

Treatment depends upon the level of symptoms and the degree of spondylolisthesis, if present at all. Without any evidence of spondylolisthesis, treatment is conservative: restriction of sports competition and a program of back- and abdominal-strengthening exercises. Hamstring spasm is common, as the muscles tighten to stabilize the spine and readjust to the center of gravity by extending the pelvis (80). Monitoring the level of hamstring spasm may help in assessing the success of treatment and progress of healing of the stress reaction or fracture. Individuals with more severe or persistent pain may require analgesic medication and a period of recumbency or an immobilization brace. The athlete may return to competition after resolution of the symptoms and appropriate reconditioning. Even though the athlete is asymptomatic, healing is usually not complete for at least several months and can continue as he resumes limited participation in competitive sports (81). If symptoms persist or recur, the physician should pursue aggressive evaluation for other possible causes of back pain or, if necessary, surgical management or stabilization.

If spondylolisthesis is detected by x-ray, treatment depends on the degree of slippage and the skeletal maturity of the athlete. A grade I spondylolisthesis is a less than 25% displacement of the body of the vertebra over the adjacent vertebra or the first sacral segment. This is treated as a spondylolysis stress reaction or fracture, and the athlete can return to full activity once he is asymptomatic. With a grade II spondylolisthesis, 25–50% of the vertebral body is displaced. The athlete should avoid sports that place a significant amount of stress on the spine or require a high level of twisting of the spine, such as wrestling and gymnastics. An athlete who is not skeletally mature should undergo close follow-up with an x-ray and evaluation of pain every 6 months until she reaches skeletal maturity, at which point the risk of further displacement is minimal (68). She should wear an anti-lordotic brace until skeletal maturity. Any degree of displacement greater than 50% usually requires surgery for stabilization (82,83). Other indications for surgical intervention (usually fusion) include progression of the displacement despite conservative management, refractive pain, neurological deficit, or an abnormal gait.

Piriformis Muscle Syndrome

The piriformis muscle originates from the anterior surface of the mid-sacrum, extends through the greater sciatic foramen, and inserts on the greater trochanter. The piriformis functions as an external rotator of the hip in a standing position and an abductor in the sitting position (84). With repetitive trauma or overstretching, the piriformis muscle may become irritated and inflamed and possibly go into spasm. The resulting low-back pain may be due to the irritation in the muscle itself or to secondary pressure and irritation of the sciatic nerve, which passes directly beneath it (84,85).

Differentiation between sciatica resulting from disc herniation and that due to piriformis syndrome may be difficult. Both cause low-back pain along the distribution of the sciatic nerve, and both can be associated with muscle spasm, limited flexion, and exacerbation of pain with straight leg raising. Piriformis syndrome is not associated with any neurological deficit, such as decreased reflexes or focal motor weakness, suggesting it is most likely a neuritis rather than an entrapment neuropathy (84). It is characterized by tenderness at the origin, body, or insertion of the muscle body of the piriformis and possibly limitation of external rotation of the hip. An increased density or spasm of the muscle may also occur. Diagnosis is usually based on the clinical examination. It has also been suggested that piriformis muscle spasm and HNP may occur together (84).

Treatment involves slow stretching of the piriformis through simultaneous forced hip flexion, adduction, and internal rotation for 1–2 minutes at a time. Manipulation and deep tissue massage of the muscle are also effective, and injection of trigger points with 1–2 mL of 1% lidocaine has been useful in some cases. For persistent or chronic pain, surgical release with exploration of the sciatic nerve may be considered as a last resort (86).

Sacroiliac Joint Injuries

Stress reaction or sprain of the sacroiliac joint may result from repetitive microtrauma or overuse, possibly related to asymmetric strength of the muscles supporting the spinal column, or a single traumatic event. Formerly considered a rare cause of sports-related low-back pain, it may well be more frequent and go either unrecognized or misdiagnosed. Diagnosis is based on a bone scan. Differentiation from other causes of low-back pain is important, since treatment requires a longer period of rest in order to avoid compensatory changes in gait, possibly increasing the risk of more serious injury (87).

In general, treatment of low-back pain in the competitive athlete involves rest, reduction of pain and spasm, and reconditioning, focusing on the muscles that help stabilize the spine. Rest is relative and can allow conditioning and strengthening as tolerated. The athlete should avoid weight training that transmits a load through the lumbar spine. NSAIDs, ice, massage, ultrasound treatment, transcutaneous electrical nerve stimulation, and mobilization can be used for pain control (34).

REFERENCES

1. Morrow RM, Seals RR, Barnwell GM, et al: Report of a survey of oral injuries in male college and university athletes. Athletic Training 26:339–342, 1991

2. Morrow RM, Bonci T: A survey of oral injuries in female college and university athletes. Athletic Training 24:236–237, 1989

3. Kumamoto DP, Jacob M, Nickelsen D: Oral trauma: on field assessment. Physician and Sportsmedicine 23(5):53–62, 1995

4. Andreasen JO, Andreasen FM: Essentials of Traumatic Injuries to the Teeth, ed 1. Copenhagen, Munksgaard, 1990

5. Andreasen JO: Traumatic Injuries of the Teeth, ed 2. Philadelphia, WB Saunders, 1981

6. Pashby TJ, Pashby RC: Treatment of sports eye injuries. In Fu FH (ed): Sports Injuries. Baltimore, Williams & Wilkins, 1994, 833–851

7. Keller AP Jr: A study of the relationship of air pressure to myringorupture. Laryngoscope 68:2015–2029, 1958

8. Davidson TM, Neuman TR: Managing ear trauma. Physician and Sportsmedicine 22(7):27–32, 1994

9. Kristensen S, Juul A, Gammelgaard NP, et al: Traumatic tympanic membrane perforations: complications and management. Ear Nose Throat J 68:503–516, 1989

10. Kelleger JC, Sullivan K, Baibak G, Dean RK: The wrestler's ear. Plast Reconstr Surg 40:540–546, 1967

11. Schuller DE, Dankle SK, Martin M, Strauss RH: Auricular injury and the use of headgear in wrestlers. Arch Otolaryngol Head Neck Surg 115:714–717, 1989

12. Schuller DE, Dankle SD, Strauss RH: A technique to treat wrestlers' auricular hematoma without interrupting training or competition. Arch Otolaryngol Head Neck Surg 115:202–206, 1989

13. Wallace RB: Application of epidemiologic principles to sports injury research. Am J Sports Med 16:S22–S24, 1988

14. Maroon JC, Steele PB, Berlin R: Football head and neck injuries: an update. Clin Neurosurg 27:414, 1980

15. Vesgo JJ, Lehman RC: Field evaluation and management of head and neck injuries. Clin Sports Med 6:1–15, 1987

16. Murphey F, Simmons JC: Initial management of athletic injuries to the head and neck. Am J Surg 98:379–383, 1959

17. Cantu RC: Head and spine injuries in youth sports. Clin Sports Med 14:517–532, 1995

18. Lehman LB, Ravich SJ: Closed head injuries in athletes. Clin Sports Med 9:247–261, 1990

19. Cantu RC: Head and spine injuries in the young athlete. Clin Sports Med 7:459–472, 1988

20. Lehman LB: The preseason athlete screening examination. Med Times 116:29–31, 1988

21. Wilberger JE Jr, Maroon JC: Head injuries in athletics. Clin Sports Med 8:1–9, 1989

22. Jennet B: Late effects of head injuries. In Critchley M, O'Leary JL, Jennet B (eds): Scientific Foundations of Neurology. Philadelphia, FA Davis, 1971, 441–451

23. Schneider RC: Head and Neck Injuries in Football: Mechanisms, Treatment, and Prevention. Baltimore, Williams & Wilkins, 1973

24. Kelley JP, Nichols JS, Filley CM, et al: Concussion in sports: guidelines for the prevention of catastrophic outcome. JAMA 266:2867–2869, 1991

25. Saunders RL, Harbaugh RE: The second impact in catastrophic contact sports head trauma. JAMA 252:538–539, 1984

26. Cantu RC: Guidelines for return to contact sports after a cerebral concussion. Sports Med 14:76–79, 1987

27. Blahd WH Jr, Iserson KV, Bjelland JC: Efficiency of the posttraumatic cross table lateral view of the cervical spine. J Emerg Med 2:243–249, 1985

28. Cantu RC: The Exercising Adult, ed 2. New York, Macmillan, 1987

29. Cantu RC: Health Maintenance through Physical Conditioning. Littleton, MA, Wright-PSG, 1981

30. Martland HS: Punch drunk. JAMA 91:1103–1107, 1928

31. Casson IR, Siegel O, Sham R, et al: Brain damage in modern boxers. JAMA 251:2663–2667, 1984

32. Gronwall D, Wrightson P: Cumulative effect of concussion. Lancet 2:995, 1975

33. Ryan AJ: Intracranial injuries resulting from boxing: a review. Clin Sports Med 6:31–40, 1987

34. Wroble RR, Albright JP: Neck and low back injuries in wrestling. Clin Sports Med 5:295–325, 1986

35. Kumano K, Uneyama T: Cervical disk injuries in athletes. Arch Orthop Trauma Surg 105:223–226, 1986

36. Simeone FA, Rothman RH: Cervical disk disease. *In* Rothman RH, Simeone FA (eds): The Spine. Philadelphia, WB Saunders, 1982, 440–472

37. Nagel DA, Koogle TA, Piziall RL, Perkash I: Stability of the lumbar spine following progressive disruptions and the applications of individual internal and external devices. J Bone Joint Surg Am 63:62–70, 1981

38. Albright JP, McAuley E, Martin RK, et al: Head and neck injuries in college football: an eight-year analysis. Am J Sports Med 13:147–152, 1985

39. Bergfield JA, Hershman E, Wilbourn A: Brachial plexus injury in sports: a five year follow-up. Orthop Trans 12:743–744, 1988

40. Watkins RG: Neck injuries in football players. Clin Sports Med 5:215–246, 1986

41. Wilbourn AJ, Hershman EB, Bergdield JA: Brachial plexopathies in athletes: the EMG findings. Muscle Nerve 9:254, 1986

42. Meyer SA, Schulte KR, Callaghan JJ, et al: Cervical spinal stenosis and stingers in collegiate football players. Am J Sports Med 22:158–166, 1994

43. Kelly JD, Clancy M, Marchetto PA, et al: The relationship of transient upper extremity paresthesias and cervical stenosis. Orthop Trans 16:732, 1992–1993

44. Goldberg MJ: Spine instability and the Special Olympics. Clin Sports Med 12:507–515, 1993

45. Martel W, Tishler JM: Observations on the spine in mongoloidism. Am J Roentgenol 97:630–638, 1966

46. Tishler J, Martel W: Dislocation of the atlas in mongolism. Radiology 84:904–906, 1965

47. Treadwell SJ, Newman DE, Lockrich G: Instability of the upper cervical spine in Down syndrome. J Pediatr Orthop 10:602–606, 1990

48. Davidson RG: Atlantoaxial instability in individuals with Down syndrome: a fresh look at the evidence. Pediatrics 81:857–865, 1988

49. Goldberg MJ: Down syndrome and other chromosome abnormalities. *In*

The Dysmorphic Child: An Orthopaedic Perspective. New York, Raven Press, 1987, 370–391

50. Peuschel SM, Scola FH: Atlanto axial instability in individuals with Down syndrome: epidemiologic, radiographic and clinical studies. Pediatrics 80:555–560, 1987

51. French HG, Burke SW, Roberts JM, et al: Upper cervical ossicles in Down syndrome. J Pediatr Orthop 7:69–71, 1987

52. Cacayorin ED, Hochhauser L, Petro GR: Lumbar and thoracic spine pain in the athlete: radiographic evaluation. Clin Sports Med 6:767–783, 1987

53. Goldstein JD, Berger PE, Windler GE, et al: Spine injuries in gymnasts and swimmers: an epidemiological investigation. Am J Sports Med 19:463, 1991

54. Hellstrom M , Jacobsson B, Sward L, et al: Radiologic abnormalities of the thoraco-lumbar spine in athletes. Acta Radiol 31:127, 1991

55. Sward L, Hellstrom M, Jacobssen B, et al: Spondylolysis and the sacro-horizontal angle in athletes. Acta Radiol 30:359, 1989

56. Sward L, Hellstrom M, Jacobssen B, et al: Disc degeneration and associated abnormalities of the spine in elite gymnasts: a magnetic resonance imaging study. Spine 16:437, 1991

57. Videman T, Sarna S, Battié MC, et al: The long-term effects of physical loading and exercise lifestyles on back-related symptoms, disability, and spinal pathology among men. Spine 20:699–709, 1995

58. Keene JS, Drummond DS: Mechanical back pain in the athlete. Compr Ther 11:7–14, 1985

59. Spencer CW, Jackson DW: Back injuries in the athlete. Clin Sports Med 2:191, 1981

60. DeOrio J, Bianco A: Lumbar disk excision in children and adolescents. J Bone Joint Surg Am 64:991–996, 1982

61. Inman VT, Saunders JB: The clinical-anatomical aspects of the lumbosacral region. Radiology 38:669, 1942

62. Mooney V, Robertson J: The facet syndrome. Clin Orthop 115:149, 1976

63. Greenan TJ: Diagnostic imaging of sports-related spinal disorders. Clin Sports Med 12:487–505, 1993

64. Sward L, Hellstrom M, Jacobssen B, et al: Acute injury of the vertebral ring apophysis and intervertebral disc in adolescent gymnasts. Spine 15:144, 1990

65. Alexander CJ: Scheuermann's disease: a traumatic spondylodystrophy? Skeletal Radiol 1:209, 1977

66. Blumenthal SL, Roach J, Herring JA: Lumbar Scheuermann's, a clinical series and classification. Spine 12:929–932, 1987

67. Wilcox PG, Spencer CW: Dorsolumbar kyphosis or Scheuermann's disease. Clin Sports Med 5:343–351, 1986

68. Kraus DR, Shapiro D: The symptomatic lumbar spine in the athlete. Clin Sports Med 8: 59–69, 1989

69. Neugebauer F: Aetiologie der sogennanten spondylolisthesis. Arch Gynak Munchen 35:375, 1882

70. Bosworth D, Fielding J, Demarest L, et al: Spondylolisthesis: a critical review of a consecutive series of cases treated by arthodesis. J Bone Joint Surg 37A:767, 1955

71. Porter R, Park W: Unilateral spondylosis. J Bone Joint Surg 64B:345, 1982

72. Jackson D, Wiltse L, Cirincione R: Spondylolysis in the female gymnast. Clin Orthop 117:68, 1976

73. Micheli L: Back injuries in gymnasts. Clin Sports Med 4:85, 1985

74. Wiltse L, Widell E, Jackson D: Fatigue fracture: the bone lesion in isthmic spondylolisthesis. J Bone Joint Surg 57A:17, 1974

75. Granhead H, Morelli B: Low back pain among retired wrestlers and heavyweight lifters. Am J Sports Med 16:530, 1988

76. Rossi F: Spondylolysis, spondylolisthesis and sports. J Sports Med Phys Fitness 18:317, 1988

77. Sherman F, Wilkinson R, Hall J: Reactive sclerosis of a pedicle and spondylolysis in the lumbar spine. J Bone Joint Surg 59A:49, 1977

78. Holder LE, Matthews LS: The nuclear physician and sports medicine. In Nuclear Medicine Annual. New York, Raven Press, 1984, 127–132

79. Teplick JG, Laffey PA, Berman A, et al: Diagnosis and evaluation of spondylolisthesis and/or spondylolysis on axial CT. Am J Neuroradiol 7:479, 1986

80. Phalen G, Dickson J: Spondylolisthesis and tight hamstrings. J Bone Joint Surg 43A:505, 1961

81. Tachdjian M: Pediatric Orthopedics. Philadelphia, WB Saunders, 1990, 289

82. Boxall D, Bradford D, Winter R, et al: Management of severe spondylolisthesis in children and adolescents. J Bone Joint Surg 61A:479, 1979

83. Hensinger R, Lang J, MacEwen G: Surgical management of spondylolisthesis in children and adolescents. Spine 1:207, 1976

84. Steiner C, Staubs C, Ganon M, Buhlinger C: Piriformis syndrome: pathogenesis, diagnosis, and treatment. Journal of Am Osteopath Assoc 87:318–323, 1987

85. Jankiewicz JJ, Hennrikus WL, Houkom JA: The appearance of the piriformis muscle syndrome in computed tomography and magnetic resonance imaging. Clin Orthop Rel Res 262:205–209, 1991

86. Barton PM: Piriformis syndrome: a rational approach to management. Pain 47:345–352, 1991

87. Marymont JV, Lynch MA, Henning CE: Exercise-related stress reaction of the sacroiliac joint. Am J Sports Med 14:320–323, 1986

Chapter 6

UPPER-EXTREMITY INJURIES

SHOULDER INJURIES

The glenohumeral joint is a ball-and-socket joint. The shallow socket, more like a saucer, allows a wider range of motion on multiple planes than any other joint in the body. Such a great arc of motion is obtained at the expense of stability in the shoulder joint. The rotator cuff muscles and joint capsule play a vital role in stabilizing the shoulder.

Only recently has the subtle instability of the shoulder joint become recognized as one of the primary causes of shoulder pain and dysfunction in athletes, especially those under 35 years of age. Athletes involved in sports requiring overhand throwing motion place repetitive mechanical stress on the shoulder, which leads to repetitive microtrauma. The force of the throw is absorbed by the ligamentous capsule and rotator cuff tendons. Chronic microtrauma may result in anterior instability, which can be subtle initially but progresses to more symptomatic subluxation and impingement as the rotator cuff tendons pass through a narrowed space between the humeral head and the acromion. Additionally, the rotator cuff plays a more important role as a dynamic stabilizer when the capsule becomes lax. As the rotator cuff is overworked to fatigue, the muscles are no longer able to shield the tendons from stress, resulting in inflammation. Tendonitis and partial tears may therefore be secondary to a subtle anterior instability in these athletes (1).

Subluxation is a broad term that refers to the abnormal movement of the humeral head out of the glenoid fossa short of complete dislocation. Both complete dislocation and subluxation can occur with one excessive force or injury (traumatic) or with usual arm motion (atraumatic) (2). *Instability* also refers to movement of the humeral head outside the glenoid fossa, but it is used to describe the direction of the movement. Instability may be present in multiple planes but most often occurs in two planes, anterior and inferior or posterior and inferior.

Traumatic Dislocation

Traumatic dislocations can occur in any direction, but anterior and posterior are the most usual. Anterior dislocations are the most common and tend to occur when the arm is driven backwards while externally rotated and hyperextended in an overhead position. The head of the humerus is levered anteriorly and may be forced completely out of the glenoid fossa, possibly tearing the capsule, labrum, or rotator cuff tendons. Two common lesions associated with traumatic dislocations are a Bankart lesion and a Hill-Sachs defect. A Bankart lesion is a tear in the anterior-inferior labrum (the structure to which the capsule attaches on the glenoid fossa). It generally occurs as the humeral head is forced out of the fossa (3,4). A Hill-Sachs defect is an impact lesion of the cartilage and underlying bone located on the posterolateral head of the humerus, occurring when the posterior humeral head impacts against the glenoid upon reduction. An individual with an acute anterior dislocation is incapable of internally rotating the affected arm or reaching the opposite shoulder with the hand of the affected side (2).

Posterior dislocations are surprisingly uncommon, accounting for approximately 2% of all shoulder dislocations (5). The mechanism involves a force that drives the humeral head posteriorly, such as falling directly on an outstretched arm. The injured athlete is incapable of externally rotating the affected arm, reaching outward, or flexing the shoulder with the arm fully adducted (6). The arm seems to be locked in internal rotation.

Initial evaluation should include an x-ray, if it can be performed expeditiously. An axillary view is usually best for diagnosis of a posterior dislocation, although it may be difficult to obtain depending on the individual's level of pain tolerance. Reduction of the dislocation is best performed as soon as possible, since secondary muscle spasm may render the reduction more difficult. Multiple methods exist for reduction of a dislocation (5,7,8). One of the simplest is to grasp the affected arm at the wrist and raise it overhead; the humeral head usually slips back into the glenoid fossa (5).

Prolonged immobilization has not been demonstrated to reduce the rate of recurrence (9,10), so the standard treatment is mobilization (as tolerated) and physical therapy to help regain full range of motion and strength. Strengthening of rotator cuff muscles may also decrease the risk of recurrence in anterior dislocations. Loss of apprehension with extreme external rotation is also recommended before the athlete returns to contact sports, which may take from 4–6 weeks to a few months.

Instability in the shoulder joint can be difficult to diagnose, given the inherent laxity and mobility in the joint itself. Instability that is atraumatic and not associated with one event of excessive stress can be particularly confusing. A careful history and physical examination may suggest a more subtle instability related to overuse or the culmination of multiple smaller episodes of stress or microtrauma. The athlete may not be aware of the instability and may not complain of the sensation of the shoulder easily giving out or subluxing. He is more likely to report shoulder pain unrelated to a particular event but associated with repetitive overhead activities such as swimming, throwing, volleyball, or tennis.

Evaluation of Shoulder Pain

Establishing the character of the pain may be helpful in determining the etiology. Burning pain is more often related to nerve irritation from a protruding cervical disc, especially if the pain radiates down the arm or is associated with paresthesias (11). Calcific bursitis can also be described as a hot, burning pain. Aching pain in the shoulder, especially at night, is suggestive of a rotator cuff tear (12). Pain with both active and passive abduction of the arm can be associated with subacromial bursitis.

Location of the pain also can be helpful in determining the etiology. Trapezial pain tends to be cervical in origin unless centered around the acromioclavicular joint. Lateral and posterior subdeltoid pain tends to be associated with rotator cuff pathology.

The relationship of the pain to specific activity, such as the phase of the throwing motion or the stroke (in swimming) that exacerbates the pain, can give helpful clues as to the etiology. Shoulder pain during the forward acceleration phase (forceful internal rotation with abduction) suggests a primary anterior instability resulting in pain in the anterior capsule and glenoid labrum resulting from excessive stress, which may lead to rotator cuff tendonitis (13). Pain at the inferomedial angle of the scapula, brought on during the cocking phase (abduction and forceful external rotation) and relieved during the follow through, is usually indicative of scapulothoracic bursitis (14). Rotator cuff tears tend to be associated with chronic aching, especially at night, whereas rotator cuff tendonitis usually develops over time with repetitive overhand motion (15). The suprascapular nerve can become impinged or irritated as it passes over the suprascapular notch, which may cause a burning or ache in the posterolateral region of the shoulder that may radiate to the arm or neck during or after the throw. Synovitis of the acromioclavicular joint, which may occur in swimmers and in weight lifters (or athletes who are weight training), produces anterior shoulder pain exacerbated when the arm is crossed in front of the chest.

The physical exam should start with inspection of the shoulder from behind. Any atrophy of the supraspinatus or infraspinatus may make the scapula appear more prominent and could indicate dysfunction or a tear of the corresponding rotator cuff tendon or, more rarely, an injury of the suprascapular nerve (11). Prominence of the acromion is sometimes seen in athletes with deltoid muscle atrophy resulting from injury to the axillary nerve, occurring in fractures, dislocations, or a direct blow to the shoulder. Lateral scapular slide is seen in conditions resulting in weakness of the scapular muscles (rhomboids). Anterior serratus muscle palsy due to injury to the long thoracic nerve results in scapular winging, which is enhanced when the athlete performs a push-up against the wall. Injury to the long thoracic nerve may result from direct trauma or lateral traction of the scapula. A cervical disc lesion at C6 may also weaken the anterior serratus muscle.

Active and passive range of motion should be observed and documented, including the following: forward flexion (arm raised directly in front of the body and the angle between the arm and thorax approximated, as viewed from the side), abduction (arm raised from the side in the plane of the thorax) with the scapula stabilized, internal rotation (documented as the level of the spinal column reached by the arm behind the back), and external rotation (arm bent to 90 degrees at the elbow, held at the side, and rotated outward). Tears of the rotator cuff, degenerative arthritis, and adhesive capsulitis, all of which tend to occur in older athletes, decrease the external rotation first, then abduction (which is compensated for by scapulothoracic motion). Experienced overhand throwers often demonstrate external rotation in the dominant arm up to 15–20% greater than that in the nondominant arm. The excess in external rotation usually is accompanied by a loss in internal rotation. These changes are not necessarily pathological (12).

The rotator cuff muscles can be isolated according to function, and the strength should be tested simultaneously with the same muscle on the opposite arm. Both the infraspinatus and teres minor externally rotate the arm and can be isolated when the athlete bends both elbows to 90 degrees flexion and holds his elbows touching the sides of his body with forearms directed forward parallel to the floor. With the thumbs pointed upward, the athlete then externally rotates his arms against resistance applied by the examiner on the lateral surface of the forearms. Any asymmetry in strength or pain should be noted. The subscapularis internally rotates the arm and can be isolated in the same position. The athlete then internally rotates his arms against resistance applied by the examiner on the medial forearms. The supraspinatus abducts the arm and can be isolated by the athlete abducting both arms to 90 degrees, then forward flexing them 30 degrees, and maximally internally rotating the arms by pointing his thumbs downward. The examiner applies a force toward the floor against the forearms while the athlete attempts to maintain 90 degrees of abduction (12,16) (figure 6.1). Since rotator cuff tears usually affect the supraspinatus to some extent, any asymmetry in strength, even if subtle, may indicate early degeneration or a small tear. If in doubt, multiple repetitions of the stress applied by the examiner may bring out a subtle weakness.

Examination of both shoulders for evidence of instability, using the unaffected shoulder for comparison, is an important part of the examination. The athlete lies supine, positioned with the shoulder to be examined off the edge of the table. To test anterior stability, the arm is then abducted 90 degrees and externally rotated. The examiner places the palm of her hand over the anterior humeral head and curls the fingers

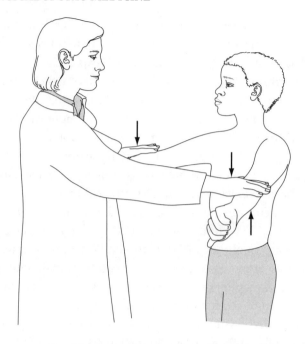

Figure 6.1. Examination of the Supraspinatus Muscle. The supraspinatus is the most common muscle of the rotator cuff to inflame or tear.

over to the posterior surface. She then uses her fingers to force the humeral head anteriorly (figure 6.2). Any subluxation of the humeral head suggests anterior instability and is usually painful. Of note, the athlete with a history of anterior subluxation often exhibits an "apprehension" in this position as the humeral head is rotated externally or with the applied anterior stress (a procedure known as the apprehension test). In this test, apprehension is defined as the involuntary contraction of the muscles supporting the humeral head to prevent an anticipated subluxation or dislocation (17). Pain with this manipulation is not considered evidence of apprehension, although it has been postulated that the pain may be suggestive of subtle instability (1,18). Posterior stress may also be applied in the test, but up to 50% posterior subluxation may be normal if symmetric (on both shoulders) (1). Abnormal subluxation can also be demonstrated by loading the

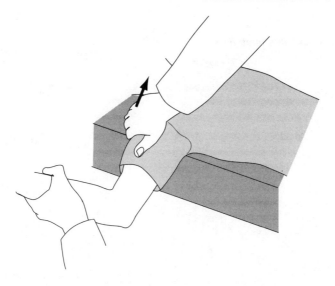

Figure 6.2. Anterior Instability Test ("Apprehension Test")

humeral head anteriorly and posteriorly while the athlete is supine with his arm in 20 degrees of abduction and forward flexion in neutral rotation. Inferior instability can be demonstrated by placing traction on the elbow while the athlete is sitting with his arms by his sides. Any "dimpling" or creation of an indentation (called a "sulcus") below the acromion may suggest laxity; it is usually reported in centimeters (18). Again, comparison with the opposite side is essential. Note that symmetric laxity may be observed in individuals with a generalized hypermobility (which may be a problem in athletes involved in sports requiring repetitive overhead motion).

The rotator cuff muscles are considered glenohumeral stabilizers, along with the joint capsule and glenohumeral ligaments (figure 6.3). Even a subtle anterior instability can lead to a narrowing of the space between the humeral head and the acromion with active motion, resulting in an impingement, or "pinching," of the supraspinatus tendon as it passes through the narrowed space. The athlete will describe an exacerbation of the shoulder pain with abduction. In the Hawkins test for the presence of impingement, the athlete places his arm in 90 degrees

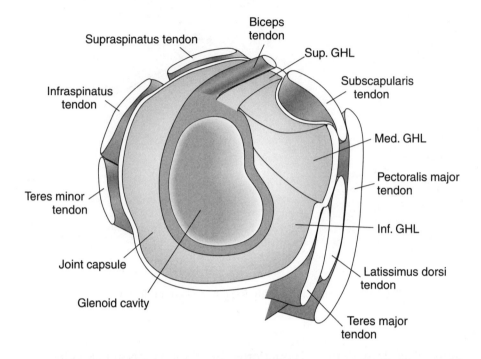

Figure 6.3. Anatomy of the Glenohumeral Joint and Relative Position of the Stabilizing Structures. The joint is shown at rest. GHL, glenohumeral ligament.

of forward flexion, and the examiner then forcibly internally rotates the shoulder (19) (figure 6.4). This maneuver narrows the subacromial space and forces the supraspinatus tendon against the acromion. Pain suggests an irritation or pathological impingement of the supraspinatus tendon. Impingement may occur without any instability, usually in individuals over 30 years of age who have some primary degenerative process already present or a pathologically narrow subacromial space as a baseline. The physician should always consider the possibility of anterior instability as the underlying problem in rotator cuff tendonitis in an athlete whose sport involves overhead motion (13,16,20).

Biceps tendonitis is another clinical presentation of a possible anterior instability. Inflammation of the biceps tendon can be determined by direct palpation for tenderness (always in comparison with the contralateral side) or by asking the athlete to flex her elbow to 90 degrees

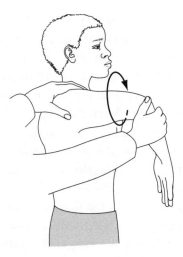

Figure 6.4. Hawkins Test for Impingement

and supinate her wrist against resistance applied by the examiner (Yergason's test) (21). Or, the athlete should fully extend the elbow, supinate the forearm, and flex the shoulder forward against resistance from the examiner (Speed's test), which can be more effective (22). The long head of the biceps tendon attaches to the superior labrum and functionally may contribute to anterior stabilization of the shoulder in abduction (23). The anterior instability resulting from repetitive throwing or overhand motions or a rotator cuff tear places repetitive traction on the biceps tendon and its attachment to the superior labrum, resulting in inflammation or tendonitis (24).

Biceps tendonitis may occur as a primary lesion, but associated pathology should always be considered in the athlete. Management involves anti-inflammatory modalities: NSAIDs or a short pulse of prednisone. The athlete's technique should also be closely reviewed for possible modification. Direct injection of the tendon sheath with steroid is not recommended. Biceps tendonitis can also be associated with a specific type of tear of the labrum, due either to a single event of compression loading of the humeral head in flexion and abduction or to repetitive microtrauma, referred to as a SLAP (superior labrum anterior and posterior) lesion (25). The superior region of the labrum, extending anteriorly and posteriorly to the midglenoid notch, may become avulsed or torn. It is not a common lesion but (in addition to the associated anterior instability) can be a significant disability to the athlete. It is best diagnosed and successfully managed by arthroscopy (26).

Posterior instability is less common and may present a diagnostic challenge. Pain usually occurs when the arm is placed in forward flexion and abduction with internal rotation, although pain during daily activities may also occur (27). For the posterior stress test, the athlete lies supine while the examiner stabilizes the athlete's scapula with one hand and applies a posterior stress to the humerus with the athlete's arm in 90 degrees of abduction and internally rotated. Posterior instability is suggested by subluxation associated with discomfort, similar to the symptoms experienced during the associated activity (28). The discomfort is similar to the apprehension associated with the anterior apprehension test and may not be painful. Because disability is often minimal, management is usually conservative and involves intensive rehabilitation to strengthen the rotator cuff muscles, primarily the infraspinatus and teres minor (27). Surgical repair is available for patients unresponsive to conservative management.

The diagnosis of instability can be established via the history and careful physical examination in 90% of cases. The MRI, especially with contrast enhancement, is a useful adjunct to determine whether any labral tears are present. Treatment for instability, with or without associated rotator cuff tendonitis, can initially be conservative, depending on the athlete's history, physical findings, and level of competition. Avoidance of overhand activity, strengthening of the rotator cuff, scapular, and back muscles, and use of NSAIDs may allow the athlete to eventually return to previous activity. The scapula provides the platform for glenohumeral function, so strengthening of scapular muscles should be included in any rehabilitation program for shoulder instability.

The MRI is a useful adjunct for determining associated labral or rotator cuff tears. The evaluation of most competitive athletes with suspected instability should include an MRI. The treatment of shoulder instability has advanced significantly with the use of arthroscopy for both visualization of the glenohumeral joint and repair of pathological lesions. Examination with the athlete under anesthesia and arthroscopic visualization of the joint may allow accurate diagnosis when physical examination is limited by pain and guarding or muscle bulk. The location of labral shredding or tears indicates the direction of subtle instability, which may then be addressed. Anterior, posterior, and multidirectional instability due to capsular tears or stretching can usually be repaired surgically or with the more recent advance of thermally assisted capsulorrhaphy, both performed by arthroscopy. Labral tears can be either resected or repaired. Primary impingement can be managed surgically by arthroscopic resection of the distal acromion, and some rotator cuff tears can be repaired. Arthroscopic treatment has become quite successful and is often the treatment of choice, especially if the injury is dealt with earlier rather than later.

Acromioclavicular Joint

The acromioclavicular (A-C) joint, which is stabilized by the acromioclavicular ligament and the coracoclavicular ligaments, functions as a radius about which the shoulder moves, with the sternoclavicular joint functioning as a pivot point (29). The A-C joint allows a moderate amount of movement for the glenoid fossa to turn in various directions. Repetitive microtrauma, commonly seen in weight lifters and athletes in sports with overhead activity, may eventually result in degenerative changes and chronic shoulder pain.

Direct impact on the acromion or a fall on the shoulder may result in a tear of the acromioclavicular ligament and possibly the coracoclavicular ligament or, if the impact is great enough, a fracture of the clavicle. The trapezius and deltoid muscles, which attach directly to the clavicle, can also be torn by sheer force, but this is much less common. With any suspected injury to the A-C joint, x-rays should be performed to rule out a fracture. X-rays taken while the athlete holds hand-weights may be helpful to evaluate the extent of A-C separation, but these films may underestimate the extent of damage if the athlete is not relaxed (30). It is also important to compare the views of the injured joint with those of the uninjured side, since many A-C joints may allow up to 50% subluxation as a normal variant (30).

Acromioclavicular joint injuries are often classified into six grades for easier description of the ligamentous damage and subluxation of the clavicle (31):

–Grade I: minimal disruption or microtears of the acromioclavicular ligament, allowing little or no subluxation of the A-C joint as viewed on x-ray.

–Grade II: tear of the acromioclavicular ligament, with the coracoclavicular ligament left intact. Deformity of the shoulder is evident on examination, and abnormal subluxation of 50% of the A-C joint is evident on x-ray.

–Grade III: tear of both the acromioclavicular and coracoacromial ligaments that allows more than 50% subluxation of the A-C joint as revealed on x-ray. Examination reveals obvious deformity and significant discomfort with any movement.

–Grade IV: posterior dislocation of the clavicle, possibly lodged into the trapezius muscle.

–Grade V: similar to grade III, associated with traumatic detachment of the trapezius and deltoid ligaments.

–Grade VI: clavicular displacement under the acromion or coracoid process. This may be associated with an injury to the brachial plexus or clavicular fracture and angulation (32).

Grades I–III sprains are generally treated conservatively with ice, NSAIDs, and a sling for comfort. Early mobilization, as tolerated, allows an earlier return to full activity (29). The period of recovery and time of return to activity are primarily based on the sport; 3–4 weeks is usually sufficient for most athletes, but resumption of overhead motion without discomfort may take up to 6 or 8 weeks. Surgical treatment of grade III sprains has not been associated with less long-term disability or earlier recovery, although some athletes are uncomfortable with the cosmetic appearance and request surgical fixation. Grades IV–VI sprains require surgical intervention and a longer recovery period. Some residual sensation of clicking or pain with overhead motions may occur in up to 30% of cases, even with a grade I sprain, but less than 5% of these are disabling. In such cases, surgical resection of the distal clavicle may be advisable, since osteoarthritis of the A-C joint has been associated with acromioclavicular sprains (29). Surgical resection of the distal clavicle at the time of primary surgical repair of an A-C joint separation is not indicated, however.

Clavicular fractures occur through the same mechanisms as sprains, only with greater force. More than 80% of clavicular fractures occur in the middle third of the clavicle and more than 15% in the distal clavicle (32). Fractures involving the middle third of the clavicle can be treated with closed reduction for approximate realignment, then immobilized with a sling or figure-eight harness. Fractures involving the distal third of the clavicle are sometimes complicated by tears of the coracoclavicular ligaments. These fractures are unstable and require surgical fixation in order to avoid significant deformity, painful non-union, or premature degenerative changes in the A-C joint (34).

Sternoclavicular Joint

Sprains of the sternoclavicular joint are rare but can occur with blunt impact on the chest wall or with transmission of an axial load on the clavicle to the sternoclavicular joint. A mild sprain remains stable with only stretching or microtears of the sternoclavicular ligaments. If the sternoclavicular ligaments are completely torn, the clavicle can be displaced anteriorly (anterior dislocation) or posteriorly (posterior dislocation). A posterior sprain can be more serious, since the clavicle may compress the trachea or tear large blood vessels (33). Dislocations may be difficult to appreciate on plain x-rays; CT scans or tomograms are often needed to clearly delineate the degree of dislocation and possible soft tissue damage. Subluxations can often be treated conservatively with ice and immobilization or arm support. Complete dislocations are usually unstable and may require surgical management (32).

ELBOW INJURIES

The elbow is a complex joint that allows not only flexion and extension but also supination and pronation (rotation). The normal range of motion is generally 140 degrees flexion from full extension and approximately 75 degrees of both supination and pronation (35). The joint is stabilized by ligaments and the bony structure.

Elbow injuries are usually associated with throwing and racquet sports. They are most commonly related to overuse and chronic stress resulting from either intrinsic or extrinsic overload forces. These repetitive forces can lead to microruptures of ligaments and tendons, stress fractures of the apophyses in the immature athlete, or frank bony stress reactions in athletes of all ages (36).

Most throwing and racquet strokes place a significant valgus stress on the elbow and the medial components of the elbow. The primary medial stabilizing component of the elbow is the ulnar (or medial) collateral ligament complex (MCL). It consists of three ligaments, the most important of which is the anterior oblique ligament, which originates from the medial epicondyle and inserts on the medial coronoid process. The posterior oblique ligament is actually more a thickening of the capsule, originating from the medial epicondyle and inserting onto the semilunar notch. The transverse ligament extends from the medial olecranon to the inferior medial coronoid process (36). Secondary stabilization is provided at the extremes of flexion (<20 degrees and >120 degrees) by the bony articulation between the humerus and ulna (37). The radiocapitellar joint is also a secondary stabilizer with valgus stress. The flexor-pronator muscles originating from the medial epicondyle provide primary dynamic stability (36).

A sudden or forceful valgus stress, with or without contact, can cause an acute and complete rupture of the MCL; however, these are relatively uncommon. The athlete generally perceives an "event" or a "pop" and subsequently finds it difficult to throw well because of pain. Medial instability and point tenderness are often present along the MCL at or distal to the medial epicondyle. If it is an isolated injury, only minimal pain occurs with wrist flexion, which helps to differentiate it from a flexor-pronator muscle rupture (36). Ecchymoses over the medial epicondyle may be evident 2 or 3 days after the event. Occasionally, an x-ray may show an avulsion fracture, and stress films may be helpful. An MRI is most commonly used to determine the extent of the disruption (well visualized on coronal T2 and fat saturation or short T1 inversion recovery [STIR]), as well as any other associated injuries. Surgical repair is recommended for the competitive athlete and those who wish to return to their previous level of play (38,39).

Medial instability is most commonly associated with repetitive valgus stress and microtrauma. The athlete with laxity of the MCL experiences a gradual-onset medial elbow pain that increases during the cocking and acceleration stages of the throw or stroke. Competitive players may describe a sudden onset of pain with a single stroke, often due to a partial tear of the MCL, although the examining physician should also consider a complete tear.

On physical examination, palpation of the MCL may elicit discomfort. Evaluation of the MCL is accomplished with the valgus stress test. The athlete stands with the affected arm by her side in external rotation and the forearm in supination. The examiner, as he faces the athlete's side, places the athlete's hand under her axilla, holding it between the chest wall and arm. With the athlete's elbow flexed to 30 degrees, the examiner applies stress on the elbow with one hand while palpating the medial joint line with the other hand. Alternatively, with the athlete lying supine holding the affected arm elevated overhead and forearm supinated, the examiner applies valgus stress to the elbow. With MCL laxity, the degree of joint separation is increased or the endpoint is indistinct compared with the findings on the unaffected side.

X-rays may reveal a bony avulsion or calcification within the ligament. MRI is presently the most widely accepted means of evaluating the integrity of the ligaments and soft tissue structures. An MRI should be obtained urgently when the onset of medial or lateral elbow symptoms is associated with trauma or an acute event. Conservative management for milder degrees of instability, with restriction of activity and strengthening of flexor-pronator muscles, at least initially, is usually reasonable, but the failure rate is over 50%. If the tear is complete or if significant chronic instability and pain are present, immediate surgical reconstruction is indicated for competitive athletes and those who wish to return to the previous level of performance.

Laxity of the MCL and medial instability, if untreated, can also lead to articular degeneration and the formation of loose bodies within the joint. With repetitive valgus stress, the medial tip of the olecranon can become impinged within the olecranon fossa. Inflammation of the tip of the olecranon due to the abnormal forces may eventually result in the formation of osteophytes and loose bodies, both of which can limit flexion and extension. Loose bodies may also result from overload forces and degeneration at the radiocapitellar joint with repetitive valgus stress. Aggressive treatment using arthroscopy to remove osteophytes and loose bodies may allow athletes to regain or maintain full range of motion, eliminate symptoms of locking or catching, and allow an earlier return to high levels of competition. The physician should always consider the possibility of MCL laxity with these types of changes and treat them appropriately to prevent further degeneration and loss of mobility.

In the skeletally immature athlete, repetitive valgus stress may cause osteochondritis dissecans on the capitellum at the radiocapitellar joint (40,41). Osteochondritis dissecans is hypothesized to be the result of a focal arterial injury resulting from compressive forces, which then leads to bone necrosis. Often known as "Little Leaguer's elbow," it is most common in children between 10 and 15 years of age; they experience a slow onset of lateral elbow pain and limited elbow extension (42). X-ray films may be normal or reveal a loose bony island(s) within the joint. Treatment is determined by the clinical exam and x-ray findings, although MRI is commonly employed for a better evaluation of the location of the lesion and possible detachment. Intact lesions can be treated with limitation of activity. Arthroscopy allows aggressive treatment of disrupted lesions with a better prognosis for return to high levels of competition.

Because the physis tends to be the weakest link in the musculoskeletal unit in the skeletally immature athlete, repetitive valgus stress may result in a medial epicondylar physeal fracture (36). Initially, the excessive valgus forces cause an acceleration in growth, but separation and fragmentation soon follow (43,44). The athlete begins to experience pain with throwing or, in racquet sports, with serving, and possibly a loss of complete extension. A widened medial epicondylar physis may be seen on x-ray. Treatment is dictated by both the age of the athlete and his symptoms.

Ulnar neuropathy may be associated with many medial elbow conditions or abnormalities. Medial instability can cause symptoms of ulnar neuropathy, due either to traction of the nerve or compression resulting from degeneration and calcification within the MCL or to soft tissue swelling or scarring. Osteophytes or thickening of the arcuate ligament may narrow the cubital tunnel and result in a compression neuropathy. Another common site of compression is between the two heads of the flexor carpi ulnaris distal to the cubital tunnel (36). Dislocation or subluxation of the ulnar nerve at the ulnar groove may also occur with elbow flexion and extension. Athletes with ulnar neuropathy usually experience pain at the medial joint, often radiating distally along the forearm. Paresthesias of the 4th and 5th digits are common, although hand weakness is uncommon. Symptoms increase with throwing or racquet swings and diminish with rest. Occasionally the location of the nerve irritation can be determined on examination, but electrodiagnostic studies (electromyogram [EMG], nerve conduction) are often helpful to establish the exact site of compression, a baseline for future reference, and possibly the need for surgery. Conservative treatment can be attempted, but surgical management, often a simple in situ decompression or a nerve transfer, is usually needed (45).

Tendonitis of the flexor-pronator muscles, primarily the pronator teres, flexor carpi radialis, and occasionally the flexor carpi ulnaris, can result from repetitive valgus stress and cause medial elbow pain. Tenderness is usually present over the medial epicondyle. The muscles of this group can tear with one event of forceful valgus stress, often accompanied by a tear of the MCL. Sudden pain and tenderness along the medial epicondyle that increases with wrist flexion, associated with a gap in the tendons and a bulge in the proximal forearm, is suggestive of a tear. An MRI is necessary to evaluate the extent of damage. Acute surgical repair is required to preserve the flexor-pronator muscles and thus medial stability. Anatomical repair may not be possible if diagnosis or surgery is delayed, since tendons will retract and are difficult to reapproximate.

Lateral elbow pain is most often due to lateral epicondylitis, which is also the most common cause of elbow pain in general. The onset of pain is insidious and is due to inflammation of the extensor-supinator muscles, primarily the extensor carpi radialis brevis (36). It is often associated with microtears or large degenerative partial tears. Pain exacerbated by wrist extension and tenderness at the lateral epicondyle are the usual manifestations.

Radial nerve entrapment can be associated with lateral epicondylitis, although it is sometimes a primary syndrome and is misinterpreted as epicondylitis. The symptoms are grossly similar to those of lateral epicondylitis, although the pain tends to radiate distally along the forearm without any paresthesias. Tenderness over the posterior interosseous nerve on the volar proximal forearm and not directly on the lateral epicondyle is indicative of primary radial nerve entrapment. Of note, the counterforce bracing band often used for lateral epicondylitis can aggravate the symptoms if radial nerve entrapment is present. In extensor tendon inflammation or tear (lateral epicondylitis), pain can be elicited by active supination, passive pronation, and resisted extension of the wrist or fingers with the elbow fully extended (36). Electrodiagnostic studies are helpful if nerve entrapment is suspected. Conservative treatment is usually successful in relieving symptoms of either nerve entrapment or epicondylitis. Surgical nerve decompression is indicated if the condition fails to improve with rest and physical therapy. Surgical intervention for epicondylitis is indicated when intensive physical therapy, local steroid injection, and rest fail to relieve discomfort or in cases of large partial or complete tendon disruption. In addition, rotator cuff tendonitis, stress overload of the olecranon, and localized lateral synovial or soft tissue impingement syndromes may all present with lateral elbow pain (36). A detailed history and precise physical exam, including localization of the point of tenderness, help differentiate the diagnosis in most cases.

Posterior elbow pain is less common than lateral or medial pain. Olecranon bursitis is most often seen in football and rugby players, occurring as an acute or chronic injury. Septic bursitis should always be considered and is suggested by tenderness and erythema over the swollen olecranon bursa. Acute bursitis (often hemorrhagic) is also painful. Treatment includes ice, NSAIDs, and compression. Aspiration is suggested if range of motion is significantly limited, although reaccumulation is possible. Elbow protection helps prevent recurrence. Occasionally, surgical removal of the bursa is required for chronic recurrent bursitis. Posterior elbow pain can also occur secondary to acute hyperextension or repetitive bony overload, often associated with posterior spur and impingement of the olecranon.

Triceps tendonitis is not common; it is characterized by posterior elbow pain with resisted elbow extension and passive flexion. Conservative treatment is recommended; local steroid injection should be avoided. Rupture of the triceps tendon is the least common of all tendon ruptures, but it can occur with an excessive counterforce during active extension of the elbow (46). This requires immediate surgical repair.

Anterior elbow pain is usually related to a stretch or tear of the anterior joint capsule or injury to the distal biceps or brachioradialis tendons, which can result from a fall on an extended elbow, resisted elbow flexion, or hyperextension. A strain of the brachialis tendon has been called "climber's elbow," due to the prolonged pronation and flexion required for climbing (47). The distal biceps tendon can rupture with a forceful overload as the elbow is in midflexion (48). This is a rare injury and may be associated with preexisting degenerative changes or inflammation in the tendon. The patient has weakness of forearm supination and pronation and displacement of the tendon proximally; surgical repair is necessary. Median nerve entrapment may cause anterior elbow pain that radiates distally along the forearm and is associated with paresthesias of the palm and first three digits. It is related to compression of the median nerve between the two heads of the pronator teres muscle upon pronation and can be confused with medial epicondylitis. Pain may be exacerbated by palpation, active pronation, passive supination, and resisted 3d-digit flexion. Weakness of the abductor pollicis brevis and flexor pollicis longus may occur. Treatment is usually conservative, but surgical release may be necessary in persistent cases.

Dislocation of the elbow joint is the second most common dislocation in adults. It usually results from a direct fall onto an outstretched arm. Pain and limited range of motion are immediate. Examination shows displacement of the olecranon posteriorly or posterolaterally. Immediate evaluation for possible intravascular compromise of the extremity is essential. Reduction can be accomplished with progressive traction on the arm with the elbow in 30 degrees of flexion. Pressure applied to the olecranon may also help. If reduction is not possible, an x-ray should be performed to confirm the dislocation and rule out any other injury. Reduction under general anesthesia may be required. A repeat evaluation of neurovascular status of the extremity should be performed after the reduction procedure. The patient requires a posterior splint to support the elbow in 90 degrees of flexion for 1 week, after which a hinged brace is used. Physical therapy with gradual rehabilitation to full flexion and extension is extremely helpful. Early mobility helps reduce the risk of flexion contractures. The decision on whether an athlete can return to activity or requires a longer course of physical therapy is determined by the stability of the joint. Persistent instability and recurrent dislocations are not common in athletes, but if present may require surgical management (49).

WRIST INJURIES

Scaphoid Fracture

The most commonly fractured carpal bone is the scaphoid. This injury results from axial impaction when the wrist is in dorsiflexion, such as when the person attempts to break a fall. The scaphoid is an important link in radiocarpal and intercarpal motion, and preservation of scaphoid function is critical for adequate wrist function (50). The injured athlete has tenderness over the "anatomic snuffbox," which is sometimes edematous. He may also have pain with movement of the wrist and thumb, but the pain is often not severe or limiting and may be considered just a sprain by both the athlete and the medical support team. The athlete may consult the physician several weeks after the initial event for persistent pain. Suspicion of a fracture should always be high, and the threshold for obtaining an x-ray low. X-rays should include posteroanterior, lateral, and ulnar deviation posteroanterior (wrist held with ulnar or lateral flexion) views of the carpals. A 45-degree pronation posteroanterior view (51) or a "clenched fist" view (which brings the wrist into dorsiflexion and ulnar deviation) (52) also allow better visualization of the scaphoid.

Even when x-rays initially show no abnormality, if the mechanism of injury and the physical exam are consistent with a fracture, the injury should be treated as a fracture, at least initially. Immobilization with a thumb spica cast or splint is recommended, with repeat x-rays 10–14 days later, at which point repair of the fracture will have started, allowing a better view with callus formation. For highly competitive athletes requiring immediate diagnosis, a CT scan gives better evaluation for a true fracture. A bone scan 3 days after injury has also been used (53).

Nondisplaced scaphoid fractures can be treated with immobilization for 4–6 weeks with a spica cast. A short arm cast is suitable for stable fractures, which allows the athlete to return to practice and competition. Displaced fractures often require surgical intervention to prevent non-union and future instability. The location of the fracture within the scaphoid is also critical in prognosis for non-union and avascular necrosis. Distal fractures have the highest rate of union, while the risk of non-union increases as the fracture becomes more proximal (53). Documentation of healing and union by 6 weeks is critical, since surgical intervention should be considered in cases of non-union.

Avascular Necrosis of the Lunate (Kienböck's Disease)

Avascular necrosis of the lunate bone is most often encountered in young adults and can be associated with a primary fracture, repetitive microtrauma, or trauma to the ligaments that provide vascular support to the lunate (54–57). The athlete presents with pain in the dorsum of the wrist, which may be associated with swelling and limited range of motion. The diagnosis is made by x-ray, which will show the range of damage from sclerosis in the earlier phases to complete collapse and arthrosis in the late stages. An MRI can be very helpful in the early stages, when changes evident on x-ray are subtle (52). Treatment is surgical. In the early stages, the radius is shortened or the ulna lengthened in an attempt to unload the lunate (58). With lunate collapse and arthrosis, limited or total arthrodesis may be useful, depending on the integrity of the joint surfaces (59).

Triangular Fibrocartilage Injury

The triangular fibrocartilage (TFC) is a cartilaginous disc located between the ulnar head and the carpal bones. It stabilizes the distal radioulnar joint and is the surface of articulation for the proximal carpals. Tears or avulsions of the TFC occur acutely from overload or impact and may be associated with distal radial fractures and dislocation of the ulna. Pain is present over the ulnar side of the wrist, possibly with deformity. Clicking and pain upon ulnar deviation of the wrist are usual. Diagnosis generally requires MRI or arthroscopy, and treatment requires surgical repair or debridement. Sprain or tear of the lunotriquetral ligament may also cause ulnar wrist pain. Clicking or clunking may be elicited with ulnar circumduction of the wrist. Diagnosis is made by MRI or arthroscopy, and treatment is surgical, either repair or fusion (51).

Dorsal Impaction Syndrome

Repetitive maximum dorsiflexion of the wrist may result in chronic dorsal wrist pain. The shearing forces resulting from compression may lead to synovitis or eventually stress fractures. Most often seen in gymnasts, dorsal impaction syndrome is characterized by pain and tenderness on the dorsum of the wrist, focused over the lunocapitate joint. X-rays may show hypertrophy and sclerosis on the borders of the scaphoid, lunate, and capitate bones, which impinge on one another during dorsiflexion. Restriction of wrist hyperextension and strengthening of the wrist flexors are the usual treatment. If symptoms persist despite treatment, complete immobilization is indicated for up to 6 weeks, with gradual return to activities. Chronic pain may be treated surgically by synovectomy and cheilectomy; however, the athlete may not be able to return to the previous level of performance (60).

HAND INJURIES

First Carpometacarpal Joint

Sprains or partial tears of the 1st volar carpometacarpal (CMC) joint due to trauma are more common than complete dislocations, which are rare (61). The volar metacarpal phalangeal (MCP) ligament complex can be disrupted by forced hyperextension or hyperabduction. The athlete will experience pain and swelling over the CMC joint. Most dislocations spontaneously reduce, but the athlete is unable to pinch with the thumb to 5th digit while the joint is dislocated. X-rays are necessary, both anteroposterior and lateral views, since fracture-dislocations are seen more often than simple dislocation. An intra-articular fracture accompanied by a displaced fracture of the metacarpal shaft, known as a Bennett's fracture, often requires open reduction and fixation (62). Stable sprains or partial tears are usually treated with 6 weeks of immobilization with a short arm spica cast, followed by an exercise program (61).

Metacarpal Phalangeal Joint

The MCP joint allows motion in multiple directions between the metacarpal head and the distal phalanx. The primary motion is flexion-extension, but abduction-adduction and some axial rotation are also possible. The joint is stabilized primarily by soft tissue structures. The collateral ligaments extend from the proximal-dorsal head of the metacarpal joint to the distal-volar periarticular surface of the distal phalanx and provide the primary stability in all planes of motion. The volar plate adds significant stability to the joint; it originates from the lateral surface of the metacarpal head and inserts onto the volar surface of the proximal phalanx (62). The volar plate tightens with extension and thus provides primarily dorsal stability.

Dorsal dislocation of the MCP joint usually occurs with forceful hyperextension. The proximal end of the volar plate is often torn with the dorsal force, allowing the proximal phalanx to sublux or dislocate. The proximal interphalangeal (PIP) joint is usually pulled into flexion. These dislocations can be reduced by firmly pressing the distal end of the phalanx back onto the head of the metacarpal bone. It is important to avoid any longitudinal traction, which may cause the volar plate to become interposed between the metacarpal head and the phalanx (61,62). Dislocation of the 1st MCP joint may be complicated by interposition of a sesamoid bone, which can sometimes be detected by a dimpling of the overlying skin on the palmar surface but may need to be documented by x-ray. Closed reduction is more difficult and involves adducting and flexing the thumb, followed by hyperextension of the proximal phalanx while forcing it dorsally (61). Complex dislocations can involve the interposition of the volar plate between the metacarpal head and proximal phalanx. These usually require surgical reduction.

Closed reductions should be followed by immobilization of the MCP joint in 60 degrees of flexion for 3 weeks. The PIP joint should be maintained in extension to avoid a flexion contracture. The athlete may return to competition using a removable splint for protection for 3 weeks. Hand therapy is also an important adjunct to rehabilitation.

Ulnar Collateral Ligament of First MCP Joint

Injury to the ulnar collateral ligament (UCL) of the thumb is often termed "skier's thumb," since it is commonly encountered in skiers who fall and forcefully abduct the thumb on the ski pole, consequently tearing the UCL. It can lead to chronic instability and disability if not recognized and treated properly.

The UCL originates from the lateral surface of the distal metacarpal head and inserts on the volar base of the proximal phalanx; it stabilizes the 1st MCP against radial deviation (63). Rupture of the UCL can occur in sports involving catching in which the thumb can be forcefully abducted by a ball. The ulnar side of the MCP is painful, tender, and swollen to some degree, and the athlete has difficulty pinching the thumb to the index finger. The stability of the joint should always be evaluated by application of radial stress to the MCP joint while it is held in full flexion and then in full extension. The UCL is the primary stabilizer of the MCP joint while in full flexion; therefore, laxity of greater than 30% compared with the non-injured side indicates a tear (64). As the MCP joint is extended, the accessory UCL adds to the ulnar stability. Laxity in full extension indicates a tear of both the UCL and the accessory UCL. Stress radiographs for confirmation of the degree of laxity of the UCL with medial stress are advisable.

Because chronic instability of the 1st MCP can be associated with long-term disability due to pain and carries the risk of early degenerative arthritis, complete UCL rupture is optimally treated with surgical intervention to ensure close approximation of the ends of the torn ligament and a stable joint (62,65). Partial tears and ruptures associated with an avulsion may be treated conservatively if the avulsion is nondisplaced. Conservative treatment involves immobilization of the MCP joint with a thumb splint to hold the MCP in mild flexion and a small amount of ulnar stress (64). The interphalangeal joint should be free and the athlete should actively attempt to maintain full range of motion. For the first 6 weeks the splint should be removed only for hand therapy sessions, which can start 3 weeks after the injury, then for the following 6 weeks the athlete can wear the splint only in situations associated with a risk of re-injury. Some physicians recommend taping for protection for 4 months after the injury (66).

Radial Collateral Ligament of First MCP

The radial collateral ligament (RCL) of the 1st MCP is injured less often than the ulnar collateral ligament. The RCL can be sprained or torn if the MCP is forcefully adducted while in flexion, which occurs most often in ball sports such as volleyball. Partial tears may heal well with immobilization in a thumb spica cast for 3 weeks. Complete tears may heal better than UCL tears without surgical repair; stabilization is best established with invasive treatment (67).

Collateral Ligament of MCP Joint

Lateral subluxations at the MCP joint usually reduce spontaneously but often sprain or tear the collateral ligament in the process. These injuries commonly occur while the MCP joint is flexed, leaving the volar plate intact and maintaining dorsal and volar stability (68). Lateral MCP instability due to collateral ligament tear is best evaluated with the MCP in flexion. The collateral ligaments are relaxed in extension, rendering evaluation difficult. X-rays may show a bony avulsion at the ligament insertion (62).

Bony avulsions without an associated fracture or significant dislocation can be treated with immobilization at 30 degrees of flexion. Taping the affected digit to the adjacent digit ("buddy taping") is acceptable for partially torn or sprained ligaments. Ruptures of the collateral ligament associated with significant instability or displaced avulsion fragment are optimally treated surgically, especially for the 5th digit. Despite appropriate treatment, chronic pain may occur, even with mild sprains. Immobilization may be helpful, but pain may recur after the splint is removed. Local injection of corticosteroids may offer relief of symptoms (68). Chronic pain rather than instability is the more common complication of these injuries.

Metacarpal and Boxer's Fractures

Fractures of the metacarpals most commonly occur in the shaft of the bone and are stable. Treatment is relatively straightforward, with a short arm cast for 4–6 weeks. Oblique or spiral fractures should be treated similarly, with buddy taping of the associated digit (61). Compound fractures or multiple fragments often require surgical fixation.

A boxer's fracture is a fracture of the distal 5th or 4th metacarpal (or both). The mechanism of injury involves a blow to the dorsum of the hand while closed in a fist. Because the bases of the 4th and 5th metacarpals are more mobile than those of the 2d and 3d, angulation of the head from the shaft of up to 40 degrees does not result in significant disability and is not usually actively reduced (61). Alignment to less than 40 degrees can usually be attained with closed manipulation; however, unstable or severely displaced fractures require open reduction. Immobilization for 4–6 weeks in a molded gutter splint, extending from the forearm to just beyond the MCP joints, usually provides enough support for adequate healing.

Intra-articular fractures of the MCP joint require reduction and close approximation of the fractured surfaces. If the surfaces are more than 1 mm out of alignment, surgery is required to maintain adequate articulation (61).

Proximal Interphalangeal Joint

The stability of the PIP joint is similar to that of the MCP joint, provided primarily by collateral ligaments and a volar plate. The volar plate functions to resist dorsal displacement of the PIP, while the extensor hood complex, composed of a central slip and two lateral bands of retinacular ligaments, prevents volar displacement (69).

Dorsal dislocation of the PIP joint is the most common dislocation in the hand in athletes and can occur with forced hyperextension. The volar plate tears from its attachment, and this may be accompanied by partial tears or splitting of the collateral ligaments. Most dorsal dislocations are easily reduced by applying steady traction to the digit with slight hyperextension of the PIP joint. The reduction is usually stable and can be treated with a splint holding the affected joint in 30 degrees of flexion for 3 weeks. The digit should then be buddy taped to the adjacent digit for 3 or 4 more weeks for protection during sports participation (69).

Injuries to the collateral ligaments of the PIP joints are also not uncommon in athletes. The radial collateral ligament tends to be affected more often than the ulnar collateral ligament, and this may be associated with injury to the volar plate. Most injuries are sprains or partial tears, although active range of motion to assess tendon integrity and stability testing in dorsal, volar, radial, and ulnar directions should always be performed in injuries involving the PIP joint. Stable sprains and partial tears with limited instability, less than 15 degrees of lateral laxity compared with the uninjured digit, may be successfully managed with either a dorsal splint in 20 degrees of flexion or buddy taping for 3–4 weeks. Complete ruptures of a collateral ligament are usually associated with a disruption of the volar plate and are unstable. Treatment recommendations for these injuries vary. Closed reduction with immobilization has been advocated if the lateral instability is evident only with passive stress applied laterally (62,70). Injuries that are unstable with both active and passive flexion without application of any lateral stress should be surgically repaired to assure stable healing (62,71).

Nondisplaced intra-articular fractures of the PIP joint can be treated with immobilization for 3 weeks, then 4–6 weeks of protection or buddy taping. Large, displaced articular fractures, fractures of the volar plate resulting in instability, or disruption of the extensor or flexor tendons all require surgical repair (61).

Rupture of Extensor Digitorum Communis (Boutonniere Deformity)

A blunt force over the dorsum of the PIP joint or active flexion against forceful resistance can result in a rupture of the central slip of the extensor digitorum communis (EDC) tendon over the PIP joint and a migration of the lateral bands toward the volar surface of the PIP. The PIP joint can then herniate dorsally through the tear resulting in a boutonniere deformity. The classical boutonniere deformity is a hyperextension of the MCP and DIP associated with flexion of the PIP. Initially, the PIP joint is swollen, tender, and rests in 15–30 degrees of flexion. Often the inability to completely extend the PIP is attributed to swelling and the digit is inappropriately splinted in semiflexion. If the central tendon remains split, a flexion contracture at the PIP can occur with a secondary hyperextension at the MCP and DIP joints. A rupture of the EDC should be considered in any injury of the PIP joint associated with a lag of more than 30 degrees of extension and tenderness at the dorsal base of the PIP. Initially, the PIP joint should be splinted in full extension while the DIP joint is allowed full motion for 6–8 weeks. The movement of the DIP joint in flexion will pull the split lateral bands of the tendon back together (72). Protective splinting should remain in place during sporting activities for 6 more weeks. In older injuries with a fixed contracture, dynamic splinting to gradually extend the PIP joint may successfully allow return of full flexion without surgical intervention.

Avulsion of the Flexor Digitorum Profundus

Avulsion of the flexor digitorum profundus (FDP) is often called "jersey finger," since a common mechanism involves forced extension of the digit while actively flexing, as in grabbing a jersey. It can be difficult to diagnose because of the lack of significant deformity. Pain and swelling are present over the affected digit, accompanied by an inability to actively flex the DIP joint. An x-ray may show a bony avulsion at the DIP. The tendon may retract past the DIP joint to the PIP joint or even into the palm, depending upon the force of extension (72). These injuries require immediate surgical repair. If the diagnosis is delayed, a second procedure may be necessary for correction of a flexion contracture (61).

Distal Interphalangeal Joint Dislocations

Dislocations of the distal interphalangeal joint can occur both dorsally and (less common) volarly, secondary to a forced hyperextension. The dislocations can be reduced easily with traction and flexion. The DIP should then be splinted with a dorsal or volar splint—a dorsal splint allows tactile sensation needed for ball handlers—for 3 weeks (73).

Extensor Tendon Disruption (Mallet Finger)

The extensor mechanism at the DIP joint can be disrupted when the DIP is forced into flexion during active extension, which can occur when trying to catch a hard-thrown ball (72). Pain and swelling are present at the affected DIP, which can be passively but not actively flexed. The DIP may passively flex at rest owing to unopposed opposition of the flexor profundus tendon, resulting in a "drop" or "mallet" finger deformity.

Five patterns of injury are possible: fracture, avulsion, rupture, stretching, or slipped epiphysis. In any mallet finger injury, the PIP joint should be examined as well. Splinting the DIP joint in extension while allowing free movement of the PIP joint continuously for 8 weeks, followed by splinting for protection during athletic activities for an additional 8 weeks, is the usual treatment. The athlete can participate in activity while splinted; ball handlers usually prefer a dorsal splint, since it allows tactile sensation. An avulsion involving more than 30% of the articular surface requires surgical intervention (61).

REFERENCES
1. Jobe FW, Bardley JP: The diagnosis and nonoperative treatment of shoulder injuries in athletes. Clin Sports Med 8:419–439, 1989
2. Zarins B, Rowe CB: Current concepts in the diagnosis and treatment of shoulder instability in athletes. Med Sci Sports Exerc 16:444–448, 1984
3. Bankart ASB: The pathology and treatment of recurrent dislocation of the shoulder joint. Br J Surg 26:23–29, 1938
4. Connolly JF: Humeral head defects associated with shoulder dislocations. *In* American Academy of Orthopaedic Surgeons Instructional Course Lectures, vol 21. St. Louis, CV Mosby, 1972, 42–45
5. Rowe CR: Shoulder girdle injuries. *In* Cave EF (ed): Trauma Management. Chicago, Yearbook Medical Publishers, 1973, 418, 420–421
6. Rowe CR, Zarins B: Chronic unreduced dislocations of the shoulder. J Bone Joint Surg 64A:494–505, 1982
7. Post M: The Shoulder. Philadelphia, Lea & Febiger, 1978, 38–39
8. Rowe CR: Acute and recurrent anterior dislocations of the shoulder. Orthop Clin North Am 11:253–270, 1980
9. Henry JH, Genung JA: Natural history of glenohumeral dislocation—revisited. Am J Sports Med 10:135–141, 1982
10. Hovelius L, Eriksson GK, Falun H, et al: Recurrences after initial dislocation of the shoulder. J Bone Joint Surg 65A:343–349, 1983
11. Howell SM, Imobersteg AM, Seger DH, et al: Clarification of the role of supraspinatus muscle in shoulder function. J Bone Joint Surg 68A:398–404, 1986
12. Yocum LA: Assessing the shoulder: history, physical examination, differential diagnosis, and special test used. Clin Sports Med 2:281–289, 1983
13. Jobe FW, Bradley JP: Rotator cuff injuries in baseball: prevention and rehabilitation. Sports Med 6:377–386, 1988
14. Sisto DJ, Jobe FW: The operative treatment of scapulothoracic bursitis in professional pitchers. Am J Sports Med 14:192–194, 1986
15. Shields CL, Glousman RE: Open management of rotator cuff tears. *In* Advances in Sports Medicine and Fitness, vol 2. Chicago, Year Book Medical Publishers, 1989, 223–242
16. Jobe FW, Jobe CW: Painful athletic injuries of the shoulder. Clin Orthop 173:117–124,1983
17. Silliman JF, Hawkins RJ: Classification and physical diagnosis of instability of the shoulder. Clin Orthop 7–19, 1993
18. Neer CS: Involuntary inferior and multidirectional instability of the

shoulder: etiology, recognition, and treatment. American Academy of Orthopaedic Surgeons Instructional Course Lectures, vol 34. St. Louis, CV Mosby, 1985, 232–238

19. Hawkins RJ, Kennedy JC: Impingement syndrome in athletes. Am J Sports Med 8:151–158, 1980

20. Neer CS, Welsh RP: The shoulder in sports. Orthop Clin North Am 8:583–591, 1977

21. Neviaser RJ: Anatomic consideration and examination of the shoulder. Orthop Clin North Am 11:187–195, 1980

22. Magee DJ: Orthopedic physical assessment. WB Saunders, 1992, 117

23. Andrews JR, Carson WG, McLeod WD: Glenoid labrum tears related to the long head of the biceps. Am J Sports Med 13:337–341, 1985

24. Garth WP, Allman FL Jr, Armstrong WS: Occult anterior subluxations of the shoulder in noncontact sports. Am J Sports Med 15:579–585, 1987

25. Andrews JR, Carson WG: The arthroscopic treatment of glenoid labrum tears—the throwing athlete. Orthop Trans 8:44, 1984

26. Snyder SJ, Karzel RP, Del Pizzo W, Ferkel RD, Friedman MJ: SLAP lesions of the shoulder. Arthroscopy 6:274–279, 1990

27. Pollock RG, Bigliani LU: Recurrent posterior shoulder instability. Clin Orthop and Related Research 291:85–96, 1993

28. Bigliani LU, Pollack RG, Endrizzi DP, McIlveen SI, Flatow EL: Surgical repair of posterior instability of the shoulder: long term results. Paper presented at the Ninth Combined Meeting of the Orthopaedic Associations of the English-Speaking World, Toronto, June 1992

29. Bowyer BL, Gooch JL, Geiringer SR: Sports medicine 2: upper extremity injuries. Arch Phys Med Rehabil 74:S433–S437, 1993

30. Waldrop JI, Norwood LA, Alvarez RG: Lateral roentgenographic projections of the acromioclavicular joint. Am J Sports Med 9:337–341, 1981

31. Tossy JD, Mead NC, Sigmond HM: Acromioclavicular separations: useful and practical classification for treatment. Clin Orthop 28:111–119, 1963

32. Neer CS II, Rockwood CA. Fractures and dislocations of the shoulder. In Rockwood CA, Green DP (eds): Fracture, ed 2. Philadelphia, JB Lippincott, 1984, 675–950

33. Rohrer MJ, et al: Axillary artery compression and thrombosis in throwing athletes. J Vasc Surg 11:761–769, 1990

34. Maday MG, Harner CD, Warner J: Shoulder injuries. In Fu F (ed): Sports Injuries. Baltimore, Williams & Wilkins, 1994, 917

35. Safran MR: Elbow injuries in athletes. Clin Orthop and Related Research 310:257–277, 1995

36. Tullos HS, Schwab GS, Bennet JB, Woods GW: Factors influencing elbow stability. In Murray DG (ed): American Academy of Orthopaedic Surgeons Instructional Course Lecture, vol 8. St. Louis, CV Mosby, 1981, 186–199

37. Conway JE, Jobe FW, Glousman RE, Pink M: Medial instability of the el-

bow in throwing athletes: treatment by repair or reconstruction of the ulnar collateral ligament. J Bone Joint Surg 74A:67–83, 1992

38. Baker BD, Bierwagen D: Rupture of the distal tendon of the biceps brachii: operative versus non-operative treatment. J Bone Joint Surg 67A:414–417, 1985

39. Bauer M, Jonsson K, Jesefsson PO, Linden B: Osteochondritis dissecans of the elbow: a long-term follow-up study. Clin Orthop 284:156, 1992

40. Shaughnessy WJ, Bianco AJ: Osteochondritis dissecans. In Morrey BF (ed): The Elbow and Its Disorders, ed 2. Philadelphia, WB Saunders, 1993

41. McManama GB, Michel LJ, Berry MV, Sohn RS: The surgical treatment of osteochondritis of the capitellum. Am J Sports Med 13:11, 1985

42. Adams JE: Injury to the throwing arm: a study of traumatic changes in the elbow joints of boy baseball players. Calif Med 102:127, 1965

43. Brodgon BG, Crow NF: Little Leaguer's elbow. Am J Roentgenol 8:671, 1960

44. Field LD, Altchek DW: Elbow injuries. Clin Sports Med 14:59–78, 1995

45. Morrey BF: Tendon injuries about the elbow. In Morrey BF (ed): The Elbow and Its Disorders. Philadelphia, WB Saunders, 1985, 452–463

46. Bollen SR: Soft tissue injury in extreme rock climbers. Br J Sports Med 22:145–147, 1988

47. Morrey BF, Askew LJ, An KN, Dobyns JH: Rupture of the distal tendon of the biceps brachii: a biomechanical study. J Bone Joint Surg 67A:418–421, 1985

48. Bradley JP: Elbow injuries. In Fu F (ed): Sports Injuries. Baltimore, Williams & Wilkins, 1994, 923–936

49. Mosher JF: Current concepts in the diagnosis and treatment of hand and wrist injuries in sports. Med Sci Sports Exerc 17:48–55, 1985

50. Griggs SM, Weiss A-P: Bony injuries of the wrist, forearm, and elbow. Clin Sports Med 15:373–400, 1996

51. Sotereanos DG, Levy JA, Herndon JH: Hand and wrist injuries. In Fu F (ed): Sports Injuries. Baltimore, Williams & Wilkins, 1994, 937–948

52. Olsen N, Schousen P, Dirksen H, et al: Regional scintimetry in scaphoid fractures. Acta Orthop Scand 54:380–382, 1983

53. Cooney WP, Dobyns JH, Linscheid RL: Fractures of the scaphoid: a rational approach to management. Clin Orthop 149:90–97, 1980

54. Beckenbaugh RD, Shives TC, Dobyns JH, et al: Kienbock's disease: the natural history of Kienbock's disease and consideration of lunate fractures. Clin Orthop 149:98–106, 1980

55. Gelberman RH, Bauman TD, Menon J, et al: The vascularity of the lunate bone and Kienbock's disease. J Hand Surg 5(3):272–278, 1980

56. Kienböck R: Concerning traumatic malacia of the lunate and its consequences: degenerative and compression fractures (translation of 1910 article). Clin Orthop 149:4–8, 1980

57. Weiss APC: Radial shortening. Hand Clin 9:475–482, 1993

58. Watson KK, Hempton RF: Limited wrist arthrodesis. I. The triscaphoid joint. J Hand Surg [Am] 5:320–327, 1980

59. Halikis MN, Taleisnik J: Soft tissue injuries of the wrist. Clin Sports Med 15:235–261, 1996

60. McCue FC III, Meister K: Common sports hand injuries. Sports Med 15:281–289, 1993

61. Isani A, Melone CP Jr: Ligamentous injuries of the hand in athletes. Clin Sports Med 5:757–772, 1986

62. Hubbard LF: Metacarpophalangeal dislocation. Hand Clin 4:39–44, 1988

63. Frickler R, Ritterman B: Skier's thumb. Sports Med 19:73–79, 1995

64. Hintermann B, Holzach PJ, Shütz M, et al: Skier's thumb—the significance of bony injuries. Am J Sports Med 21:800–804, 1993

65. Brown AP: Ulnar collateral ligament injury of the thumb. *In* Clark GL, Shaw Wilgis EF, Aiello B, et al (eds): Hand Rehabilitation: A Practical Guide. New York, Churchill Livingstone, 1993, 261–267

66. Camp RA, Weathernox RJ, Miller EB: Chronic post-traumatic radial instability of the thumb metacarpophalangeal joint. J Hand Surg [Am] 5:221–225, 1980

67. Minami A, An KN, Cooney WP, et al: Ligament stability of the metacarpophalangeal joint: a bio-mechanical study. J Hand Surg [Am] 10:261–264, 1985

68. Greene DP: Dislocations and ligamentous injuries of the hand. *In* Evarts CM (ed): Surgery of the Musculoskeletal System. New York, Churchill Livingstone, 1983, 141–151

69. Vicar AJ: Proximal interphalangeal joint dislocations without fractures. Hand Clin 4:5–13, 1988

70. Redler I, Williams JT: Rupture of a collateral ligament of the proximal interphalangeal joint of the finger. J Bone Joint Surg 49A:322, 1967

71. McCue FC III, Wooten SL: Closed tendon injuries of the hand in athletics. Clin Sports Med 5:741–755, 1986

72. Brunet ME, Haddad RJ Jr: Fractures and dislocations of the metacarpals and phalanges. Clin Sports Med 5:773–781, 1986

73. McCue F, Meister K: Common sports hand injuries. Sports Med 15(4): 281–289, 1993

■ ■ ■ ■ ■ ■ ■ ■ ■ ■ Chapter 7

LOWER-EXTREMITY INJURIES

KNEE INJURIES

Disruption of the Anterior Cruciate Ligament

The anterior cruciate ligament (ACL) originates from the posteromedial aspect of the lateral femoral condyle and inserts on the anterior tibial eminence. Its primary function is to stabilize the knee joint by preventing anterior translation of the tibial plateau, restraining varus and valgus angulation and preventing tibial rotation. The ligament is the most lax when the knee is in 20 degrees of flexion and tightens as the knee is flexed further. It tends to be injured in sports requiring deceleration, twisting, and cutting movements. The most common mechanism is a valgus force while the knee is in external rotation and flexion. The most common noncontact mechanism of injury is hyperextension on deceleration.

Snow skiing is the sport with the highest incidence of ACL tears, estimated to be more than 100,000 per year (1), although incidence is also high in contact sports. In one study of college football teams, the average incidence of ACL ruptures was 2.4 per team each season (2). Interestingly, injuries to the ACL have been shown to occur almost twice as often in female athletes as in male athletes who compete in the same sport at the same level of competition (such as soccer and basketball) (3). The etiology of this trend has yet to be established; however, it may be related to abnormal knee kinematics and functional instability (i.e., imbalance of hamstring vs. quadriceps strength), which is magnified with cutting, pivoting, and jumping. Many institutions are beginning to use different training for female athletes, focusing on hamstring and quadriceps strength balance and jumping techniques in an attempt to decrease the incidence of ACL tears. The success of these new techniques remains to be seen. A smaller ACL confronted with a higher load has also been considered as a factor in the higher incidence in women (4).

Athletes who have ruptured the ACL usually describe either feeling or hearing a "pop" in their knee as they land with a valgus force on the affected side, with the knee in flexion and external rotation. The level of pain varies greatly, which may also be related to any associated injuries or hemarthroses. Common associated injuries include bone contusions, meniscal tears, and sprain or tear of the medial collateral ligament. Disruption of posterolateral soft tissues is also possible. Hemarthrosis tends to occur quickly, often within an hour (5). Examination of the knee immediately after the injury is preferable, since effusions and pain can limit the ability to detect abnormal findings. The integrity of the ACL can be assessed by the Lachman test, the anterior drawer test, and the presence of a pivot shift.

The Lachman test is the easiest and most reliable test in an acute situation. The knee is placed in 30 degrees of flexion while supported by one of the examiner's hands. It is important that the athlete is relaxed and lies with his head resting on the table. If he has difficulty relaxing the knee, which is not uncommon due to apprehension of pain with manipulation, placing a pillow or blanket beneath the knee for support in flexion is helpful. The examiner grasps the tibia just below the joint line with one hand and grasps the femur above the joint line with the other. With the knee in 30 degrees of flexion, the tibia is forced anteriorly (figure 7.1). Both the amount of anterior translation and the qual-

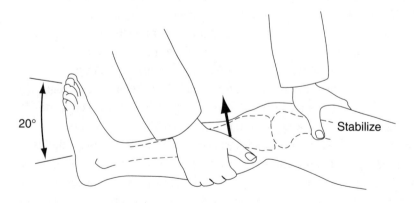

Figure 7.1. Lachman Test

ity of the endpoint, which should be firm and solid, should be noted. Comparison with the uninjured knee is critical, since the baseline of ligament laxity varies in different individuals. The Lachman test is considered the most sensitive and reliable maneuver for assessment of injury to the ACL (6).

In the anterior drawer test, the examiner places the athlete's knee in 90 degrees of flexion with the foot resting on the table, with the athlete reclined and relaxed or sitting with his foot over the edge of the table. The examiner then places an anterior force on the tibia and notes the amount of anterior placement, comparing it with the opposite knee (7). The pivot shift test is difficult to assess, especially acutely, and is not necessary with a positive Lachman test and a detailed history.

Magnetic resonance imaging can be extremely helpful in confirming the diagnosis, especially if the examination is difficult or indeterminate, and also in determining the extent of any associated injuries. Partial tears of the ACL sometimes occur, usually involving the anteromedial bundle, which provides more than 90% of the restraining capability of the ACL (8). A partial tear may well be functionally equivalent to a complete tear (9). In fact, studies suggest that many knees initially thought to have a "partial" ACL tear, on the basis of an examination showing increased anterior translation but a good endpoint, eventually progress to symptomatic ACL deficiency (10). Examination may reveal an endpoint for a ligament that has only a few intact fibers, but a ligament that is biomechanically incompetent may subject the knee to further, irreversible damage of the articular surface when it does fail. MRI is extremely useful in these cases. Treatment depends upon an early diagnosis, and MRI is very specific and sensitive to ACL pathology.

Current treatment of ACL tears involves reconstruction by arthroscopy, using either a bone–patellar tendon–bone autogenous or allogenic graft from a cadaver. An Achilles tendon from a cadaver is the most popular allograft presently used. Surgery for the isolated ACL tear does not need to be performed urgently and should be delayed until swelling has resolved. Some associated injuries may require more urgent surgery, such as repairable meniscal tears, other ligament tears, or fractures. It is the athlete's decision as to whether an allograft or autograft is used. Both have a low incidence of rupture, although the incidence is slightly lower for an autograft (4% vs. 6%), which may be critical for the elite or professional athlete. The autograft does carry a higher risk (about 10%) of fibrosis of the infrapatellar tendon where the graft is removed, and since it is a more invasive procedure, the rehabilitation time is longer, usually 4–5 months with return to full sports activity at 6 months. Rehabilitation for an allograft is approximately 2–3 months, which is preferred by some athletes. Both types of grafts require the use of a brace for 6 months after return to full activity. Allografts are frozen after removal from the cadaver, which prevents host rejection and has no effect on the structural integrity of the ligament (11,12). In addition, avascular tissues such as ligaments have been shown to carry an infinitesimally low risk of transmission of HIV (13).

Some athletes may function without reconstruction of the ruptured ACL. However, the ACL-deficient knee is at higher risk for further meniscal damage and traumatic arthritis because of the lack of stability. Selection of candidates for surgery may be challenging. Pivotal considerations should include the present activity level (including the athlete's occupation), age, future expectations, motivation to participate in postoperative rehabilitation, and the presence of any associated meniscal or ligamentous injury (4). Braces may help, but the added stability is limited.

The role of ligamentous instability in the development of osteoarthritis is unclear. ACL resection is a commonly used method of inducing osteoarthritis in dogs (14). In humans, the role of ACL reconstruction in preventing or retarding the development of osteoarthritis is complicated by the association of more than 50% of ACL ruptures with meniscal tears (5). In general, preservation of the meniscus is critical in the prevention of articular degeneration in ACL-deficient knees (15). Removal of the meniscus at the time of ACL repair has been correlated with an increase in the degeneration observed in follow-up serial radiographs (5).

The goal in ACL reconstruction is to restore stability. Accepted indications for surgery include any instability that interferes with daily activities or prevents participation in sports. In addition to stability, the condition of the meniscus must be determined. The incidence of secondary meniscal tears in ACL-deficient knees has been found to be as high as 25% over 5 years, whereas the incidence in ACL-reconstructed knees was 4% (5). Re-injury may also lead to laxity of other ligaments (4).

Meniscal Tears

Injuries to the meniscus are among the most common knee injuries, either as solitary lesions or in association with other injuries. Both the lateral and medial menisci are critically important in absorbing and dissipating a large portion of the force imparted to the articular cartilage. They protect the articular cartilage by increasing the contact area on the tibial plateau of the femoral condyles, thus preventing focal areas of stress. The menisci have been shown to transmit up to 50% of the applied stress load across the knee in flexion and up to 80% in extension (4).

Given the critical role of menisci in normal knee physiology, it is understandable that an injury to either meniscus can have serious consequences. In the past, torn menisci were treated surgically by a total meniscectomy. The absence of a meniscus results in a smaller area of contact between the tibia and femur, which can double or triple the force applied to a much smaller area (16). Total meniscectomy has now been abandoned, following multiple long-term studies that showed an accelerated incidence (up to 40%) of degenerative changes in articular cartilage (17).

Mechanisms of meniscal tears vary but often involve some twisting of the knee with a valgus or varus stress applied. Pain level can vary as well; some athletes return to play after an injury and do not experience pain or swelling until several hours later. Clues to a meniscal injury include a locking, clicking, or catching with weight bearing. A knee effusion may or may not be present. Findings on physical examination can vary widely. No one particular test or manipulation is considered uniformly sensitive or specific, although joint-line tenderness is highly suggestive of meniscal derangement. The definitive diagnosis of meniscal tears requires MRI or arthroscopy. MRI is reported to have a 5–10% incidence of false-positive readings and about 10% false negatives. Arthroscopy is the procedure of choice for delineating the exact morphology of the tear and for treatment.

Various types of tears exist, and treatment is based not only on the type of tear but also on the athlete's symptoms, age, and activity level, the chronicity of symptoms, and any associated injuries. The major types of meniscal injuries are degenerative, horizontal, transverse (radial), oblique (flap), and vertical longitudinal (4) (figure 7.2).

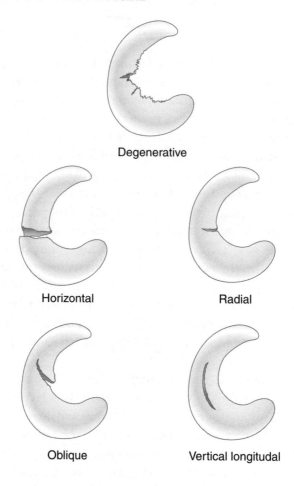

Figure 7.2. Meniscal Tears

Degenerative meniscal tears are most commonly encountered in individuals over the age of 40 years and are associated with degenerative changes within the meniscus and the joint, including the cartilage. Treatment for degenerative tears is based on the type and chronicity of the individual's symptoms—that is, whether the symptoms are associated with a specific insult. Determining the contribution of a degenerative meniscal tear to pain in a joint with degeneration of the articular cartilage may be difficult, and perhaps possible only after the degenerated and torn meniscus is removed.

Horizontal tears of the meniscus extend from the center of the meniscus to the periphery. The meniscus can then move in and out of the joint, causing pain and mechanical symptoms (4). Treatment depends on the extent of the tear. Resection of the meniscus peripherally until the rim is stable is a common procedure. Some of these tears may be candidates for repair, using one of the methods currently available.

Radial and oblique tears can have severe consequences. If the tear extends far enough peripherally, it may disrupt the collagen fibers that extend circumferentially to enclose the entire meniscus. These collagen fibers play a vital role in dissipating an axial load horizontally (like a "hoop"); if they are torn, the meniscus cannot function. These injuries are usually treated with resection of the torn area to leave a balanced rim of meniscus, but some may be repaired, which is preferable, especially if the tear is large (4).

Vertical tears can be complete, extending partially or completely through the entire meniscus. Arthroscopy allows the best visualization of these types of tears, with probing to determine the extent and stability of the injury. Stable, smaller tears are treated by simple observation or with abrasion of the meniscal surface, which stimulates vascularization (4,18). Larger or unstable tears may be either repaired or resected. Large, vertical longitudinal, or "bucket-handle," tears are commonly associated with ACL tears. These are usually unstable and symptomatic. If possible, repair is the optimal treatment, since resection often requires removal of a significant portion of the meniscus (4).

During the last decade, research has shown that the menisci, previously considered avascular, are supplied by branches of the geniculate arteries, which supply the outer 10–25% of the lateral meniscus and the outer 20–30% of the medial meniscus. Although the blood supply is limited, both menisci do have the capacity to heal (16). Experimental studies have shown that even tears in the avascular portions, if they communicate with the perimeniscal capillary complex, can heal with surgical repair (17). In fact, repairs of the meniscus performed at the same time as ACL reconstruction yield the highest success rates of all.

Removal of even 16–39% of the meniscus increases joint surface contact forces by more than 300% (17). Moreover, the degree of articular cartilage degeneration is thought to be directly proportional to the amount of meniscus resected. Repair of central and peripheral meniscal tears up to 5 mm deep can preserve the cartilage (16). A variety of surgical techniques has been developed to repair different types of tears. For flap tears, complex tears, and tears in locations where healing is unlikely, debridement of the injured portions of the meniscus back to a smooth and continuous rim of cartilage allows maximal protection of the articular surfaces while removing a minimal amount of tissue to maintain stability of the meniscal rim (16).

Other factors also need to be considered when deciding whether a meniscal tear should be treated by removal or repair or left alone. Meniscal tears that are mechanically and clinically stable but have not healed completely, if they are asymptomatic, do not necessarily require removal of the meniscus. The remaining meniscus may still function to protect the articular surfaces and dissipate load forces, depending upon other biomechanical factors such as degree of valgus and varus angulation of the knee (17). One concern, however, is that a tear can enlarge over time. Some degenerative tears are asymptomatic, and knee pain may be secondary to articular cartilage degeneration rather than the meniscal tear itself (4). Activity status and chronicity of symptoms may also play a role. The athlete's age, however, does not seem to be a significant factor in the healing of repairs or the functional outcome postoperatively (16,17).

Meniscal tears and ACL injuries seem to be intricately related. Many studies have shown that the most significant factor influencing the outcome of meniscal repair is the status of the ACL (17,19–22). In ACL-deficient knees, the rate of re-injury of the meniscus approaches 50%.

Medial Collateral Ligament

The medial collateral ligament contains superficial and deep layers. The deepest layers are actually a fibrous thickening of the medial midportion of the joint capsule attached to the medial meniscus. The more superficial layers extend from the medial femoral epicondyle to the medial tibia, within 4 cm distal to the joint line (4). The MCL functions as a restraint to valgus stress on the joint. It is also a secondary restraint to anterior tibial translation, which becomes more important after any injury to the ACL. The MCL is most lax at 25–30 degrees of flexion, and with extension it functions as a primary stabilizer, allowing decreasing degrees of joint-space opening in response to applied valgus stress (4,23).

Injuries to the MCL can occur alone or associated with meniscal and/or ACL injuries. With excessive valgus force, the MCL can stretch (grade 1), partially tear (grade 2), or completely tear (grade 3). The athlete generally experiences pain, tenderness, and swelling along the medial aspect of the knee, above or below the joint line. Rarely, some degree of ecchymosis may also be present 1–2 days after the injury, depending on the extent of the tear. Pain does not correlate with the degree of injury, as the most serious injuries "decompress" the joint thus decreasing the level of pain.

The examiner should assess the integrity of the MCL while the athlete lies supine and relaxed on the examining table. The examiner supports the injured knee with one hand placed under the thigh, just proximal to the joint line. The other hand grasps the tibia, just distal to the joint line and applies a valgus stress. The MCL should be assessed with the knee in both 30 degrees of flexion and in full extension. The grade can be estimated by the medial opening as stress is applied with the knee in 30 degrees of flexion: grade 1 injury is associated with up to 5 mm of opening or laxity, grade 2 with 5–10 mm of laxity, and grade 3 or complete tear with greater than 10 mm of laxity. Only complete tears allow a detectable laxity while the knee is in full extension (4).

Treatment for grades 1 and 2 MCL injuries is primarily conservative, with limited activity, early rehabilitation, and the use of a lateral hinged brace to prevent valgus stress. Isolated grade 3 (complete) MCL tears, in which the posteromedial capsule is intact, may be treated without surgical repair, possibly allowing earlier return to full activity (4,24,25). The rate of healing and contraction of the ligament seems to be genetically determined to a large extent. MCL injuries associated with ACL tears are often repaired surgically, although nonoperative treatment of complete MCL tears with ACL reconstruction may be an alternative, which is not associated with any significant valgus laxity (4,26).

Posterior Cruciate Ligament

The posterior cruciate ligament (PCL) has been described as the strongest ligament in the knee. It originates from the central posterior region of the tibia, extending for more than 1 cm below the joint line and extending superiorly to insert onto the medial wall of the femoral notch. The primary function of the PCL is to prevent posterior translation of the tibia, although it also provides secondary stabilization for the collateral ligaments with varus and valgus stress. The PCL also functions with the ACL and collateral ligaments to provide static stability to the knee in full extension (27).

Posterior cruciate ligament injuries were once considered rare, but with the improved diagnostic methods now available they are found to account for up to 20% of injuries to ligaments in the knee (4,28). Isolated PCL injuries are most often caused by a direct posterior force on the tibia with the knee in flexion. Other mechanisms of injury to the PCL include hyperextension with or without an associated valgus or valgus stress (these may be associated with injuries to other ligaments in the knee) (4,29).

The physician should suspect damage to the PCL following injury by any of the mechanisms mentioned above and by any high-impact collision. A mild effusion usually occurs soon after the injury, often within 2 hours. Pain is often present in the popliteal space, and weight bearing is difficult. The athlete commonly feels an instability with full extension of the knee as the tibia subluxes posteriorly. Examination of the knee in 90 degrees of flexion often reveals a posterior "sag" sign, in which the tibial tubercle cannot be seen on lateral view due to gravity-assisted posterior displacement of the tibia (27). Quadriceps muscle spasm sometimes supports the tibia and prevents a sag. The most sensitive clinical test to detect a PCL injury is the posterior drawer test. This test should be performed with the athlete relaxed and lying supine. The knee is flexed to 90 degrees, with one of the examiner's hands supporting the thigh posteriorly. A posterior sag may be evident. If the tibial tubercle seems to be placed posteriorly (not in the usual neutral position, with an 8 mm anterior step-off between the tibial tubercle and the femoral condyle), it is critical to relocate the tibia to the neutral position. Of note, relocating the tibia involves anterior subluxation, which should not be confused with a positive anterior drawer sign (suggestive of an ACL tear). After relocation to the neutral position, a posterior force that allows posterior subluxation suggests a PCL injury (4). This test may also be performed with the athlete sitting, legs hanging over the side of the table. Another test for PCL integrity is the "quadriceps active test," in which the athlete is able to anteriorly sublux the tibial tubercle into neutral position by activating the quadriceps muscle. This can be performed with the knees in 90 or 20 degrees of flexion and the thighs supported either by the examiner or by a rolled towel. The athlete must be able to relax the quadriceps completely prior to activation (30).

Radiographs of the injured knee should be performed to rule out fracture or a bony avulsion associated with a PCL tear. MRI is useful not only to confirm the existence of a PCL tear but also to detect any other associated injuries. Treatment depends on whether any other ligamentous injuries are present. Although isolated mid-substance tears are rarely repaired or undergo grafting acutely, a PCL tear with a bony avulsion requires acute surgical intervention for open reduction and internal fixation; this generally has a good result (4,27). Isolated PCL tears with an associated laxity of less than 5 mm can usually be treated conservatively with intensive rehabilitation, which will allow earlier return to sports activity. The quadriceps muscle can compensate for posterior laxity. However, tears associated with other ligamentous laxity may be candidates for acute repair or grafting with an autograft or allograft. Functional symptomatic instability due to chronic PCL tear is uncommon. It responds well to surgical intervention, though passive stability testing rarely returns to normal. The posterior subluxation and laxity associated with chronic PCL tears that are not well compensated by quadriceps activity or grafting have been shown to contribute to early osteoarthritis, especially in the medial compartment (31–33). The abnormal stress placed on the patello-femoral joint may result in both patello-femoral pain and degeneration (34). In general, PCL surgery is not as dependable or nearly as commonly required as ACL reconstruction. However, it is usually effective in the cases requiring it.

Lateral Collateral Ligament

The lateral and posterolateral region of the knee are stabilized by the lateral collateral ligament (LCL), the popliteus tendon, the popliteofibular, arcuate, and short lateral ligaments, and the posterolateral joint capsule, collectively referred to as the posterolateral joint complex (4). Disruption of the LCL allows increased varus opening of the joint throughout knee flexion, maximally at 30 degrees of flexion. Rupture of the PCL results in a larger degree of varus opening. Because posterolateral laxity is most often associated with other ligamentous injuries, especially damage to the popliteofibular, the integrity of all ligaments should be assessed. The close proximity of the peroneal nerve places it at risk for traction, including rupture, with any injury to the LCL, and this should be evaluated as well (4). LCL injury can be assessed by the same maneuver used for MCL evaluation, with the application of varus stress. Some degree of external tibial rotation may be present at 30 degrees of flexion. The examiner should compare the injured and opposite sides and also assess the PCL. MRI can be very useful in evaluating the extent of the damage. Surgical intervention for repair of a completely torn LCL is the usual treatment, whereas partial tears respond to conservative treatment and rehabilitation (4,35).

Patellar Dislocation

Acute primary dislocations of the patella occur predominantly in younger athletes, mostly between the ages of 14 and 20 years (36). Dislocation or subluxation is the result of the strong lateral force produced by a fixed foot and internal rotation of the femur coupled with contraction of the quadriceps muscle (37). Other mechanisms include a direct blow to the medial patella driving it laterally or a valgus force to the lateral surface of the knee.

Even complete dislocations usually reduce spontaneously. If necessary, manual reduction can be performed by fully extending the knee and applying a medial force on the lateral patella. A component of direct pressure on the lateral patella elevates the medial rim, allowing the patella to slide back into place more easily. If the patella spontaneously relocates, the athlete often cannot identify the event that made the knee "give out" or "buckle." A somewhat vague history may mimic the history of a ligament injury, so the examination is critical to diagnosis. Postreduction examination reveals pain and apprehension with manipulation of the patella and some degree of swelling. Tenderness with or without disruption of the vastus medialis or lateral retinaculum may also be present. Comparison with the uninjured knee is important, since evidence of hypermobility or a high-riding patella increases the probability of a dislocation or subluxation.

Certain predisposing factors seem to place an athlete at higher risk of patellar dislocation; these factors include malalignment, abnormal patellar or femoral trochlea configuration (38), hypermobility, and a history of recurrent subluxations or previous dislocations (36). Much controversy exists about the treatment for a primary patellar dislocation, since the recurrence rate may be as high as 60% (36). Nonsurgical, conservative treatment seems to be most successful in athletes without any of the predisposing factors mentioned above and with only minor skeletal soft tissue laxity. Those with one or more predisposing factors may be candidates for more aggressive, earlier surgical stabilization (36,39).

X-rays including a skyline and tunnel view should be performed in every case of suspected patellar dislocation, because the presence of an osteochondral fragment, particularly of the articular surface, may require arthroscopy for better evaluation of the fragment and possible fixation or removal (39). MRI may help clarify the primary injury as well as demonstrate any fragments and bone impact or contusions on axial STIR or fat saturation. An athlete with an osteochondral fragment and any predisposing factor is at a significantly higher risk of recurrence, and surgical stabilization should be considered. In fact, athletes with acute traumatic dislocations should undergo primary soft tissue repair. Unfortunately, even with surgical intervention, 30–50% of athletes may experience persistent instability and chronic anterior knee pain as a result of primary osteoarthritis of the patello-femoral joint (chondromalacia) or posttraumatic arthritis (39).

Patellar Tendon Rupture

Complete rupture of the patellar tendon is relatively rare and is most commonly associated with systemic disease such as diabetes mellitus (40,41). Anabolic steroid use is considered a predisposing factor, since these drugs allow abnormally intense training and possibly alter the integrity of tendon strength. Complete ruptures may be associated with rupture of the medial and lateral retinaculum. Partial tears are more common and tend to occur in athletes who have a history of chronic infrapatellar tendonitis and participate in sports requiring explosive movements, such as jumping, bending, and cutting (42). MRI may be helpful in establishing the diagnosis. Complete ruptures of the patellar tendon require surgical repair. Partial tears may initially be managed conservatively with anti-inflammatory medication and rehabilitation. If symptoms persist after conservative management, surgical intervention may produce favorable results (42). Injection of corticosteroid into the patellar tendon should be carried out rarely and cautiously; the steroid may weaken the tendon for several weeks after injection and thus increase the risk of rupture with even minimal stress.

ANKLE INJURIES

Sprains and Instability

The ankle is the most frequently injured region of the body, accounting for up to 45% of all athletic injuries (19). More than 80% of these injuries are sprains, involving either a stretch or tear of one or more of the multiple ligaments of the ankle. Most sprains are considered minor; the athlete may not seek evaluation or treatment, at least initially. Unfortunately, this often leads to a predisposition for re-injury, which can occur in up to 40% of cases (19). Chronic instability of the ankle and possibly early degeneration are common sequelae.

Three major ligament groups support and stabilize the ankle joint: the deltoid ligament complex (including the posterior talotibial ligament) located medially, the lateral ligament complex (composed of the calcaneofibular and anterior and posterior talofibular ligaments), and the tibiofibular ligaments (figure 7.3). More than 85% of ankle sprains are inversion sprains, affecting the lateral ligament complex. These injuries occur when the athlete's weight lands on the ankle while it is in both plantar flexion and internal rotation, the least stable position of the ankle mortise (19). This commonly happens during poorly executed cutting or when landing on an uneven surface, such as another player's foot (as in basketball). In the lateral ligament complex, the anterior talofibular ligament seems to be the most vulnerable to injury, since it lies perpendicular to the long axis of the talus and is stressed particularly

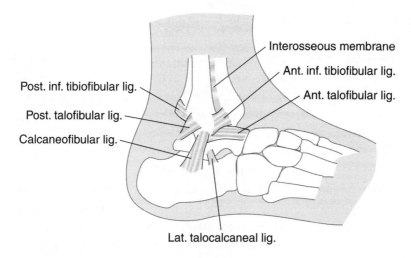

Interosseous membrane

Ant. inf. tibiofibular lig.

Post. inf. tibiofibular lig.

Ant. talofibular lig.

Post. talofibular lig.

Calcaneofibular lig.

Lat. talocalcaneal lig.

Figure 7.3. Ligamentous Structures of the Ankle (Lateral View)

with plantar flexion and inversion. The remaining 15% of ankle sprains involve the deltoid ligament complex and the syndesmosis (tibiofibular ligaments; this type of sprain is discussed separately below).

The incidence and type of ankle injuries vary with geographic region and the popularity of particular sports; in the United States, almost 50% of all ankle sprains occur in basketball (19). Examination as soon as possible after injury is always optimal. The physician should ascertain the mechanism or movement just before the injury—that is, inversion versus eversion—and the athlete's ability to bear weight. The location of swelling, tenderness, and discoloration should be noted. Location of the area of tenderness is particularly helpful in identifying which ligaments are injured.

Assessment of ankle stability should be attempted, although it may be limited by swelling and pain. The anterior drawer test is commonly used but is not always sensitive. The examiner grasps the athlete's distal tibia with one hand, while the other hand holds the heel with the ankle in neutral position and the foot resting on the examiner's forearm. An anterior stress is then placed on the ankle by the hand grasping the heel. Subluxation of more than 4 mm or the appearance of a sulcus at the anterior joint line suggests some degree of ligamentous laxity or tear of the anterior talofibular ligament and possibly the calcaneofibular ligament.

The syndesmotic ligaments, which join the tibia to the fibula, should be assessed by the "squeeze test," in which the tibia and fibula are compressed together just below the knee. The resulting stress on the syndesmotic ligaments will elicit pain above the ankle if any of the ligaments are torn or strained (21). Pain at the site of compression over the proximal fibula may indicate a fracture, called a Maissoneuve fracture, commonly associated with ankle injuries (43).

Ankle sprains, both lateral and medial, are often graded from 1 to 3, depending on the clinical presentation and the extent of injury. In a grade 1 sprain, the ankle is mildly swollen and tender over a ligament, without any associated ecchymosis. Range of motion is mildly limited, often by pain, and no instability can be demonstrated. The athlete can usually tolerate some weight bearing. In these sprains, one ligament, most often the anterior talofibular ligament, has been stretched, with some degree of microtears of the ligament fibers (19).

In a grade 2 lateral sprain, moderate swelling and a significantly limited range of motion are present. Ecchymosis over the injured ligament suggests a complete tear, usually of the anterior talofibular ligament. The calcaneofibular ligament may also be partially torn. Mild instability may be present and the athlete cannot do a toe raise or hop on one foot (19).

Complete tears of the anterior talofibular and calcaneofibular ligament are present in a grade 3 sprain, which may be accompanied by a tear of the posterior talofibular ligament (a complete dislocation). The ankle is diffusely swollen, tender, and ecchymotic, especially over the lateral surface of the ankle. Although moderate to severe instability is present, it is often not evident on examination because of the significant swelling and pain. Radiographs should be obtained to rule out the possibility of an avulsion fracture. Stress films can detect instability in the acute setting (43).

The primary goal in the acute management of an ankle sprain is to minimize pain and swelling and to provide ankle support, which will limit the amount of hemorrhage and soft tissue fibrosis as well as minimize pain, allowing earlier rehabilitation. The popular mnemonic "RICE"—rest, ice, compression, elevation—is very useful (21). NSAIDs help decrease inflammation. The grading system to describe sprains also helps in determining the appropriate management. A grade 1 sprain can be treated by functional support with a brace or taping and early weight bearing as tolerated. Functional rehabilitation should allow return to play within a week to 10 days, assuming no previous injury. A grade 2 sprain requires more conservative management after the acute phase. Weight bearing should be limited until swelling has begun to subside. Rehabilitation with strengthening of the surrounding muscle groups and restoration of proprioception are critical and need to be aggressively pursued. Complete ankle support such as a posterior splint or a walking boot should be worn at all times, at least initially. Aggressive rehabilitation should allow return to play in 2–3 weeks (19).

Management of grade 3 sprains (i.e., multiple torn ligaments) remains controversial. Both surgical and conservative treatments have been reported as successful. Studies that suggested early surgical repair as more successful were poorly controlled (19). Conservative management is aided by the use of a splint, cast, or walking boot (starting with a period of complete non–weight bearing for at least 1–2 weeks) until acute pain and swelling have cleared. Athletes undergoing aggressive functional rehabilitation with taping for support often recover and return to a pre-injury level of play in a significantly shorter period of time than with a surgical approach (44). Both surgical and conservative management with intense early rehabilitation produce excellent results in up to 90% of sprains.

The recurrence rate of ankle sprains is high, and prevention is the key to keeping the athlete active. Ankle braces can give excellent support and can be superior to taping, since tape can loosen and lose its rigid support after 20 minutes. The athlete can choose from a wide variety of braces to find the most comfortable and appropriate type. The ASO brace, one of the more comfortable types, is made of soft fabric, laces up anteriorly, and has wrap-around straps for added support. Some athletes prefer taping; it must be done by someone who is familiar with the appropriate technique. The final taping should place the ankle in relative dorsiflexion and eversion, which limits the degree of plantar flexion and inversion. Both taping and bracing increase proprioception, adding to stability by stimulating the supporting ankle muscles (19). After a grade 3 sprain, an ankle brace during all athletic activities is strongly recommended.

Chronic lateral ankle instability is frustrating to both the athlete and the physician. The athlete usually has a long history of recurrent ankle sprains, often without adequate rehabilitation. Ankle pain, with or without swelling, after activities and a sensation of the ankle "giving out" are common. On physical exam, instability can be demonstrated by an anterior drawer test. A moderate degree of talar tilt may be evident on inverting the calcaneus while stabilizing the tibia. It is important to perform these maneuvers on both ankles, using the uninjured ankle as an internal control, since athletes with a generalized ligamentous laxity will have an abnormal examination as baseline. Other causes of ankle pain, such as posttraumatic arthritis and osteochondritis dissecans, need to be considered as well. The increasing use of MRI has allowed these alternative diagnoses to be made more easily.

Instability may be aggravated by the loss of muscle strength that often accompanies repetitive sprains. Treatment of chronic ankle instability should include rehabilitation focusing on the restoration of range of motion, strengthening of supporting muscles (especially the peroneus brevis), and training to achieve adequate proprioception. Surgical management for chronic instability is an option if conservative treatment is unsuccessful and the athlete is not willing to limit activity. More than 30 different techniques have been described for correcting chronic instability. According to several studies comparing the various techniques for lateral reconstruction, surgery is successful in 68–96% of cases, regardless of the specific surgical technique (19).

Lateral ankle instability may be mimicked by instability of the peroneal tendons. The tendons of the peroneus longus and brevis pass beneath a tendon sheath or retinaculum as they extend inferiorly around the lateral malleolus. The tendon sheath can be injured with an inversion (lateral) sprain. As the tendons sublux across the malleolus with plantar flexion, the athlete senses frequent episodes of instability or "giving out," often misinterpreted as joint instability. Tendon instability should be considered in cases of perceived "instability" while walking on flat surfaces with minimal stress on the joint, occurring with increasing frequency. Rehabilitation has nothing to offer. Surgical reconstruction of a retinaculum to prevent subluxation of the tendons successfully eliminates symptoms.

Syndesmotic Sprains

The syndesmosis of the ankle, the distal articulation of the tibia and fibula, is stabilized by four separate ligaments: the anterior and posterior tibiofibular ligaments, the transverse tibiofibular ligament, and the interosseous membrane. These ligaments function to maintain the ankle mortise (figure 7.4). Medial stability to the ankle is provided by the deltoid ligament, which attaches the tibia to the talus and calcaneus.

Sprains of the syndesmosis are uncommon, making up approximately 10% of all ankle sprains, but they are commonly underdiagnosed. The most usual mechanism of injury involves a forced external rotation of the foot with the leg internally rotated, which forces the talus against the distal fibula, stressing the entire mortise (45). Forced hyperdorsiflexion of the foot can also place excessive stress on the mortise and has also been associated with injury to the syndesmosis (46).

Syndesmotic sprains are not commonly encountered in basketball players and runners, tending to be more frequent in athletes in contact sports such as football and hockey. The syndesmotic ligaments are quite strong and thus require significant force to produce an injury (47). In fact, the excessive force required to injure the syndesmosis often results in concomitant fractures of the tibia or fibula (48).

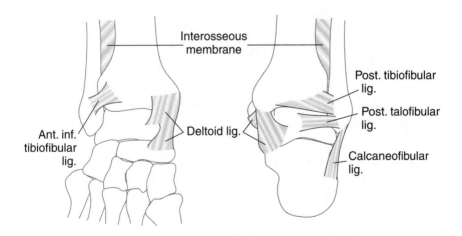

Figure 7.4. Anatomy of the Syndesmosis of the Ankle

Possible injury to the syndesmotic ligaments should be considered, at least initially, in all ankle sprains. The athlete may describe pain in the Achilles tendon without any tenderness on the tendon itself (actually referred pain from the posterior syndesmosis) or a diffuse pain in the ankle. Examination findings that suggest an injury to the anterior talofibular ligament include exquisite tenderness over the ligament (just distal to the anterior joint line at the medial edge of the fibula and the lateral edge of the tibia), limited range of motion, and minimal swelling (which can mislead the examiner as to the severity of the injury). Dorsiflexion of the foot exacerbates pain as the syndesmosis is forced apart. The external rotation and eversion test involves the application of a firm external rotation force on the ankle while it is in neutral position and the knee is flexed to 90 degrees. Increased pain over the anterolateral aspect of the ankle proximal to the joint line is highly suggestive of an injury to the syndesmosis (49). The Hopkinson squeeze test is another maneuver that stresses the syndesmosis by squeezing the tibia and fibula together in the middle of the calf. Increased pain distal to the point of pressure at the ankle suggests injury to the syndesmosis (50). Pain at the site of pressure may indicate a fracture of the fibula, a Maissoneuve fracture.

Radiographs can be helpful in making the diagnosis and in ruling out any associated fracture. Radiographic evidence of injury to the syndesmosis depends upon the view:

–mortise view: widening of the anterior tibial tubercle–fibular space by more than 5 mm
–anteroposterior view: widening of the posterior tibial tubercle space or medial ankle joint space by more than 5 mm
–lateral view: asymmetry of the tibiotalar crescents (51)

If the clinical exam is suggestive of a syndesmotic injury and the x-ray results are normal, eversion stress views under the fluoroscope may be useful to demonstrate an instability. If a mortise view taken while an external rotation and abduction force is applied to the ankle reveals a widening of the medial joint space of more than 1 mm compared with the uninjured side, this is consistent with a syndesmotic injury (46). Radiographs taken 2 or 3 weeks after syndesmotic injury show heterotopic ossification (HTO) of the interosseous membrane in more than 50% of cases (50,52). HTO has not been shown to affect long-term ankle function or stability after recovery from the initial injury (47,52).

Associated tears of the syndesmosis and the deltoid ligament that widen the mortise should be managed aggressively. Surgical intervention with a screw holding the tibia and fibula together to reduce the diastasis and help restore the mortise has proved successful (49). Failure to reduce the mortise contributes to development of osteoarthritis. Conservative management, with a removable support cast to allow early motion, should be considered only for injuries without any mortise displacement (53,54). Ankle injuries have been shown to have a significant neural component; if neural function is maintained at some level with early motion and proprioception training, the athlete may return to play earlier with a decreased risk of recurrent injury (55,56)

Athletes with a syndesmotic injury typically require a longer period of rehabilitation before returning to play (up to 6 or 8 weeks) at the previous level of performance. The increased recovery time is probably related to the greater amount of soft tissue damage than in a more common lateral ankle sprain, as well as the constant strain placed on the syndesmotic ligaments during regular daily activities. Unfortunately, since plain x-rays often have normal findings and the amount of swelling tends to be minimal, these sprains sometimes go unrecognized and are considered mild, uncomplicated ankle sprains. The athlete then returns to full activity too soon (and may be considered to be malingering), further prolonging the recovery period (50). After recovery, either a functional brace or taping of the injured ankle is recommended for at least a year to minimize stress while the ligaments recover completely. An added two or three circumferential tape straps 3 or 4 cm above the joint line may further support the syndesmosis and decrease the stress to these ligaments (57).

All types of ankle injury may be associated with chronic pain or soreness. The most common cause is residual scar tissue or granulation, which is easily removed arthroscopically. Other causes of chronic discomfort include traumatic arthritis, periarticular tendon injuries, and sinus tarsi syndrome. Sinus tarsi syndrome occurs after a lateral sprain and is associated with a tear of the tarsal canal ligaments. It is usually treated with local steroid injections into the canal, but may require surgery (58).

MUSCLE INJURIES

Strains and Tears

Muscular pain is the most common type of pain in the athlete. In most cases the pain is benign and limited, usually related to overexertion in the preceding 24–48 hours, and improves with gentle stretching and perhaps a decrease in exertion for a day or two.

Muscle injuries are divided into two categories: strains or tears and contusions. Muscle strains are the result of excessive stretching of the muscle fibers, sometimes referred to as a "pulled muscle." Mild strains involve only microscopic tears or stretching and are described as first-degree strains. More severe stretches resulting in larger, macroscopic tears of the muscle fibers are second-degree strains, or partial tears. A third-degree tear is a complete tear of the muscle body (59,60). Strains tend to occur more often in the lower extremities and to involve muscles that extend across two joints, such as the rectus femoris and the hamstring muscles (muscles of the posterior thigh, including the semimembranosus, semitendinosus, gracilis, sartorius, and biceps femoris). The usual mechanism is a forced stretch when the muscle is in active contraction. The stretch or tear most commonly occurs at the musculotendinous junction, the weakest point of the musculotendinous unit (61).

Depending upon the grade of the strain and the extent of the tear, the athlete will experience some degree of pain along the entire muscle with tenderness over the area of the strain or tear. Pain can also be elicited with both active and passive stretching of the involved muscle. Significant swelling due to a hematoma may be present over the area of the strain, especially if a significant tear has occurred. A palpable defect or indentation in the muscle body at the site of a tear may be evident. Loss of strength also correlates somewhat with the extent of the tear, although motion may be limited because of pain. A complete inability to contract the affected muscle should alert the examiner to a possible complete tear.

Radiographs are not necessarily indicated unless a complete tear is suspected, in which case they can be used to evaluate a possible avulsion fracture. MRI can be very useful in the evaluation of injuries involving possible significant tears, as in athletes who demonstrate a significant loss of function following a muscle injury. It is critical to determine the extent of the tear in order to determine the treatment and prognosis. A complete tear cannot be surgically repaired unless it is associated with a tendon or bone avulsion (62).

For elite or professional athletes, evaluation with MRI to determine the extent of the injury will help in planning the optimal rehabilitation program for the earliest return to competition without excessive risk to the athlete. A muscle strain is best appreciated as high-intensity signal images on a T2-weighted image, which signify edema within the muscle. The high-intensity signal may last for up to several weeks, but intensity is greatest after the first 24 hours and for the following 4 days (63). A "rim sign," or high-intensity signal around the edge of the muscle involved, may also be present (64). The T1-weighted images will show a high-intensity signal if a significant amount of hemorrhage has occurred. A discontinuation of the muscle signifies a tear; some intact muscle fibers will be evident if the tear is not complete. In a complete tear some retraction of the muscle can occur. The T1-weighted signal shows high-intensity signals if the hemorrhage is acute, and these will fade as the hemoglobin is broken down. The T2-weighted signal is also of high intensity because of the associated edema and inflammation. In cases of deep muscle injury, an ultrasound may show an area of intramuscular fluid as well. Aspiration of the fluid and injection of corticosteroid can speed rehabilitation.

The focus of immediate treatment is to minimize swelling and bleeding as much as possible, with local icing, compression, and elevation initially. Application of heat is not advised, because it may increase any associated muscle hemorrhage. The use of NSAIDs, at least in the first 24 hours, may also increase bleeding. Acetaminophen or other analgesics can be used initially for pain. Early passive motion and muscle stimulation treatment (with an external unit) can contribute to a faster recovery and rehabilitation. After the acute phase, NSAIDs may be useful for any associated inflammation. Second- and first-degree strains can be treated with NSAIDs and aggressive rehabilitation and physical therapy to restore range of motion and then strength.

Muscle Contusion and Myositis Ossificans Traumatica

Direct impact on a muscle, if forceful enough, may result in a contusion within the muscle itself. In contrast to a hematoma, which is a local collection or pool of blood, a contusion is characterized by capillary rupture, edema, infiltrative hemorrhage, and local inflammation. The severity of the contusion is related to the degree of hemorrhage and the extent of crush injury to the surrounding muscle and is often assessed by the amount of passive flexion possible 24 hours after injury (65). Contracted muscle fibers tend to incur less severe injury with impact than relaxed muscle fibers (66).

Early treatment is critical to minimize rehabilitation time and avoid complications. Ice should be applied immediately and for 20 minutes every hour over the following 24 hours, as far as possible. Constant local compression and maintenance of maximal passive flexion (as with a continual passive motion [CPM] machine) are also helpful. In order to minimize bleeding, NSAIDs, local heat, and massage should be avoided immediately following the injury. Recommendations for imaging and possible aspiration or injection are identical to those for muscle strain management. As with a muscle strain, strengthening exercises should begin once range of motion has been regained. Return to activity is allowed when range of motion and strength are in symmetry with the uninjured side (65).

Myositis ossificans traumatica (MOT) is the occurrence of non-neoplastic bone or cartilage within soft tissue as a complication of a muscle contusion. The etiology of MOT is still not well understood, but the many hypotheses include organization of a local hematoma, proliferation of osteoblasts released from damaged periosteum, and metaplasia of intramuscular connective tissue into bone and cartilage (67). MOT develops relatively rapidly, and calcification can be seen on an x-ray within 3 weeks after the injury (65). Calcification occurs in a rimlike pattern, spreading from the outer edges toward the center as the MOT matures.

Myositis ossificans traumatica is more likely to develop following moderate to severe muscle contusions and is most common in the quadriceps muscle (68). Factors associated with a higher risk of MOT include the following:

–failure to apply ice within the first 24–48 hours following injury

–application of heat or massage during the initial phase (first 5–6 days)

–excessively aggressive rehabilitation with active stretching or strengthening too early during recovery

–re-injury of a contusion before healing occurs

–return to competitive activity too soon

–the presence of an intramuscular hematoma or seroma, especially in athletes with bleeding diatheses, such as hemophilia (69)

The development of MOT should be suspected when local swelling, tenderness, and overlying warmth and erythema persist or increase for longer than 3 or 4 days after blunt injury to a muscle. A significant loss in range of motion of adjacent joints occurs, due to pain and stiffening in the muscle (67). Active, developing MOT is characterized by an increase in the induration of the overlying tissue, persistent or worsening tenderness, and muscle atrophy during the 2–3 weeks following the injury. A definitive, firm mass can usually be palpated by 3 weeks, at which point calcification can be detected radiographically. Triple-phase bone scan may show activity prior to any x-ray evidence of calcification. MRI can be useful in localizing the area of calcification and the affected soft tissues and for athletes who may not recall a specific injury (70). The appearance on MRI depends on the age of the lesion. Acutely, the intramuscular mass shows a high-intensity signal only in T2-weighted images. As the lesion develops and begins to ossify, the center has a high-intensity signal on T2-weighted images; however, a rim of low-intensity signal surrounds it, signifying the area of early mineralization. An established MOT shows a high-intensity signal on T1 images of the center, corresponding to high fat content, and a surrounding area of low-intensity signal, corresponding to cortical bone (71).

Once an MOT lesion has developed, treatment should be directed toward regaining pre-injury strength and function, but this needs to proceed slowly in order to minimize additional trauma. The initial phase of treatment should focus on restoration of range of motion. These exercises may be active but should be relatively pain-free, as the extremes of the range are gradually increased. Any recurrence of erythema, warmth, swelling, or worsening of pain signifies excessive stress and should be managed with local ice therapy, NSAIDs (and possibly a short course of corticosteroids, depending on the situation), and no physical therapy until the inflammation has resolved. Physical therapy should then be restarted at the initial level and progress even more slowly. Once the range of motion has significantly advanced, the athlete can progress to resistance exercises. As strength increases, exercise for speed, agility, proprioception, and balance can be added. In general, the calcium deposits are resorbed over time, but this may take several months. The athlete should not return to full activity until the extremity has regained full range of motion and strength is symmetric with that of the contralateral side; unfortunately, this may take up to 6 months (69). Of note, no studies have shown that radiotherapy, ultrasound, hyaluronidase, proteolytic enzymes, long-term corticosteroids, or short-term diathermy reduce the length of disability (72).

Surgical intervention for the removal of an MOT lesion is not usually necessary. If the calcified mass is so large that it predisposes the athlete to further injury or prevents restoration of range of motion, thus producing significant loss of function, or if pain or weakness is persistent, excision should be considered. Surgery should not be performed until at least 6–12 months after injury, since local reossification may occur (67).

Any moderate to severe muscle contusion can potentially develop into an MOT, resulting in several weeks of disability. Therefore, to minimize this risk, it is critical that medical personnel caring for athletes be knowledgeable about the conservative approach to management of muscle contusions. Proper conservative management initiated immediately after injury will prevent long-term functional disability in the majority of cases (67).

FOOT INJURIES

Traumatic injuries to the 1st metatarsal phalangeal (MTP) joint increased significantly with the advent and growing popularity of artificial turf in the 1970s. The term *turf toe* refers to an injury to the capsuloligamentous complex of the 1st MTP joint, an injury that often leads to osteoarthritis and spurring, leading to decreased range of motion and inciting a cycle of recurrent injury.

The primary stabilizing components of the 1st MTP joint are the joint capsule and the musculotendinous structures, which also lend dynamic support. Medial and lateral sesamoid bones are present beneath the plantar surface of the joint and are contained within the double tendon of the flexor hallucis brevis. Congenital variants of the sesamoids consisting of bipartite or tripartite parts that failed to fuse occur in up to 30% of the population (73). The sesamoids act as a fulcrum to improve mechanical function of the flexor hallucis brevis tendon, elevating it away from the axis of motion. They also are weight-bearing points for the 1st MTP joint (74). Stress fractures, frank fractures, and avascular necrosis of sesamoid bones may also lead to pain in the same area.

The 1st MTP joint is subjected to more than twice the force placed on the remaining MTP joints in the foot. Up to 60% of total body weight is carried on the 1st MTP joint during normal walking (75). This force increases two- or threefold during running, and a running jump can increase the force to eight times total body weight (76). Factors related to a turf toe injury, besides artificial turf, include flexible shoes, restricted motion of the 1st MTP joint, decreased ankle motion, and the athlete's position. The higher incidence of injury to the 1st MTP joint on artificial turf is thought to be related to the greater surface friction, which fixes the forefoot on the turf more readily and thus promotes injury to the MTP joint when external forces are applied to the athlete's body (77). The multi-cleated flexible shoes used for better traction on artificial turf also contribute to turf toe, since stress placed on the forefoot is directly passed to the MTP joints (78). Athletes with a greater range of dorsiflexion of the ankle are known to have a higher incidence of turf toe injuries (79). Football players seem to have the highest incidence of turf toe, although soccer and lacrosse are also commonly played on artificial turf (80).

Hyperextension of the MTP joints is the most common mechanism producing a turf toe injury. The foot is dorsiflexed, the forefoot is on the ground, and the heel is raised. An external force that produces a further hyperextension of the MTP joint can stretch or tear the joint capsule at the neck of the metatarsal. A forced hyperflexion of the 1st MTP joint may also injure the joint capsule, which is somewhat less common.

Injuries to the 1st MTP joint are often graded from first to third degree, similar to ankle sprains. A first-degree sprain involves stretch of the capsuloligamentous complex and is characterized by some tenderness along the medial or plantar surface of the joint, mild swelling, and no ecchymoses. Range of motion is usually only mildly limited and the athlete is able to bear weight without much difficulty. Athletes with first-degree sprains may return to play, with or without taping, as long as symptoms are minimal. Local icing intermittently for 24 hours after the injury helps minimize any further swelling. A second-degree sprain is a partial tear of the capsuloligamentous complex. Symptoms are more severe than in a first-degree sprain, and more swelling occurs. Ecchymoses are present, the range of motion is more limited, and the athlete walks with a limp. Return to play is not usually possible and is not advised until symptoms resolve, since the player will be at a higher risk of further injury. A complete tear of the capsuloligamentous complex is described as a third-degree sprain. The 1st MTP joint is severely painful, swollen, and tender with significantly reduced range of motion (77). Radiographs are useful if swelling or pain is significant in order to rule out fracture or avulsion and possible associated injury to the sesamoid bones.

Management of injury to the MTP joints should always include initial local icing, compression, and elevation. Early mobilization has been shown to decrease the period of disability and should be encouraged. However, the athlete should not misconstrue this as permission to return to previous activities, since returning to competition too soon may extend the recovery period. NSAIDs and compression dressing or tape help to minimize swelling. Stiff inserts for the forefoot part of the shoes decrease the amount of flexion of the forefoot and may help prevent further injury or re-injury upon return to activity. These inserts may be custom made for maximum comfort (77). Athletes with a first-degree injury can continue to compete, either with shoe inserts or with taping of the 1st MTP joint. Athletes with second-degree injury should reduce their activity and return gradually to competition, which may take 1–2 weeks. A third-degree sprain requires a few days of non–weight bearing, after which return to activity is slow, often requiring up to 6 weeks to regain full range of motion and weight bearing without discomfort. Most sprains heal well within 3 or 4 weeks. Surgery is rarely required unless a possible intra-articular loose body or chronic instability leads to persistent pain and disability.

Previous turf toe injury may be associated with persistent pain and restricted motion, especially if re-injury occurs. Long-term sequelae include hallux valgus and rigidity (76). One long-term follow-up study showed a 50% incidence of some level of chronic discomfort (78). Longer-term management may include taping, orthotics, anti-inflammatory medications, modalities such as ultrasound and corticosteroid injections. Surgery for debridement may help in patients with chronic symptoms unresponsive to other management methods.

Injuries to the sesamoids should always be considered when evaluating an athlete with pain in the 1st MTP joint area. The sesamoid bones can fracture or separate, if bipartite or tripartite, with the same mechanism as (or in association with) a turf toe injury. Radiographs should be carefully examined for evidence of sesamoid fracture: the edges of the fragments will be sharp and the fragments appear to "fit" together. With a bipartite sesamoid, edges are smooth and round (81). Treatment is symptomatic, including rest, orthotic support, and rarely, injection of corticosteroid. For chronic pain, surgery is sometimes useful.

REFERENCES

1. Feagin J, Lambert K, Cunningham R, et al: Consideration of the anterior cruciate ligament injury in skiing. Clin Orthop 216:13, 1987

2. Hewson G, Mendini R, Wang J: Prophylactic knee bracing in college football. Am J Sports Med 14:262, 1986

3. Arendt E: Orthopaedic issues for active and athletic women. Clin Sports Med 13:793, 1994

4. Swenson TM, Harner CD: Knee ligament and meniscal injuries. Orthop Clin North Am 26:529–546, 1995

5. Daniel D, Stone M, Dobson B, et al: Fate of the anterior cruciate ligament injured patient: a prospective study. Am J Sports Med 22:632, 1994

6. Donaldson W, Warren R, Wickiewicz T: A comparison of acute anterior cruciate ligament examinations. Am J Sports Med 10:100, 1992

7. Feagin JA: The office diagnosis and documentation of common knee problems. Clin Sports Med 8:453–459, 1989

8. Guan Y, Butler DL, Dormer SG, et al: Contribution of anterior cruciate ligament subunits during anterior drawer in the human knee. Trans Orthop Res Soc 16:589, 1991

9. Furman W, Marshall JL, Girgis FG: The anterior cruciate ligament: a functional analysis based on postmortem studies. J Bone Joint Surg 58A:179–185, 1976

10. Noyes FR, Moorar LA, Moorman CT III, et al: Partial tears of the anterior

cruciate ligament: progression to complete ligament deficiency. J Bone Joint Surg 71B:825–833, 1989

11. Barad S, Cabaud HE, Rodrigo JJ: The effect of storage at –80°C as compared to –4°C on the strength of rhesus monkey anterior cruciate ligament. Trans Orthop Res Soc 7:378, 1982

12. Meyers JF: Allograft reconstruction of the anterior cruciate ligament. Clin Sports Med 10:487, 1991

13. DiStefano V: Anterior cruciate ligament reconstruction. Clin Sports Med 12:1–11, 1993

14. Brandt K, Braunstein E, Visco D, et al: Anterior (cranial) cruciate ligament transection in the dog: a bona fide model of osteoarthritis, not merely of cartilage injury and repair. J Rheumatol 18:436, 1991

15. Ferretti A, Contduca F, Decarli A, et al: Osteoarthritis of the knee after anterior cruciate ligament reconstruction. Int Orthop 15:367, 1991

16. Awbrey BJ: Arthroscopic management of meniscal injuries. Curr Opin Rheumatol 5:309–316, 1993

17. Meara P: The basic science of meniscal repair. Orthop Rev 22:681, 1993

18. Metcalf R: Arthroscopic meniscal surgery. In McGinty J (ed): Operative Arthroscopy. New York, Raven Press, 1991, 203–236

19. Liu S, Jason W: Lateral ankle sprains and instability problems. Clin Sports Med 13:793, 1994

20. Miller D: Arthroscopic meniscus repair. Am J Sports Med 16:315, 1989

21. Ryan J, Hopkinson W, Wheeler J, et al: Office management of the acute ankle sprain. Clin Sports Med 8:477, 1989

22. Sherman M, Lieber L, Bonamo J, et al: The long-term follow-up of primary anterior cruciate ligament repair. Am J Sports Med 19:243, 1991

23. Sullivan D, Levy IM, Shesker S, et al: Medial restraints to anterior-posterior motion of the knee. J Bone Joint Surg 66A:930, 1984

24. Woo SL-Y, Inoue M, McGurk-Burleson E, et al: Treatment of the medial collateral ligament injury. II. Structure and function of canine knees in response to different treatment regimens. Am J Sports Med 15:22, 1987

25. Reider B, Sathy MR, Talkington J, Blyznak N, Kollias S: Treatment of isolated medial collateral ligament injuries in athletes with early functional rehabilitation. Am J Sports Med 22:470–477, 1993

26. Shelbourne KD, Porter DA: Anterior cruciate ligament–medial collateral ligament injury: non-operative management of medial collateral ligament tears with anterior cruciate ligament reconstruction. Am J Sports Med 20:283, 1992

27. Kannus P, Bergfield J, Jarvinen M, et al: Injuries to the posterior cruciate ligament of the knee. Sports Med 12:110–131, 1991

28. Clendenin M, Heckman J: Interstitial tears of the posterior cruciate ligament. Orthopaedics 3:764, 1980

29. Wascher D, Markolf K, Shapiro M, et al: Direct in vivo measurement of

forces in the cruciate ligaments. Part I. The effect of multiplane loading in the intact knee. J Bone Joint Surg 75A:377, 1993

30. Staubli H-U, Jakob RP: Posterior instability of the knee in near extension. J Bone Joint Surg 72B:225–230, 1990

31. Dejour H, Walch G, Peyrot J, Eberhard PH: The natural history of rupture of the posterior cruciate ligament. Rev Chir Orthop 74:35–43, 1988

32. Longnecker SL, Hughston JC: Long-term follow-up of isolated posterior cruciate injuries. Am J Sports Med 15:628, 1987

33. Parolic JM, Bergfeld JA: Long-term results of nonoperative treatment of isolated posterior cruciate ligament injuries in the athlete. Am J Sports Med 14:35–38, 1986

34. Torg JS, Barton TM, Pavlov H, Stine R: Natural history of the posterior cruciate ligament-deficient knee. Clin Orthop 246:208–216, 1989

35. Palmer I: On the injuries to the ligaments of the knee joint: a clinical study. Acta Chir Scand 81(suppl 53), 1938

36. Cash JD, Hughston JC: Treatment of acute patellar dislocation. Am J Sports Med 16:244–249, 1988

37. Hughston JC: Reconstruction of the extensor mechanism for subluxing patella. J Sports Med 1:6–13, 1972

38. Wiberg G: Roentgenographic and anatomic studies on the femoropatellar joint. Acta Orthop Scand 12:319–410, 1941

39. Hawkins RJ, Bell RH, Anisette G: Acute patellar dislocations. Am J Sports Med 14:117–120, 1986

40. Kelly DW, Carter VS, Jobe FW, et al: Patellar and quadriceps tendon ruptures—jumper's knee. Am J Sports Med 12:375–380, 1984

41. Maddox PA, Garth WP: Tendonitis of the patellar ligament and quadriceps (jumper's knee) as an initial presentation of hyperparathyroidism. J Bone Joint Surg 68A:288–292, 1986

42. Karlsson J, Lundin O, Lossing IW, Peterson L: Partial rupture of the patellar ligament. Am J Sports Med 19:403–408, 1991

43. Johnson K, Teasdall R: Sprained ankles as they relate to the basketball player. Clin Sports Med 12:363, 1993

44. Smith R, Reischl S: The influence of dorsiflexion in the treatment of severe ankle sprains: an anatomical study. Foot Ankle 9:28, 1988

45. Brosky T, Nyland J, Nitz A, Caborn DNM: The ankle ligaments: consideration of syndesmotic injury and implications for rehabilitation. J Orthop Sports Phys Ther 21:197–205, 1995

46. Edwards GS, DeLee JC: Ankle diastasis without fracture. Foot Ankle 4:305–312, 1984

47. Boytim MJ, Fischer DA, Neumann L: Syndesmotic ankle sprains. Am J Sports Med 19:294–298, 1991

48. Pankovich AM: Fractures of the fibula proximal to the distal tibiofibular syndesmosis. J Bone Joint Surg 60A:221, 1978

49. Miller CD, Shelton WR, Barrett GR, Savoie FH, Dukes AD: Deltoid and syndesmosis ligament injury of the ankle without fracture. Am J Sports Med 23:746–750, 1995

50. Hopkinson WJ, Pierre PS, Ryan JB, Wheeler JH: Syndesmosis sprains of the ankle. Foot Ankle 10:325–330, 1990

51. Sclafani SJA: Ligamentous injury of the lower tibiofibular syndesmosis: radiographic evidence. Radiology 156:21–27, 1985

52. Taylor DC, Englehardt DL, Bassett FH III: Syndesmosis sprains of the ankle: the influence of heterotopic ossification. Am J Sports Med 20:146–150, 1992

53. Cass JR, Morrey BF, Yoshihisa K, Chao EYS: Ankle stability: comparison of primary repair and delayed reconstruction after long-term follow-up study. Clin Orthop 198:110–117, 1985

54. Cox JS: Surgical and nonsurgical treatment of acute ankle sprains. Clin Orthop 198:118–126, 1985

55. Jackson JP, Hutson MA: Cast brace treatment of ankle sprains. Injury 12:251–255, 1986

56. Linde F, Hvass I, Jurgensen U, Madsen F: Early mobilizing treatment in lateral sprains. Scand J Rehabil Med 18:17–21, 1986

57. Roy S, Irvin R: Sports Medicine Prevention, Management, and Rehabilitation. Englewood Cliffs, NJ, Prentice Hall, 1983

58. Klausner VB, McKeigue ME: The sinus tarsi syndrome. Physician and Sportsmedicine 28(5):75–80, 2000

59. Fleckenstein JL, Shellock FG: Exertional muscle injuries: magnetic resonance imaging evaluation. Top Magn Reson Imaging 3:50–70, 1991

60. Speer KP, Lohnes J, Garrett WE: Radiographic imaging of muscle strain injury. Am J Sports Med 21:89–96, 1993

61. Ryan JB, Wheeler JH, Hopkinson WJ, et al: Quadriceps contusion: West Point update. Am J Sports Med 19:299–304, 1991

62. O'Donoghue DH: Treatment of Injuries to Athletes, ed 4. Philadelphia, WB Saunders, 1984, 51–63

63. Fleckenstein JL, Canby RC, Parkey RW, et al: Acute effects of exercise on MR imaging of skeletal muscle in normal volunteers. AJR Am J Roentgenol 151:231–237, 1988

64. Fleckenstein JL, Weatherall PT, Parkey RW, et al: Sports-related muscle injuries: evaluation with MR imaging. Radiology 172:793–798, 1989

65. Young JL, Laskowski ER, Rock MG: Subspecialty clinics: physical medicine and rehabilitation. Mayo Clin Proc 68:1099–1106, 1993

66. Kuland DN. The Injured Athlete, ed 2. Philadelphia, JB Lippincott, 1988, 428–453

67. Booth DW, Westers BM: The management of athletes with myositis ossificans traumatica. Can J Sport Sci 14:1, 10–16

68. Rothwell AG: Quadriceps hematoma: a prospective clinical study. Clin Orthop 171:97–103, 1982

69. Danchik JJ, Yochum TR, Aspegren DD: Myositis ossificans traumatica. J Manipulative Physiol Ther 16:605–614, 1993

70. DeSmet AA, Norris MA, Fisher DR: Magnetic resonance imaging of myositis ossificans: analysis of seven cases. Skeletal Radiol 21:503–507, 1992

71. Tuite MJ, DeSmet AA: MRI of selected sports injuries: muscle tears, groin pain, and osteochondritis dissecans. Semin Ultrasound CT MR 15:318–340, 1994

72. Connor JM: Soft Tissue Ossification. New York, Springer-Verlag, 1983

73. Frankel J, Harrington J: Symptomatic bipartite sesamoids. J Foot Surg 29:318–323, 1990

74. Van Hal ME, Keene JS, Lange TA, et al: Stress fractures of the great toe sesamoids. Am J Sports 10:122–128, 1982

75. Stokes IAF, Hutton WC, Stott JRR: Forces under the hallus valgus foot before and after surgery. Clin Orthop 142:64–72, 1979

76. Clanton TO: Etiology of injury to the foot and ankle. In Delee JC, Drez D (eds): Orthopaedic Sports Medicine: Principles and Practice. Philadelphia, WB Saunders, 1994, 1642–1704

77. Clanton TO, Ford JJ: Turf toe injury. Clin Sports Med 13:731–741, 1994

78. Clanton TO, Butler JE, Eggert A: Injuries to the metatarsophalangeal joints in athletes. Foot Ankle 7:162–176, 1986

79. Rodeo SA, O'Brien S, Warren RF, et al: Turf toe: an analysis of metatarsophalangeal joint sprains in professional football players. Am J Sports Med 18:280–285, 1990

80. Ekstrand J, Nigg BM: Surface-related injuries in soccer. Sports Med 8:56–62, 1989

81. Rodeo SA, Warren RF, O'Brien SJ, Pavlov H, Barnes R, Hanks GA: Diastasis of bipartite sesamoids of the first metatarsophalangeal joint. Foot Ankle 14:425–434, 1993

Chapter 8

OVERUSE SYNDROMES

Overuse syndromes, such as tendonitis, commonly occur in adult athletes. Estimates suggest that up to 50% of all athletes have some sort of injury and at least half of those injuries are related to overuse (1). In general, the term *overuse* refers to an "overload" or repetitive microtrauma to the musculoskeletal system (2). Microtrauma results from tension or shear force that damages various components of the musculotendinous unit at the molecular and microscopic level.

Microtrauma may result from a single episode of excessive stress, but it becomes more significant with repetitive loading forces on the musculotendinous unit that are actually within the physiological limit. The components of the musculotendinous unit are bone (the site of attachment), the tendons and ligaments, and the muscle itself. Each of these components tends to adapt to an applied load or force differently. Bone adds greater mass to the site of attachment in order to accommodate the increase in loading force, tendons and ligaments increase collagen content and cross-linking to reinforce the tensile strength, and muscle hypertrophies. Over time, these adaptations function collectively to increase the strength and flexibility of the entire unit. Repeated load (and microtrauma) to the musculotendinous unit, without allowing time for these adaptations and for repair, causes disruption, inflammation, and possibly weakening of the unit (1).

Both intrinsic and extrinsic factors may compound overuse syndromes. Intrinsic factors include muscle imbalance, malalignment, and instability; for example, high arches may be associated with Achilles tendonitis and patellar tendonitis. Extrinsic factors include training errors and poor technique, demonstrated to be involved in up to 60% of injuries in runners (2). Many studies have shown a direct relationship between increased mileage or intensity in runners and the incidence of injury (3). Even minor improper training techniques can eventually lead to muscle imbalance, usually of a particular group of muscles, which can strain other musculotendinous units. In addition, weakness or loss of contractility due to fatigue limits the ability to absorb shock or stress (2).

All components of the musculotendinous unit are susceptible to injury. Injury generally occurs at the weakest point in the unit, which varies with the age of the athlete. In younger athletes, excessive stress tends to result in an avulsion fracture. In athletes over the age of 25 years, the tendon is the most susceptible to traumatic and overuse injuries, in part because of the progressive degeneration of collagen fibers and perhaps a diminishing ability to withstand repetitive stress. Muscle injuries and tears are more common in older athletes. In addition to age, the demands of various sports contribute additional stress to the pre-existing intrinsic and extrinsic factors (see below).

One of the most important aspects of sports medicine is the perception of "overuse." Non-orthopedists, especially rheumatologists, are familiar with inflammation and often view it as a primary entity. It is easy to classify an overuse injury as secondary to repetitive motion and treat it with relative rest and anti-inflammatory medication. As has become evident recently, however, inflammation associated with overuse may actually be a symptom of a larger or underlying biomechanical abnormality or imbalance. When treating overuse injuries in general, the sports physician must not only treat and control the inflammation but also carefully evaluate the patient for muscle imbalance, ligamentous laxity, and joint abnormalities (either congenital or acquired). Exogenous factors such as poor training programs, inadequate techniques, and poor, ill-fitted equipment may also play a role. A classic example is biceps tendonitis, which can easily be considered an overuse injury resulting from repeated overhead motion. However, biceps tendonitis has been closely associated with superior labral tears and instability of the glenohumeral joint. Recognition of the associated biomechanical abnormality is critical to preventing recurrence of the overuse syndrome and possible irreversible injury.

SHOULDER INJURIES: IMPINGEMENT AND ROTATOR CUFF TENDONITIS

The most common overuse injury to the shoulder in adult athletes who participate in throwing and racquet sports is rotator cuff tendonitis (RCT), or inflammation of the rotator cuff. In order to achieve the wide range of motion inherent in the shoulder, stability is primarily provided by soft tissue structures. The capsuloligamentous structures are the primary static stabilizers (i.e., at rest). The muscles of the rotator cuff, the teres minor, infraspinatus, supraspinatus, and subscapularis, provide most of the dynamic stability, functioning to accelerate, decelerate, elevate, and depress the humeral head during motion. Other muscles around the shoulder also contribute to some extent (see Chapter 6).

The etiology of RCT can be complex and related to the interaction of multiple factors; for simplicity these are divided into extrinsic and intrinsic factors. Extrinsic effects are the result of structures outside the joint itself. The most important extrinsic factor influencing the rotator cuff is the acromion or coracoacromial arch (4). The tendons of the rotator cuff are confined in a limited space between the humeral head on one side and the acromion on the other (supraspinatus outlet). The tendons of the rotator cuff, primarily the supraspinatus, may become "impinged" or caught between these two structures. Repetitive overhead motion can cause irritation, inflammation, and eventual degenerative changes of the tendons as they become crushed between the humeral head and the acromion, referred to as "impingement syndrome" (5) (figure 8.1). The area of impingement of the supraspinatus is also considered to be a focus of minimal vascularity, which may contribute to degenerative changes associated with irritation. The level of impingement is directly related to the size and shape of the acromion, which has numerous morphological variants but may also degenerate and form enlarging osteophytes with aging (4,6).

Impingement may also be a secondary effect. Secondary impingement occurs when the supraspinatus outlet decreases in size secondary to instability of the glenohumeral joint (7). Secondary impingement is more often encountered in younger athletes. The instability may be due to a genetic ligamentous laxity or a repetitive microtrauma on the labrum (the ring of fibrocartilage that forms the glenoid cavity of the

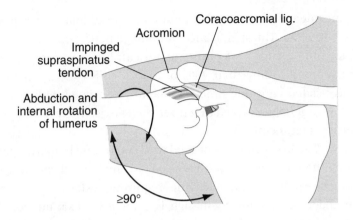

Figure 8.1. Impingement of the Shoulder Joint

scapula) and the capsular ligaments. Even with mild ligamentous laxity, increased stress is placed on the muscles of the rotator cuff as they attempt to stabilize the shoulder in lieu of adequate passive stabilizers. As the rotator cuff muscles fatigue, the humeral head can shift anteriorly, allowing impingement of the supraspinatus tendon. If the instability is not treated, tendonitis and eventually degeneration result in microtears and "tendinosis" (see below), possibly leading to partial tears of the tendons (4). Musculoscapular support also contributes to humeral stability. Weakened or inflexible scapulothoracic muscles, especially the trapezius, rhomboids, and serratus anterior, can alter the required scapulothoracic rhythm and synchrony with the glenohumeral joint during overhead motion. The asynchronous motion can allow the coracoacromial arch to impinge the rotator cuff (8).

Intrinsic factors contributing to rotator cuff tendonitis are most often related to fatigue, weakness, and muscle strength imbalance. Traumatic injuries to the rotator cuff may also result in asymmetric weakness and contribute to tendonitis by allowing the anterior and superior translation of the humeral head and subsequent impingement. The vascular supply of the tendons of the rotator cuff is an important factor. As mentioned above, an area of relatively low vascularity exists near the insertion of the supraspinatus tendon. Any irritation or inflammation in this area could potentially progress because its blood supply is inadequate for the reactive hypermetabolism necessary for repair (4).

Impingement and subsequent tendonitis can ultimately progress to rotator cuff tears. The significance of impingement, both primary and secondary, in overuse tears of the rotator cuff has been recognized for several years (9). More than 90% of rotator cuff tears, not including those associated with one-time trauma, are associated with impingement. It is generally accepted that three stages exist in the development of overuse rotator cuff tears.

Stage 1: The first stage is associated with edema and hemorrhage surrounding the tendons. The athlete usually complains of shooting pain radiating down the arm after activities requiring flexion or abduction of the shoulder. An impingement sign is evident on examination. The presence of pain when the examiner exerts forward flexion and internal rotation of the athlete's arm while the scapula is stabilized is a positive impingement sign, as the supraspinatus tendon is forcibly compressed between the greater tuberosity of the humerus and the anterior acromial surface (10). Range of motion of the affected shoulder is full and normal.

Stage 2: Pain is similar in location to stage 1 but becomes persistent and worsens at night. The pain is exacerbated with overhead motion. Impingement sign is present and tenderness may be present around the shoulder. Active range of motion is usually limited by pain, but passive range of motion is full.

Stage 3: Symptoms are similar to stage 2 but usually have become chronic. Athletes may experience weakness from pain, disuse, or possible partial tear of a rotator cuff tendon. Because of the chronic inflammation, the tendon(s) undergoes attrition and degeneration and may tear or stretch more easily with minor trauma or stress. Rotator cuff tears associated with impingement usually involve the supraspinatus tendon, so even subtle changes in strength can be associated with partial tears. The examiner can evaluate the strength of the supraspinatus muscle as the athlete abducts both arms to 90 degrees then flexes the arms forward 30 degrees and internally rotates them with the thumbs pointing down. This position isolates the supraspinatus muscle. (See the section on shoulder injuries in Chapter 6 for a description of maneuvers for evaluating the integrity of the rotator cuff.) Resistance to forced adduction simultaneously on both sides allows comparison for symmetry of strength (10).

Physical examination of the shoulder can be helpful in determining the integrity of the rotator cuff. Wasting of the supraspinatus muscle (with or without wasting of the infraspinatus muscle), a painful arc of motion at 90 degrees of abduction or flexion, and a greater passive than active range of motion are all suggestive of rotator cuff tears or weakness, as is severe pain or a history of a traumatic event involving the shoulder. Evaluation of the strength of each muscle of the rotator cuff may help determine the involved tendons. Testing of supraspinatus muscle strength is described above. The remaining rotator cuff muscles can be evaluated by asking the athlete to place her elbows, flexed to 90 degrees, close to her sides, with the hands held anteriorly in a thumbs-up position. Resistance to forced internal rotation (provided by the examiner) isolates the infraspinatus and teres minor muscles and resistance to external rotation isolates the subscapularis muscle. The subscapularis can also be isolated with maximal internal rotation of the shoulder coupled with extension (raising the hands behind the back) and evaluation of symmetry of extension. A complete tear of the rotator cuff is suggested by the inability to slowly lower the arm from 90 degrees of abduction ("drop arm test") (11). Maneuvers for evaluating instability should also be included in the evaluation.

Radiographs can be helpful in some cases to visualize any irregularities or degenerative changes on the undersurface of the acromion, the acromioclavicular joint, and the glenohumeral joint. A narrowing of the distance between the undersurface of the acromion and the head of the humerus (<6 mm) is suggestive of a rotator cuff tear. Calcification of one or more of the tendons of the rotator cuff may occur with prolonged inflammation. Although an arthrogram is more sensitive for detecting rotator cuff tears, MRI is the best method for evaluating the integrity of the rotator cuff tendons and the surrounding soft tissue structures. MRI can also detect inflammation within soft tissue and areas of abnormal bone stress. The vast amount of information gained from an MRI can then be used to determine the diagnosis and assess contributing abnormalities, and thus ensure that appropriate treatment is delivered as early as possible.

The differential diagnosis of shoulder pain includes subacromial bursitis and acromioclavicular osteoarthritis (especially in older patients), both of which may be aggravated with overuse and repetitive motions.

The physician should be aware that bursitis may be associated with rotator cuff inflammation. Forced horizontal adduction or resistance to horizontal abduction with the arm starting at 90 degrees of elevation near the midline of the body both compresses the acromioclavicular joint and exacerbates pain in acromioclavicular arthritis or synovitis. Pain on palpation of the involved structure can help with the differentiation. When differentiation is difficult, local injections of lidocaine into each structure followed by reevaluation of the athlete's pain is quite useful.

Stage 1 overuse can usually be managed conservatively with avoidance of the overhead activity and the use of NSAIDs and intensive physical therapy. Physical therapy should focus on strengthening the individual rotator cuff muscles, particularly for internal and external rotation. The use of intra-articular steroids is somewhat controversial; if used, but one injection does not give substantial relief and allow completion of a physical therapy program, or if the pain recurs, more aggressive evaluation using either an MRI or arthroscopy should be considered. Most cases of stage 1 tendonitis are reversible, unless a primary factor such as an inherent capsular laxity is present. Instability from overuse can often be reversed with rehabilitation and strengthening of the muscles of the rotator cuff (11).

Stage 2 tendonitis usually has progressed to a fibrotic supraspinatus tendon, and the athlete experiences persistent pain. Conservative treatment initially may be an option, but these athletes usually have a more significant level of instability. Early aggressive management can allow an earlier return to high-level activity and a better prognosis. Arthroscopy is the preferred option. It provides direct visualization of the glenohumeral joint and subacromial area, as well as the rotator cuff and joint capsule, and allows successful management of most rotator cuff problems. One of the most recent advances in management is thermally assisted capsulorrhaphy for capsular laxity, performed by arthroscopy, which involves the use of a heat source such as a laser or radiofrequency probe to shrink the capsule. Both labral tears and small tears of the rotator cuff can be repaired arthroscopically. Removal of subacromial spurs and subacromial decompression can be performed for athletes who have primary impingement due to acromial derangement. This procedure, known as an acromioplasty, allows increased movement of the humeral head without abutting the acromion. More than 90% of patients experience significant relief and are able to participate in most activities (12).

A fibrotic tendon resulting from chronic inflammation, or "tendinosis," has a high risk of rupture or tear, which can either progress gradually, starting as a partial thickness tear, or occur suddenly with a small amount of force. A tear might be considered a stage 3 injury.

Early aggressive pursuit of both the diagnosis and primary cause of rotator cuff pathology and surgical management with arthroscopy are presently the preferred method of management, especially for competitive athletes. Athletes with small to moderate tears are treated arthroscopically with debridement, repair, and an acromioplasty. Athletes with large partial rotator cuff tears are best treated with early repair, which results in improved function and relief of pain and, more importantly, prevents progression to complete tears. Complete tears of the rotator cuff should be repaired in virtually all patients. Small tears are repaired more easily and have a better functional outcome (12). If the repair is delayed, the tear will enlarge and make repair far more difficult, if not impossible. The prevention of complete rotator cuff tears also decreases the incidence and severity of secondary glenohumeral arthritis. The chronic pain of rotator cuff pathology can lead to adhesive capsulitis, which poses a serious management problem for both the athlete and the orthopedist. It may require a manipulation under anesthesia to restore the full range of motion—another procedure that must be followed by aggressive physical therapy. Medical conditions such as diabetes place certain athletes at a higher risk of adhesive capsulitis.

The most important factors contributing to a poor prognosis, even with surgical management, are the size of the rotator cuff tear and the duration of restricted motion before treatment, both of which support the argument for early and aggressive surgical management (12). There are numerous surgical procedures for managing shoulder pain, depending on the etiology.

ELBOW INJURIES: EPICONDYLITIS

Epicondylitis, inflammation of the tendons that insert along the medial and lateral epicondyle, is the most common overuse injury to the elbow.

These injuries tend to occur in athletes in throwing or racquet sports. Inflammation in the tendons and eventual degeneration (tendinosis) are the result of repetitive shearing forces and chronic tension overload over the epicondyle of the humerus. These forces are related to the grip size and the weight of the racquet (or club), an extensive range of motion of the arm during the swing or throw, and the long duration of eccentric muscle contractions around the elbow joint (13). The vibrations and energy generated from the sudden impact of high-velocity balls on the racquet are transferred to the arm, producing overload and microtrauma. The repetitive microtrauma eventually results in stiffness and weakness from inflammation in the wrist extensors and supinators (in lateral epicondylitis) or wrist flexors and pronators (in medial epicondylitis). The weakness, muscle imbalance, and lack of flexibility resulting from the inflammation further irritate and inflame the tendons by increasing the shearing forces (13).

Lateral epicondylitis, commonly referred to as "tennis elbow," involves the tendons of the wrist extensors and supinators. It is more common than medial epicondylitis and is estimated to occur in 40–50% of all athletes involved in racquet sports at some point in their careers, often after the age of 30 years (14). The athlete experiences pain on the lateral surface of the elbow with any activity involving resisted wrist extension, such as a racquet backhand stroke. The pain may radiate distally along the lateral aspect of the forearm; it improves with rest but recurs upon return to the inciting activity. Persistent pain and morning stiffness will develop if the athlete continues to play despite symptoms (15).

Physical examination reveals tenderness along or just distal to the lateral epicondyle with flexion of the elbow. Resisted wrist extension produces pain in the same location. No loss of range of motion occurs; swelling or erythema may be present over the lateral epicondyle or the forearm. It is important to differentiate epicondylitis from degenerative changes of the radiocapitellar joint, which can be accomplished by applying an axial load to the forearm combined with gentle passive supination and pronation. This maneuver compresses the radiocapitellar joint without stressing the surrounding tendons and therefore should not elicit pain in lateral epicondylitis. Calcific deposits may occur with chronic epicondylitis, but x-ray findings are usually negative (15).

Medial epicondylitis, or "golfer's elbow," is an inflammation at the origin of the wrist flexor and pronator tendons. Pain and tenderness are present over the medial epicondyle and are exacerbated with resisted wrist flexion and pronation or with finger flexion. Swelling and erythema are absent and the athlete has full range of motion. Medial epicondylitis tends to be associated with overhead racquet strokes and some golf strokes. These strokes produce an overload force from the tension of the pronator and flexor tendons and a valgus stress on the soft tissues surrounding the elbow. Differentiation from a tear of the elbow's medial collateral ligament is important. Application of a valgus stress to a slightly flexed elbow with a pronated forearm and flexed wrist stresses the medial collateral ligament but will not produce pain in medial epicondylitis or if ligaments are intact.. Medial epicondylitis may be associated with impaired conduction of the ulnar nerve, ulnar neurapraxia. The presence of pain radiating along the medial forearm and 5th digit along with medial epicondylitis suggests ulnar neurapraxia, which is usually reversible. One study found almost 60% of patients undergoing surgery for chronic medial epicondylitis showed some signs or symptoms of ulnar nerve involvement (15). It may also be associated with compression of the median nerve by the pronator-pronator syndrome, resulting in diffuse volar and midforearm pain and tenderness over the nerve. Electrophysiological studies can assist in determining the possible involvement of nerve compression in epicondylitis.

Management for both medial and lateral epicondylitis is similar. Initially, the stroke or throwing motion should be avoided. NSAIDs, or a short course of oral prednisone followed by NSAIDs, are useful for pain and inflammation; the NSAID should be taken regularly for at least 3 weeks. Passive range-of-motion exercises help maintain muscle and tendon flexibility while the inflammation is still active. Once the inflammation and pain are controlled, strengthening exercises, using light forms of resistance, can begin. Counterforce bracing or bands put pressure over the involved tendons and help relieve symptoms for some athletes. The pressure of the band is thought to constrain muscle expansion, which decreases the contractile tension and distributes the forces to the surrounding tissues rather than to the involved tendon (15).

Novice tennis players have a higher risk of developing lateral epicondylitis. In order to minimize recurrence, the other critical component of rehabilitation is a close review of stroke or throwing technique. For example, it is well established that a one-handed backhand stroke requires greater strength and coordination than a two-handed stroke. One popular hypothesis involves the linking of body parts. The one-handed backhand links five body parts prior to impact—hips to trunk to shoulder to elbow to wrist. The two-handed backhand links only two body parts before impact with the ball—hips to trunk, since the trunk, arms, and racquet move as one unit. No movement occurs in the wrist and elbow (assuming the stroke is performed correctly), which helps the entire arm absorb the force of the impact. The energy of the ball impact is transmitted through the elbow and wrist rather than absorbed by the soft tissues around it (15). Proper equipment can also play a role. Racquets with a larger head (but not heavier) decrease the vibrations and number of missed hits, thus diminishing the microtrauma to the soft tissues of the elbow (14).

The completion of a well-designed rehabilitation program and correction of poor technique is imperative for the athlete's complete recovery and successful return to prior level of competition. Previous injury can play a significant role in the overall prognosis. For athletes with incomplete rehabilitation of a previous episode of epicondylitis, the risk of recurrence is close to 70%, especially if the technique is not corrected (13). Surgery may be considered for treatment of epicondylitis, but only if conservative treatment fails and the symptoms become chronic or if an ulnar or median neurapraxia is present and has not resolved. Local steroid injection can be a part of the rehabilitation program, but the athlete should not return to play too soon after the injection because of the risk of tendon rupture, which can persist for up to 4 weeks. Surgery involves local debridement of the abnormal granulation tissue (which forms with prolonged inflammation) and abrasion at the site of the involved tendons to stimulate healing. Release or translation of the ulnar or median nerve may also be necessary (13).

KNEE INJURIES

Patello-femoral Dysfunction and Patellar Tendonitis

Anterior knee pain is the most common complaint seen by the sports medicine physician. Overuse contributes in the majority of cases, especially in athletes participating in sports requiring running and stopping, jumping, and turns or pivots. Abnormal patellar tracking (maltracking), due either to malalignment of the patella with the sulcus of the femur (patello-femoral dysfunction) or to variation in the shape of the patella, can result in chronic overload. In fact, symptomatic patello-femoral dysfunction is estimated to occur in up to 25% of the general population and to have an even higher incidence in athletes, most likely because of overuse and excessive lateral forces on the joint (16).

The patella is the largest sesamoid bone in the body. It functions as a "lever arm" to the quadriceps muscle during extension, increasing the force of extension of the knee by up to 50% throughout the entire range of motion (17). It also distributes the loading force of the quadriceps to the trochlear surface of the femur. Forces on the patello-femoral joint per unit area are among the highest of any joint in the body. The undersurface of the patella is protected by the thickest layer of cartilage of any joint surface, allowing it to repeatedly withstand forces that can exceed seven times body weight during squatting (18).

Articulation of the patella with the femur occurs within the sulcus, or trochlea (the indentation between the two condyles), of the anterior femur and initiates when the knee is in 20 degrees of flexion (full extension is 0 degrees). Abnormalities in articulation are related to several factors, including the size and shape of the patella, which is known to have numerous variants (some of which are named after the physicians who first described them), and the shape of the femoral condyles and the sulcus, since a shallow groove allows a greater degree of malalignment and varying degrees of subluxation. The tracking of the patella through the range of motion is not in a straight line. The patella is positioned somewhat laterally in full extension and is pulled medially during flexion. An excessively tight lateral retinaculum can prevent or decrease the medial movement of the patella during flexion, thus increasing the pressure on the lateral facet of the patella. The eventual degeneration can lead to symptoms and is commonly referred to as lateral patellar compression syndrome, a variant of patellar malalignment (19). The quadriceps muscle influences patellar tracking as well. The quadriceps muscle group favors lateral deviation of the patella, since the vastus medialis tends to be weak and does not counterbalance the force of the lateralis well. The position of insertion of the infrapatellar tendon at the tibial tubercle also affects tracking. Lastly, abnormal limb alignment, such as knee valgus or foot pronation, and general ligamentous laxity can contribute to abnormal tracking (20).

The term *chondromalacia* refers to lesions of the articular cartilage of the patella and historically has been used loosely to mean any patello-femoral pain. Abnormal patellar tracking, increases in the compressive forces on the patella, and changes in the articular cartilage are causally linked, because malalignment decreases the area loaded while the forces remain the same. Arthroscopy has allowed a close examination of the condition of cartilage and staging of chondromalacia: grades 1 (mild) to 4 (severe with bone exposed). Interestingly, a direct correlation between the extent of chondromalacia and clinical symptoms of patello-femoral pain has not been demonstrated. Cartilage degeneration certainly can cause pain when bone becomes exposed, but other factors related to patellar malalignment, such as a chronic strain on the lateral retinaculum (which is richly innervated) or reactivity of osteochondral bone to overload, may result in similar pain. Chondromalacia is presently believed to be the result of chronic patello-femoral dysfunction, but it is considered a gross pathological diagnosis and should be reserved for findings from surgery or arthroscopy (21–23). Primary osteoarthritis of the patello-femoral joint is usually associated with degeneration of the other compartments of the knee, especially in the presence of an angular deformity of the knee, but isolated osteoarthritis of the patello-femoral joint can produce symptoms similar to patello-femoral dysfunction.

The diagnosis of patello-femoral dysfunction is not always easy, since symptoms can be vague and physical findings subtle. The athlete typically describes a dull ache in the subpatellar or peripatellar region. The onset of the discomfort is gradual and initially is associated with activities involving running, especially long-distance, and with jumping, squatting, and quick stops and turns. The ache resolves with cessation of the activity, but it may eventually become constant and prevent participation in athletic activities. One knee may be more affected than the other. Certain daily activities such as squatting, walking up and down stairs, and kneeling also tend to exacerbate symptoms. Prolonged flexion is painful as well, such as sitting for long periods of time; moving the knee from flexion to extension often alleviates some of the discomfort.

Some athletes can feel a grinding, popping, or catching sensation beneath the patella.

Physical examination may reveal relative atrophy of the vastus medialis and tight hamstring muscles. Tight hamstring muscles can lead to patello-femoral pain by preventing full knee extension during running, thus increasing the patello-femoral joint forces (24). These are important observations in the physical exam because simple rehabilitation can alleviate discomfort related to muscle imbalance.

Patellar stability should then be evaluated with the athlete supine with her knee flexed to 20 degrees over a pillow. She should be relaxed, with her head flat against the examining table. The examiner then pushes the edge of the patella medially and laterally. The degree of mobility is often estimated by quadrants of the patella extending beyond the joint line, described as 1+ to 4+ (complete dislocation). Medial displacement limited to less than 1 quadrant indicates a tight lateral retinaculum (19). Displacement to either side of greater than 3+ (75% of the width of the patella) indicates an increased risk of subluxation and patellar instability. Both findings indicate patello-femoral dysfunction or malalignment (20).

The presence of crepitus, which is often felt by the athlete, is only significant if it is associated with pain, swelling, catching, or giving out (25). An effusion does not occur with simple patello-femoral dysfunction. Observation of the patella as the knee moves from complete extension to flexion can be useful. A lateral glide of the patella as the quadriceps is contracted or the knee is fully extended suggests patello-femoral dysfunction or malalignment.

An apprehension sign, which can be elicited with the application of lateral pressure on the patella while the knee is flexed to 20 degrees, suggests recurrent subluxation. A high-riding patella (patella alta) or a patella that exhibits a lateral rotation over the trochlea is also at a higher risk for subluxation. Manual compression of the patella while the knee is passively flexed may elicit crepitus and pain in athletes with severe cartilage degeneration and exposure of bone, which may accompany chronic patellar malalignment (20).

Radiographs may be helpful to evaluate patellar alignment and thickness. An inferior patellar tendon that is longer than the patella is indicative of a high-riding patella, which increases the risk of subluxation and is associated with chondromalacia (20). A merchant's (or sunrise) view allows evaluation of the patella while engaged in articulation with the femoral condyles. The thickness, shape, and tilt of the patella are also evident. Low femoral condyles or a shallow groove contribute to poor patellar stability and tracking (18).

Treatment for patello-femoral dysfunction primarily involves aggressive physical therapy, and good results often depend upon above-average skills and management on the part of the physical therapist. Stretching of the iliotibial band, lateral retinaculum (if it is tight), and hamstring muscles can give significant relief. Strengthening of the vastus medialis can help minimize the dynamic lateral tracking of the patella and improve the shock absorption for the patella and for the entire knee. Patellar stabilization braces, usually neoprene sleeves with a central hole for the patella, may be useful. Several months of physical therapy and muscle strengthening may be required before the athlete experiences maximal improvement in symptoms. She can use NSAIDs for pain relief, though inflammation is not usually a significant component of patello-femoral pain. Nonloading exercise for maintenance of cardiovascular fitness, such as bicycling and swimming, should be encouraged. The physician should try conservative management before recommending surgery in all but the most severe cases, unless frank subluxation or dislocation is involved.

Corrective surgery for patello-femoral malalignment may be performed arthroscopically. Lateral release of a tight retinaculum by arthroscopy improves patello-femoral alignment and may also contribute to pain relief through denervation of the retinaculum itself and patellar decompression. This procedure is useful for athletes with mild malalignment or subluxation leading to patellar overload due to a tight retinaculum. Those with more advanced malalignment or patellar instability may not improve significantly with only a lateral release (26) and require more complex surgical procedures to alter both the position and dynamics of the patella. These procedures include medial retinacular tightening and tibial tubercle anteromedialization, which are useful for recurrent subluxation or significant patellar tilting and degeneration (22). Additional procedures to address an arthritic surface of the patella may also be necessary.

Tendonitis of the patellar tendon is another cause of anterior knee pain also associated with overuse or repetitive strain. The pain is usually located in the infrapatellar tendon, although the inflammation resulting from the repetitive microtrauma may be present anywhere along the knee extensor mechanism, from the quadriceps tendon to the infrapatellar tendon insertion onto the tibial tubercle. Patellar tendonitis tends to occur in athletes involved in sports requiring running, jumping, and kicking, as well as quick stops and starts—the same activities that can aggravate symptoms of patello-femoral dysfunction. In fact, patellar malalignment is commonly associated with infrapatellar tendonitis. Pain is often gradual in onset, and initially it occurs after activity has ceased. If the inciting activity is continued, the pain eventually occurs at the beginning of the activity then disappears after warm-up, only to recur after the activity has stopped; later, it becomes constant and may predispose the athlete to partial or complete tendon rupture due to chronic inflammation and degeneration (27). Athletes with patello-femoral dysfunction often describe pain walking up and down stairs and after sitting for prolonged periods of time. Recent changes in sport, footwear, activity level and intensity, or terrain (e.g., from flat terrain to hills or from a soft to a hard floor surface as in basketball) can also be contributing factors.

Tenderness at the insertion of the patellar tendon at the inferior edge of the patella is the most significant finding, although tenderness may also be present along the entire infrapatellar tendon or at the insertion at the tibial tubercle. Prepatellar bursitis may also be associated with tendonitis. Radiographs are not usually helpful, although radiography may show irregularities at the distal pole of the patella and ossicles within the tendon in cases of patellar tendonitis (28). Ultrasound has been used for assessment of the patellar tendon; involved areas appear irregular and show decreased echogenicity (29). MRI is far more useful for evaluating patellar tendonitis and possible partial tears. T2-weighted images reveal increased signal intensity in areas of inflammation and fibrinoid necrosis (30). The STIR images may show associated areas of stress in the surrounding bone.

Conservative management is appropriate in mild to moderate cases. Physical therapy for strengthening of quadriceps (to assist in impact absorption, as in jumping), stretching of hamstrings, and ultrasound and ice treatment are important. The athlete should initially avoid activities associated with pain, usually jumping, pivots, and quick stops. NSAIDs help to alleviate inflammation while the primary malalignment or muscle imbalance is corrected. Infrapatellar compression bands may help redistribute the load on the tendon to the surrounding soft tissues. Corticosteroid injection into the tendon is virtually always contraindicated, since it significantly increases the risk of tendon rupture (31). Chronic inflammation may result in irreversible changes within the tendon tissue that compromise the function of the tendon, leading to persistent pain, disability, and degenerative tears. Surgical intervention for excision and debridement of the areas of degeneration and necrosis has been successful, but this is usually reserved for recalcitrant cases (32).

Plica

Another source of anterior knee pain that needs to be considered in athletes who complain of a gradual onset of pain without a history of injury is a plica. It is commonly misdiagnosed as chondromalacia, especially in adolescents. A plica is a redundant fold of synovial tissue, estimated to be present in almost 60% of the general population. It is considered a normal variant and represents an embryonic septum that persists in an adult knee. The plica is often crescent shaped; it extends from the medial fat pad and loops around both femoral condyles as it crosses below the patello-femoral tendon to insert on the lateral retinaculum. Occasionally, the folds may impinge on the medial femoral condyle or, with overuse and stress on the knee, may become inflamed, fibrotic, and symptomatic (33).

The athlete with a symptomatic plica most often describes the gradual onset of anterior knee pain, somewhat localized over the area of the plica. Pain is usually associated with activity such as running, but it may also occur after sitting for prolonged periods, increase in intensity upon rising, then diminish after walking 8 or 10 steps. This phenomenon is probably related to entrapment of the plica over the femoral condyle in flexion, impingement of the plica with extension of the knee, then extraction by the action of the articularis genus muscle—though this may require a few steps before the plica is sufficiently elevated (24). The athlete may also sense a "snap" in the knee upon extension as the plica moves across the femoral condyle (33). A feeling of buckling or "giving out" can occur as well.

The physical exam may be helpful, revealing tenderness over the medial femoral condyle (where the plica lies, although the plica itself cannot often be palpated). Crepitus may be present, but this is a nonspecific finding; an effusion is uncommon (33). Loss of motion or quadriceps atrophy may be seen in extreme, chronic cases. The diagnosis can be made from the history alone, but often the symptoms are vague and the clinical exam is unremarkable. In these cases, diagnosis can be made with an MRI. The sensitivity of the MRI is increased by an intra-articular injection of sterile saline prior to the imaging, which outlines the shape of the plica, especially on the axial views. Arthroscopy is the gold standard for diagnosing a plica and also facilitates removal of the plica using a laser or other coagulating instrument (33). Medial plicas that become chronically impinged may contribute to the degeneration of the subpatellar cartilage (34). Differentiation from patello-femoral syndrome and maltracking may be difficult and may require an MRI. Though a course of physical therapy for quadriceps strengthening and hamstring stretching generally alleviates symptoms of a plica, once present, the symptoms tend to recur with resumption of the inciting activity. Thus, early arthroscopic intervention is justified.

Iliotibial Band Syndrome

The iliotibial band (ITB) is a part of the fascia lata, sometimes referred to as the tensor fascia lata. It originates from the anterior superior iliac spine, extends distally to join the fascia lata, and inserts on the lateral tibial tubercle (Gerdy's tubercle). It is attached to the lateral femur by the intermuscular septum, which ends just proximal to the femoral condyle. Actually, the only place that the distal ITB is not attached to bone is between the lateral femoral condyle and the tibial tubercle. The ITB functions as a ligament to stabilize the knee laterally (35).

The distal ITB is located anterior to the lateral femoral condyle during extension and slides posteriorly as the knee is flexed. With repetitive flexion and extension, such as in long-distance running or cycling, the bursa between the ITB and the femoral condyle can become inflamed, resulting in lateral knee pain commonly referred to as ITB syndrome (35). The athlete with ITB syndrome most often describes diffuse lateral knee pain associated with running or cycling. The pain arises after a certain distance has been covered and usually does not occur with walking. Climbing up and down stairs and running downhill also aggravate symptoms. Dedicated runners often continue to run despite the discomfort, which is not usually disabling but more of an annoyance.

Findings on physical examination of the knee are unremarkable. Tenderness to palpation is present over the lateral femoral epicondyle or Gerdy's tubercle on the tibia and is usually not located over the lateral joint line. Manual pressure exerted over the lateral epicondyle while the athlete actively flexes and extends the knee can also reproduce the pain (36). The diagnosis is usually based on the history and the clinical exam. In unclear cases, MRI may reveal a thickening of the ITB and increased intensity with T2-weighted and gradient echo images deep to the ITB, consistent with edema or fluid in the bursa (36). ITB syndrome has been estimated to account for 1.6–12% of all overuse injuries in runners (37). It is more common in runners who run between 20 and 40 miles a week and also in men (possibly because of the greater ligamentous laxity and higher percentage of general body fat in women) (38). Predisposing factors include a tight ITB but also excessive mileage, a sudden increase in mileage, running on roads with a gradient, and worn-out or poorly supportive running shoes (37). Biomechanical factors that may contribute to the development of ITB syndrome include pes cavus (high arches), genu varum, leg length discrepancy, and rearfoot or forefoot varus (39,40).

Treatment should emphasize a reduction in stress to the lateral knee and ITB, such as reducing the weekly mileage and changing to new running shoes more often. The physician should individualize management to consider both external factors and biomechanics. Any leg length discrepancy or malalignments can be helped with orthotics. Regular stretching of the ITB is very helpful and should be encouraged, but athletes often need instruction in this exercise since it can be difficult to perform. Local ice and NSAIDs may be useful, and local steroid injection, into the bursa under the ITB between the femoral condyle and the tibial tubercle, might be considered in cases unresponsive to other, more conservative approaches (35). Surgery for partial release has been attempted but is not a common technique for general management (41).

LOWER-LEG AND FOOT INJURIES

Achilles Tendonitis

Achilles tendonitis has been estimated to account for 15% of all overuse injuries associated with running (42). It is more common in male athletes, both recreational and elite, in sports requiring constant running and jumping.

The Achilles tendon arises from the medial and lateral heads of the gastrocnemius muscle and the deeper layers of the soleus muscle. All these layers combine to form an oblong tendon that inserts on the proximal calcaneal tuberosity (43). During running, it withstands tensile loads of eight times the body weight, probably among the highest forces exerted on any part of the body. Blood supply to the Achilles tendon also plays a role in the development of inflammation. A watershed area approximately 2–6 cm proximal to the calcaneal insertion is the site of most noninsertional overuse injuries of this tendon (44).

Overuse injury to the Achilles tendon occurs in stages, defined by the areas affected by inflammation. Initially, the paratendon (tendon sheath) becomes inflamed and edematous with repetitive trauma and stress or overuse, referred to as paratendonitis. If the stress continues, the paratendon thickens and the inflammation spreads to the tendon itself, causing tendonitis. Continuous inflammation eventually may lead to tendinosis, a focal area of poorly organized fibrous tissue and degeneration that tends to weaken the tensile strength of the tendon. Complete or partial rupture of the Achilles tendon may be the eventual consequence of chronic overuse tendonitis. A common mechanism is an eccentric contraction of the gastrocnemius, overloading and exceeding the tensile capacity of the tendon. The stages of tendonitis can be differentiated histologically, but clinical differentiation may be difficult despite its importance in determining therapeutic options (43,45).

Most cases of Achilles tendonitis have a multifactorial cause, a combination of poor body mechanics, training errors (which allow fatigue in muscles that function in shock absorption), and other extrinsic factors resulting in malalignment of the hip, knee, ankle, or foot. One common extrinsic factor is the athletic shoe, which either does not sufficiently stabilize the hind foot, resulting in excessive varus or valgus rotation or excessive pronation, or does not provide sufficient shock-absorbing material. The exercise surface can also add to the stress placed on the Achilles tendon, such as a particularly firm surface with minimal absorbing capacity (46). Poor warm-up before exercise and abrupt changes in exercise intensity, frequency, or duration all can contribute to overload and stress on the tendon and result in inflammation (42).

In the earliest stage, the athlete notices pain in the Achilles area after strenuous activity. With continued training, the pain occurs during the activity, most often associated with running and jumping. Pain becomes localized to the inferior posterior calf. The athlete may sense weakness during activity (42). Morning stiffness occurs in some chronic cases.

Findings on physical examination can vary depending on the extent and duration of the inflammation. Decreased ankle dorsiflexion and tight hamstring muscles are common. Palpation of the tendon usually reveals tenderness in the area 2–6 cm above the insertion of the tendon on the calcaneus. If the inflammation includes paratendonitis, a more focal area of tenderness and swelling is present near the calcaneus, which is fixed and thus will move as the ankle is flexed. The presence of a firm, thickened area, often nodular, indicates involvement of the tendon itself (43). Paratendonitis and tendinosis often occur simultaneously. Swelling and tenderness located between the tendon and the posterior edge of the calcaneus are characteristic of a retrocalcaneal bursitis, produced as the inflamed Achilles tendon impinges on the superior angle of the calcaneus (46).

Both MRI and ultrasound are used to evaluate the extent of Achilles tendon injuries. Ultrasound can quickly and easily demonstrate the extent of paratendon and tendon thickening and degeneration. MRI is more effective in determining the degree of tendon injury and degeneration, including the extent of a possible rupture, as well as any abnormalities in the surrounding tissues (46).

Conservative, noninvasive treatment is usually advocated initially, but the response can vary, probably related to the extent of tendon involvement and the duration of symptoms. The primary focus of conservative treatment is stretching and progressive resistance strengthening of calf muscles, while avoiding the inciting activity. The use of orthotics can be helpful, as can the correction of any existing limb malalignment. Heel wedges may help alleviate symptoms during daily activities, but their use should be closely monitored: regular use without any rehabilitation program may contribute to further tendon contracture and inflexibility (46). Injection of corticosteroid is not advised, because the Achilles tendon is not covered with a true sheath and thus there is a high risk of intratendinous injury and subsequent rupture. In some cases, the use of a splint or cast for a short period of time is helpful to minimize ongoing irritation. A short course of oral corticosteroids often can control acute symptoms so that the rehabilitation program can progress. Once pain and tenderness have resolved and flexibility and strength have improved, athletes may gradually return to their previous activities.

Surgical intervention is sometimes an option if symptoms do not respond well to conservative management. The timing is controversial, however, ranging between 2 and 6 months (42,46). Chronic fibrotic paratendonitis is best managed with surgery; without surgery, symptoms always recur with resumption of activity owing to the irreversible tightness of the paratendon (47). In cases of chronic tendinosis, surgical release of the fibrotic posterior fascia and debridement of the areas of focal degeneration within the tendon are the usual procedures (46). Of note, on further exploration, many athletes diagnosed with chronic tendinosis are found to have partial tears that were not detected by MRI. In these cases the necrotic areas are excised and the tendon is repaired and reinforced. Up to 75% of athletes who undergo surgical intervention for chronic Achilles tendinosis unresponsive to conservative management return to high performance levels, and 90% of recreational athletes return to their previous level of activity (43).

Overuse and chronic tendinosis can ultimately result in the rupture of the Achilles tendon, partial or complete. Complete ruptures occur most often in middle-aged men participating in recreational sports. Elite athletes between 20 and 30 years of age are more susceptible to partial ruptures (42,45). The mechanism involves sudden eccentric loading of the Achilles tendon while the knee is extended and the ankle is flexed. The athlete may sense a "pop" in the calf, which is not always particularly painful, but he will not be able to continue the activity because of significant weakness and swelling due to hemorrhage and edema (42).

A palpable gap in the tendon at the site of rupture may be evident acutely, but after several hours the area tends to fill with a hematoma. The injured athlete usually has difficulty in performing a single-toe calf-raise due to profound weakness. It is important to remember that active plantar flexion is still possible with a complete rupture of the Achilles tendon, because the posterior tibialis, peroneals, and long toe flexor muscles are still intact. The most reliable indication of a complete rupture is a positive finding on Thompson's test. The Thompson test involves squeezing the posterior calf muscle of the involved leg while the athlete lies prone on the examining table with his feet off the edge of the table. The absence of plantar flexion with this maneuver indicates a discontinuity between the muscle and the foot (42). Both MRI and ultrasound can assist in confirming the presence of complete and partial ruptures.

Recent studies support the use of early surgical repair of ruptures; 75% of elite athletes and more than 90% of recreational athletes return to previous levels of athletic performance following surgery (45). Nonsurgical management is associated with a higher rate of re-rupture and a lower level of subsequent athletic performance. A fibrous band does form between the two ends of the tendon without surgery, but only 10–30% of athletes are able to return to previous levels of performance (42).

Medial Tibial Stress Syndrome (Shin Splints)

Medial tibial stress syndrome (MTSS) is exercise-induced pain along the anterior tibia, especially along the medial edge of the distal third of the tibia, commonly referred to as "shin splints." The pain may also radiate to the soft tissues posterior to the lateral edge of the tibia (48). The source of the pain in MTSS is still under debate. The most popular hypothesis is overuse resulting in inflammation along the insertion of the soleus at the posteromedial edge of the tibia. Periostitis beneath the posterior tibialis muscle also seems to contribute to symptoms (49). MTSS is estimated to occur in up to 10% of athletes. Runners (especially sprinters and hurdlers), basketball players, and athletes in ballistic sports seem to be the most susceptible (50).

The pain of MTSS, most commonly bilateral, is exacerbated by exercise and, initially, resolves with rest. If the athlete continues the inciting activity, the pain can become persistent and occur even with walking. On physical examination, tenderness is commonly detected along the edge of the distal tibia, occasionally associated with mild swelling. The neurological examination is normal, and passive movement of the foot and ankle does not elicit pain. Plain radiographs also reveal no abnormality. The differential diagnosis includes stress fracture and medial compartment syndrome (see below). A triple-phase bone scan can be helpful; this has three consecutive phases: angiogram, blood pool, and delayed image (or delayed uptake). Findings are normal in chronic compartment syndrome, abnormal in all three phases in stress fractures, and abnormal only in the delayed-uptake phase in MTSS (48). MRI is even more specific and just as sensitive and allows visualization of surrounding soft tissues.

Various treatments have been used, and the results seem contradictory. The success of conservative management most often depends on the duration of the symptoms. Symptoms of MTSS associated with a newly initiated training program often resolve with a short period of rest followed by gradual return to activity. A regular warm-up program with stretching is also useful. Symptoms present for more than 3 months require a longer period of rest from the inciting activity. A cross-training program will help the athlete maintain cardiovascular fitness, and participation in the original activity at a lower level of intensity is allowed, as long as symptoms do not recur. Biomechanical evaluation for excessive pronation and abnormal subtalar mobility, which can be corrected by custom orthotics, is also useful. Bracing and local corticosteroid injections have not been shown to be particularly useful. Return to activities should be gradual to prevent recurrence (49).

Some athletes experience chronic MTSS. If symptoms do not improve with conservative management, surgery may be considered: posteromedial fasciotomy with release of the fascial bridge of the soleus muscle and the fascia of the deep posterior compartment (49). This procedure generally improves symptoms, but athletes' level of sports performance after the procedure and rehabilitation is variable (50).

Compartment Syndromes

Many muscle groups are covered by a common fascia, to form what are referred to as "compartments." With intense exercise, the intracompartment pressure increases as intracellular and extracellular fluid accumulates. If the surrounding fascia is noncompliant, the increased intracompartment pressure leads to an increased venous pressure, which may cause ischemia of the compartment tissues. The resulting pain and weakness of the muscle group, or compartment syndrome, is reversible. If any nerves within the compartment are compressed, dysesthesias may result (49,51).

Compartment syndrome can occur in the upper and lower extremities, but in athletes it most commonly involves the anterior compartment of the calf, which is divided into four compartments. The anterior compartment is bordered posteriorly by the interosseous membrane, medially by the tibia, laterally by the intramuscular septum, and superficially by the crural fascia. It contains the anterior tibialis, extensor hallucis longus, and extensor digitorum muscles and the deep peroneal nerve. Athletes with anterior compartment syndrome experience an aching or cramping pain in the anterolateral lower leg, during or immediately after exercise. Chronic anterior compartment syndrome occurs repeatedly, usually after a certain distance or period of time. Runners account for more than 70% of athletes with chronic anterior compartment syndrome (50). During the earliest stages, the symptoms resolve completely with rest, but if the athlete continues to train, the symptoms persist during rest. Compression of the peroneal nerve will cause numbness between the 1st and 2d toes. Symptoms are often bilateral (49,51).

Diagnosis can be elusive, due to the lack of findings on physical examination, especially if the athlete was not exercising immediately prior to the exam. The best time for the physical exam is when the athlete is experiencing symptoms. A palpable fullness and tenderness may be present over the anterolateral leg (51). Distal pulses are normal, even while symptoms are present. Radiographic findings are normal, and a bone scan helps to rule out MTSS (shin splints) and stress fractures. Referred pain from a herniated disc should also be considered in the differential diagnosis. Normal MRI and bone-scan results often make diagnosis difficult.

Definitive diagnosis is made by measuring the pressure of the compartment before, during, and after exercise (which has induced symptoms). Both invasive and noninvasive devices are available to determine compartment pressure. In chronic compartment syndrome, pre-exercise pressures are greater than 15 mm Hg, increasing to more than 30 mm Hg 1 minute after the exercise associated with symptoms has ceased. Levels greater than 15 mm Hg usually persist for 5 minutes after exercise. Some physicians make the diagnosis based on one measurement of compartment pressure in a symptomatic athlete immediately following exercise (51). The documentation of at least one compartment pressure is important, especially if the symptoms persist despite conservative management.

Initial management is rest and avoidance of any activity associated with symptoms. After 4–6 weeks, the athlete may gradually advance activity level. Return to the previous level of performance may require several weeks, but more likely, symptoms will recur at a certain level of duration or intensity (51). A second period of rest from activity and gradual advancement should be attempted, but failure to reach the previous level of performance is likely. In these cases, the goals of the athlete need to be seriously reconsidered. If she is comfortable limiting activity to tolerable levels, then further intervention is not necessary. Most athletes, however, are not satisfied with the limitation of activity and opt for surgical intervention. Surgery for chronic compartment syndrome is a decompression procedure with fasciotomy. More than 90% of athletes who undergo surgical treatment experience some improvement and often complete resolution of their symptoms (49). Despite resolution of pain with surgery, a fasciotomy may result in up to 20% loss of strength. A stress fracture should always be considered in the differential diagnosis of lower-extremity pain with exercise (see below).

Plantar Fasciitis

The plantar fascia originates as a thick and narrow band from the medial tubercle of the calcaneus and spreads out distally along the sole of the foot. It becomes thinner and wider as it extends distally and divides into five branches, each of which then inserts onto one toe (52). The plantar fascia provides static support for the longitudinal arch, often described as a "bowstring" on the sole of the foot. Repetitive and excessive loads can lead to microtears and inflammation, referred to as plantar fasciitis. Certain conditions, such as pes planus (flat feet), pes cavus (high arches), limited subtalar motion, inadequate dorsiflexion (usually associated with a tight Achilles tendon), and weakness of the plantar flexor muscles, can alter the biomechanics of normal gait, thus increasing the tensile stress on the plantar fascia. These stress factors are compounded by the forces incurred by running, jumping, sudden changes in training programs, or poor shoe support (52).

Plantar fasciitis is characterized by the gradual onset of heel pain where the plantar fascia inserts onto the calcaneus. The sensation of burning or aching in the heel area is common and often radiates to the arch. The athlete typically describes a worsening of the pain in the morning, which then resolves after warming up. After the initial improvement during the morning, however, the pain recurs or increases with activity during the day, especially on exercise. Runners may be able to run through the discomfort during the early stages, but if training continues, the pain will intensify and become chronic, eventually preventing prolonged running or weight-bearing activities (53). If the symptoms become severe, the athlete may begin to walk on the ball of the foot in an attempt to minimize discomfort (52).

On physical examination, tenderness is evident at the insertion of the plantar fascia on the medial calcaneal tubercle. The pain may extend distally toward the longitudinal arch. Branches of the medial calcaneal nerve that serve to innervate the heel pad and periosteum of the calcaneal tubercle may become impinged and result in heel pain, but the area of tenderness from fasciitis is located on the medial heel pad, just proximal to the insertion of the plantar fascia (52). Of note, inflammation from the fasciitis may also irritate these nerves, causing tenderness in the heel fat pad as well. Swelling is occasionally present. In chronic cases, a nodule of fibrotic tissue may be palpable just distal to the calcaneal tubercle. Passive dorsiflexion, eversion of the foot, and extension of the 1st toe, maneuvers that stretch the plantar fascia, usually exacerbate symptoms (52,53).

Routine radiographs may reveal a calcaneal spur, especially if the fasciitis is chronic. The clinical significance of a calcaneal bone spur is a controversial topic. Calcaneal spurs have been demonstrated in asymptomatic individuals, with an estimated prevalence of 20% in the general population. On the other hand, incidental heel spurs found on x-ray were symptomatic in 10% of random patients. Additionally, 50% of patients complaining of heel pain, not necessarily due to plantar fasciitis, were found to have a heel spur on x-ray (53). Therefore, whether a heel spur is the cause or the result of plantar fasciitis is still unclear. Given the uncertainty regarding the significance of heel spurs, their surgical removal is not advocated as strongly as in the past. A bone scan or MRI can be useful to exclude a stress fracture of the os calcis of the calcaneus, which can be misdiagnosed as plantar fasciitis. An MRI can very precisely define the extent and severity of the fasciitis and determine whether any fascial tear exists. The triple-phase bone scan in cases of plantar fasciitis demonstrates uptake at the medial calcaneal tubercle in both the blood-pool and delayed-uptake phases, most likely due to local inflammation at the origin that extends into the periosteum of the calcaneus (52).

Initial treatment, as in all overuse syndromes, includes ceasing the inciting activity and taking NSAIDs for control of inflammation. The only rehabilitation modality shown to be beneficial is careful instruction in proper stretching of the plantar fascia and encouragement to stretch it regularly in association with an Achilles tendon stretch. The best stretching technique is to lean forward against a wall while keeping the feet flat on the floor and flex the knees. The amount of stretch is determined by the distance from the wall. Ultrasound applied before the stretch can help by raising the temperature of the tissue. Use of heel cups to absorb some impact by dispersing it over a larger surface is not considered beneficial for most affected individuals, although many athletes do like the soft surface offered by the newer gel heel pads. Orthotics for correction of biomechanical abnormalities are particularly helpful for most athletes. Repetitive running up steep hills has been associated with the development of plantar fasciitis and should be avoided, especially during the return to activity.

More chronic symptoms sometimes respond to a corticosteroid injection into the origin of the fascia; however, as with all local steroid injections near connective tissue, the risk of rupture increases for a few weeks. Avoidance of exercise is advised during this period, for at least 3 or 4 weeks. Even more risky is a second injection, which should be performed only in particularly refractory cases; not only does the risk of rupture increase but the heel fat pad may atrophy, further complicating the case (52). These risks are reduced (but not eliminated) with the use of short-acting soluble steroids such as dexamethasone. A rigid splint that holds the foot in a neutral position, worn during the night, is another means of passively stretching the plantar fascia. Heel wedges may eventually be added to hold the foot at a small angle of dorsiflexion to further stretch the fascia. Early diagnosis and aggressive stretching improve the long-term prognosis. Athletes should be aware that recovery is often a slow process, especially in chronic cases, and may take up to a year (53).

Given the slow recovery, surgical treatment generally should not be considered unless the athlete has tried at least 6–8 months of conservative treatment or a partial tear is not responding to treatment. Various surgical techniques exist, and consensus on the best technique is not uniform. The most common procedure is a fasciotomy and release of the fascial origin. Excision of a calcaneal spur, if present, is often performed as well. More recently, the involvement of branches of the medial calcaneal nerves has gained wider recognition, and decompression is advocated if any such involvement is suspected. The athlete usually can return to activity 3 months after surgery (52).

The acute onset of pain on the sole of the foot may indicate a partial or complete tear of the plantar fascia. Tears of the fascia often follow a sudden movement of the foot while planted in dorsiflexion, such as in running or jumping. Of note, the fibrosis and degeneration that accompany chronic fasciitis predispose the athlete to rupture or tear of the weakened tissue, especially at the origin on the calcaneus. Physical examination typically reveals tenderness of the sole and localized swelling at the site of the tear. A loss of the rigid fibrous band on the sole of the affected foot is evident when the examiner compares it with the opposite foot. Initially, the athlete should avoid weight bearing, apply ice locally, and take NSAIDs to control inflammation and swelling. Partial weight bearing with the use of a walking boot for 4–6 weeks allows faster healing; return to activities should be gradual and dictated by pain tolerance (53).

Tarsal Tunnel Syndrome

Tarsal tunnel syndrome (TTS) may be mistaken for plantar fasciitis, especially since the incidence of TTS has increased with the growing popularity of running. The tibial nerve passes through the tarsal tunnel, a fibro-osseous tunnel located posterior to the medial malleus of the ankle (figure 8.2). The roof of the tunnel is formed by the flexor retinaculum, a fibrous band of tissue up to 10 cm wide, extending from the medial malleolus to the calcaneus and abductor hallucis muscle. The tibial nerve passes through the inelastic tunnel and branches into the medial calcaneal and medial and lateral plantar nerves at the distal end of the tunnel. Compression of the tibial nerve or its branches due to any inflammation within the tunnel may produce symptoms (54).

The etiology of TTS in athletes, primarily runners, seems to vary. Abnormal biomechanics are considered to be a major contributing factor. Excessive pronation or a valgus deformity of the foot, compounded by the repetitive stress of running, especially without sufficient support, may stretch the tibial or medial calcaneal nerves. Inflammation (tendonitis) of the abductor hallucis longus muscle tendon secondary to repetitive stress or stretching resulting from malalignment may lead to dynamic compression of the tibial nerve and subsequent symptoms (55).

Symptoms of TTS occur in the same area as plantar fasciitis, which

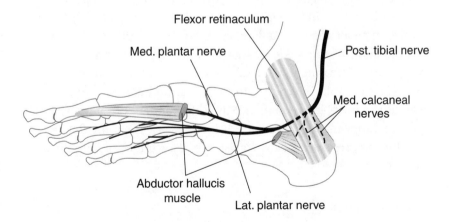

Figure 8.2. Medial View of the Ankle, Showing the Flexor Retinaculum and Posterior Tibial Nerve. The tibial nerve travels through the tarsal tunnel.

probably explains the common confusion between the two syndromes. Initially, the athlete with TTS begins to experience paresthesias, burning or loss of sensation, around the medial malleolus, heel, or sole of the foot. The discomfort is more often located in the medial arch of the sole rather than the heel, as in plantar fasciitis. It may also radiate proximally to the calf. Flexion of the 1st toe may be weakened. During the initial stages, symptoms of TTS arise at the start of exercise such as running and improve as the exercise continues. As training continues, the pain becomes chronic, even at rest, and worsens with exercise. The pain tends to be less in the morning, increasing during the day, as opposed to plantar fasciitis, in which pain is worse in the morning (54,55).

The physical examination is helpful. The athlete often cannot localize the pain, which may reflect early loss of two-point discrimination. The discomfort can be reproduced by passive dorsiflexion and eversion of the foot. Tapping over the tarsal tunnel posterior to the medial malleolus can reproduce the discomfort or induce shooting pain or tingling (Tinel's sign) (54). Valleix's sign, tenderness to palpation either distal or proximal to the point of nerve entrapment, is not present as often as Tinel's sign (56). The diagnosis of TTS is confirmed by an EMG study to evaluate both motor and sensory nerves of the foot and leg. The EMG must include the medial and lateral plantar nerves. Denervation potentials should be present only in the distribution of the tibial nerve distal to the flexor retinaculum in order to diagnose TTS (55). The use of MRI to demonstrate the soft tissues of the ankle is gaining in popularity and can add critical information about anatomy and inflammation within the tarsal tunnel.

Evaluation of the ankle or foot for malalignment is an important component of treatment, which should also include rest and NSAIDs. A local corticosteroid injection into the tarsal tunnel may also be quite helpful to control inflammation. Surgical treatment can be considered if conservative management fails. It involves release of the flexor retinaculum and resection of any connective tissue bridges within the tunnel (54,55).

GROIN INJURIES

Groin injuries compose approximately 2–5% of all sports injuries (57). The affected muscle groups include the hip abductors and flexors and the trunk flexors and rotators. The tenuous nature of the abdominal muscles seems to predispose them to injury. The internal and external oblique muscles function in trunk rotation. Both insert diffusely along the iliac crest bilaterally, but only the internal oblique inserts directly into the inguinal ligament and thus the pubis. The external oblique muscle inserts as an aponeurosis to the linea alba rather than directly onto the pubis (58). The rectus abdominis, a major trunk flexor, extends from the xiphoid and costal cartilage of ribs 5 through 7 to insert directly onto the pubic symphysis and also expands to join the inguinal ligament. Because the abdominal muscles join to form the cremaster and external and internal spermatic fascia, strains of these muscles may appear as scrotal pain (58).

Strains of the abdominal muscles most often occur in athletes in racquet or throwing sports. The trunk is initially extended and rotated to create potential energy, and as the athlete follows through on the stroke or throw, the rectus abdominis flexes the trunk and the contralateral internal and external oblique muscles counter the rotation. This movement must be synchronized and smooth. Any asynchrony of the relaxation and activation of the involved muscles or sudden halt of the motion can result in the muscle flexing against a force of momentum and ultimately lead to a strain or partial or complete tear of the muscle (58).

The hip adductor muscles include the adductor longus, magnus, and brevis and the gracilis and pectineus. The adductor longus is the most likely muscle of the adductor group to be injured athletically. In some individuals, the tendon of the adductor longus muscle may be particularly short or the muscle may insert directly onto the pubic bone, thus increasing the risk of strain (58). The rectus femoris, one of the primary hip flexors, is also commonly injured but seems to be susceptible more to rupture than to strain. A strain of any of these muscles can also result in groin pain (59).

Knowing the mechanism of injury, as well as the activity that tends to enhance discomfort, is helpful in making the diagnosis. Strains involving the abdominal muscles tend to be exacerbated by coughing or sneezing and performing sit-ups. Strains of the adductors or flexors of the hip can be associated with limited range of motion of the hip and increased pain with resisted flexion of the affected muscle. Passive stretching of the muscle can also be uncomfortable. The physician should perform a full neuromuscular examination, since groin pain may result from a herniated disc.

Non-musculoskeletal causes of groin pain should always be considered. Inguinal and femoral hernias, testicular torsion, and epididymitis are not uncommon in young males and should be ruled out, either by clinical exam or by further testing if any suspicion exists. Pathology involving the hip joint may also present as groin pain. Acute arthritis or synovitis, slipped epiphysis, and Perthes disease should be considered in the proper clinical setting. Plain radiographs may help rule out these diagnoses or may reveal an avulsion fracture, which can accompany a groin muscle injury. A bone scan or MRI can be useful to rule out a stress fracture of the inferior ramus of the pubic bone or the femoral neck as well as osteitis pubis (inflammation of the symphysis pubis; see below).

Magnetic resonance imaging can be useful in determining the extent of soft tissue injury, including any possible ruptures. Local inflammation and edema resulting from microruptures (strains) show up as high-intensity signals on T2-weighted or fat-suppression images (60). Disruption of the muscle fibers or tendon in partial or complete ruptures is easily visualized and is also associated with fluid accumulation. Ultrasound is another diagnostic test that has gained popularity, due to the ease and availability of studies and the ability to compare the affected side with the contralateral side. Locating the exact site of discomfort is also easier and results are available sooner. New linear high-resolution probes have advanced the sensitivity of ultrasound findings. Tendon injuries and tears are easily demonstrated as hypoechoic regions with possible disruption of fibers (61). Muscle injuries have a similar appearance but may also show a local area of hematoma (62).

Acute treatment for groin strains includes avoidance of any pain-producing activity for at least 24–48 hours. The athlete may need crutches initially for mobilization. Local ice and NSAIDs help minimize inflammation. Rehabilitation begins with passive stretching, eventually followed by a strengthening program. Avoidance of the inciting activity for at least a week is essential. The athlete must not return to the inciting activity too soon (before full range of motion and total strength and coordination have been restored), since re-injury can lead to longer rehabilitation and chronic pain. Treatment is primarily conservative, and surgery is rarely considered (59).

Osteitis pubis is another cause of groin pain in athletes that is gaining wider recognition. It is a noninfectious inflammation of the pubic symphysis resulting from stress overload of the pelvis; it may extend to the perichondrium and periosteum (63). It tends to occur in athletes in kicking and running sports, such as soccer, ice hockey, football, and rugby. The pubic symphysis is an amphiarthrodial joint, not lined with a synovium, located between the two pubic bones. Biomechanically, the pelvis allows the transfer of the weight of the trunk from the sacrum to the hips. The pubic symphysis connects the two weight-bearing arches of the pelvic rim. Osteitis pubis is thought to be related to a shearing stress at the symphysis secondary to repeated kicking or running (63–65). Osteonecrosis of the symphysis pubis may also play a role (63).

The athlete experiences a gradual onset of aching and vague discomfort in the anterior pubic area, which may radiate to the groin and possibly the perineum (63,66). Physical activity, especially kicking and one-legged pivoting, exacerbates the pain. Rest relieves the discomfort to some degree. During pelvic movement, such as walking on an uneven surface or rising from sitting, the athlete may feel a "click" in the pubic area (63). The pain may be severe enough to cause him to walk with a waddling gait in an attempt to minimize the stress on the pubic symphysis.

The pubic symphysis is tender to palpation in more than 70% of cases of osteitis pubis (67). The inner aspect of the symphysis tends to be exquisitely tender on palpation, which is performed rectally or vaginally (63). Pain may limit abduction or rotation of the hips. Pain may also be elicited by applying pressure to the iliac wing while the athlete is in the lateral decubitus position, often called the lateral compression test. Although it is nonspecific, this test is positive in almost 50% of affected athletes (68). The "cross leg test," in which the examiner presses against the iliac wing while stressing the ipsilateral crossed extremity, may also elicit pain in the pubic area.

Plain radiographs are usually unremarkable during the early stages of osteitis pubis (63), but after several months may begin to show fraying of the pubic periosteum, widening of the symphysis due to erosions, and subarticular sclerosis (69). A bone scan may demonstrate increased uptake at the symphysis and pubic bones, often before changes are evident on x-ray. Notably, the uptake is symmetric, unlike the bone-scan findings in a pelvic stress fracture, tumors, tendonitis, and strains (70). MRI shows disruption of the cartilage, periosteum, and possibly the bone (63).

When the diagnosis of osteitis pubis has been made, treatment should be aggressive. Strengthening and stretching of the hip rotators, flexors, and adductors is an important component of rehabilitation. Cross-training activity such as swimming, pool running, or cycling is permitted, as tolerated. Kicking and running should be avoided. NSAIDs may help, but intra-articular corticosteroid injections have not proved particularly useful (66,67). A significant majority of athletes respond well to rehabilitation and conservative treatment. A wedge resection of the pubic symphysis that leaves the anterior and posterior ligament intact has relieved symptoms in patients who have failed to respond to conservative management. Athletes are able to resume all activities after surgery, probably because the symphysis plays only a small role in overall pelvic stability (68). Pathological examination of the affected tissue removed during surgery has not been helpful in determining the etiology of osteitis pubis, showing only fibrosis and chronic inflammation (63,68).

Other musculoskeletal causes of groin pain in athletes include pelvic stress fractures and gracilis syndrome. Pelvic stress fractures involving the pubic ramus make up only a small percentage of all stress fractures in athletes, but should be ruled out in an athlete with asymmetric groin pain. Female runners are most often affected; they describe a gradual onset of groin and thigh pain and significant discomfort while standing and supporting full weight on the leg on the ipsilateral side of the stress fracture (71). Palpation of the affected pelvic ramus usually reveals significant tenderness. Plain radiographs often have normal findings in the initial stages, and diagnosis is aided by a bone scan demonstrating increased uptake over the affected pubic ramus.

Pelvic stress fractures differ from other stress fractures. They tend to occur after a long-distance run (such as a marathon) or with intensification of a training schedule, rather than with initiation of running after a long period of inactivity or a change in running surface or training equipment, as with other stress fractures. A stress fracture of the pelvis in a single area rather than in combination with a contralateral fracture, as is typical in pelvic fractures resulting from trauma (due to the ring-like structure of the pelvis), suggests a response to tensile stress rather than a compressive force. The tensile stress is most likely delivered by the muscles on the lateral aspect of the ramus and ischium during hip extension (69). The higher incidence of pelvic stress fractures in female athletes cannot easily be explained by biomechanical differences between men and women. Osteoporosis may play a role, but this is not a consistent finding. Other factors, such as gender differences in gait, may play a role (69). Treatment of a pelvic stress fracture is similar to that for other stress fractures: rest and avoidance of pain-inducing activities. Non-union may result if the athlete continues to train.

The gracilis syndrome has recently been recognized as a separate entity from osteitis pubis; it is an avulsion fracture at the origin of the gracilis muscle on the lower half of the symphysis pubis. This is considered to be an overuse syndrome, related to the repetitive force inflicted by the gracilis muscle at the pubic symphysis during activities such as kicking, but it may also result from a single traumatic event. Detection of a small bone fragment or an irregular area at the lower margin of the pubis or asymmetric uptake in a bone scan can help differentiate the syndrome from osteitis pubis. Treatment is conservative, with rest. The rare associated chronic pain often resolves with surgical removal of the bone fragment (70).

STRESS FRACTURES

Stress fractures are overuse injuries of bone. Repetitive nonviolent force from exercise, usually overtraining, can produce microfractures in trabecular bone, which, if not allowed to repair, can culminate in a partial or complete fracture of the bone (72). Stress fractures tend to occur in the lower extremities and are most often associated with running. A stress fracture should always be included in the differential diagnosis of continuous focal pain in an athlete.

In addition to facilitating movement and providing strength, muscles also function as shock absorbers, absorbing energy when loaded and gradually transmitting it to the bone. With prolonged exercise, as muscle fatigues and its capacity to absorb energy diminishes, impact forces are transmitted directly to the bone. According to one hypothesis, this results in increased stress and microfractures at focal areas; if these are not allowed to heal, a stress fracture forms (73). A less accepted hypothesis attributes stress fractures to the dynamic force of muscles on the bone: the repetitive pull of contracting muscle on the bone may create microfractures. The occurrence of stress fractures in non-weight-bearing bones is the strongest argument for this hypothesis (73,74). Both mechanisms may play a role to some extent.

Several extrinsic factors are associated with stress fractures, but the most important is the training regimen. A rapid increase in either the mileage or the intensity of workouts in a set unit of time correlates directly with an increased incidence of stress fractures (75). Other risk factors include malalignment of the lower extremities, abrupt changes in running surface, and poorly absorbent shoes or running surfaces (72). The incidence of stress fractures is up to 12 times higher in female than in male athletes under similar training conditions. Multiple explanations for this discrepancy have been proposed, such as gait, diminished cortical bone thickness, and different biomechanics due to a wider pelvis in females (72). The high incidence of amenorrhea in female athletes, especially long-distance runners, and the secondary osteoporosis are contributing factors to some degree. With the diagnosis of a stress fracture, the physician should conduct a complete evaluation of all possible contributing factors, including training habits, athletic technique, biomechanics, and menstrual function (72).

Diagnosis of a stress fracture is not always easy. The affected athlete characteristically experiences a gradual onset of localized pain. In the earlier stages, she notices pain after activity, usually running, but if training continues she also experiences pain during activity, which eventually limits her tolerance of exercise (76). Findings on the physical exam are often unremarkable but may reveal localized tenderness and swelling in the later stages.

Plain radiographs show no abnormalities in the early stages in almost 60% of cases, and only half of affected individuals ever develop any radiographic change related to the fracture, even after healing. Periosteal new bone formation, endosteal thickening, and a radiolucent line are all consistent with a stress fracture (72). A bone scan is considered the most sensitive imaging technique for diagnosis of a stress fracture, particularly early in the course of the injury. Bone scans are capable of detecting small areas of new bone formation and can reflect the area of accelerated bone turnover stimulated by the microfractures. Bone scans may also help determine the age of the stress fracture. During the earlier stages the scan reveals diffuse uptake in the region of the stress reaction, but as the fracture advances, a more fusiform area of uptake is evident (76).

A bone scan, especially a triple-phase scan, is also very helpful in differentiating a stress fracture from common soft tissue overuse injuries. Shin splints, which can be a cause of pain in the anterior shin, show uptake only in the delayed-image phase, whereas a stress fracture shows uptake in all three phases. Other soft tissue disorders, such as plantar fasciitis, also have characteristic patterns on bone scan (76).

Stress fractures can occur in any bone, the location and incidence depending on the particular sport. Running is associated with a significantly higher incidence of stress fractures, close to 70% of all stress fractures in athletes in one study (76). Other activities associated, though less frequently, with stress fractures include basketball, dancing, and racquet sports. A significant majority of stress fractures involve the lower extremities.

Although not the most common, a stress fracture of the head of the femur is one of the most serious locations. The athlete's symptoms are somewhat vague and nonspecific, often groin pain and painful motion of the hip. Because the microfractures occur perpendicular to the lines of stress and tensile forces, displacement is a major complication. The risk of avascular necrosis, non-union, and malunion is high if the diagnosis is delayed, so the physician must always have a high index of suspicion. Often the preferred treatment is internal fixation with multiple threaded pins, whether or not displacement has occurred (76).

The tibia, fibula, and metatarsals are more commonly affected in runners. Almost half of all stress fractures in runners involve the distal third of shaft of the tibia (76). Most of these fractures heal well with treatment. Activities that involve jumping, such as basketball and ballet, may be associated with stress fractures of the anterior midshaft of the tibia. These stress fractures have a higher incidence of complications, such as delayed union or complete fracture, and may require a bone graft to allow complete healing. The pathogenesis of the higher complication rate is not clear but may be related to the poor vascularity of the tibial cortex.

Stress fractures of the tarsal navicular bone are not common; they tend to occur in basketball players. The diagnosis must be made as early as possible in order to avoid complications and chronic disability. The relatively avascular central core of the tarsal navicular bone places it at a higher risk for avascular necrosis. The athlete may experience only mild discomfort, but it is insidious and unrelenting. Tenderness may be found over the tarsal navicular bone, and dorsiflexion and subtalar motion may be present. The preferred treatment is immediate cast immobilization and non–weight bearing for 6–8 weeks (73). A stress fracture of the proximal 5th metatarsal (Jones fracture) is another uncommon stress fracture encountered in both football and basketball players, which also has a higher rate of complications due to malunion or nonunion. Again, poor local blood supply most likely plays a key role in complications from a stress fracture. Early bone scan is advocated for any athlete with pain in either of these areas to rule out a potential stress fracture. Prolonged immobilization to prevent non-union is advised but not always successful. A high incidence of re-fracture with nonoperative treatment has been reported (73).

The proper management of stress fractures depends upon the location, duration, and associated activities. Conservative treatment is appropriate and successful with early diagnosis. Initial management involves the use of NSAIDs and physical therapy focusing on stretching and flexibility. The athlete should avoid the inciting activity and sport, but weight bearing as tolerated during daily activity is permitted. After 2 or 3 weeks, once the athlete is pain-free at rest, she is allowed to return gradually to the previous activity, possibly starting every other day. Progress in rehabilitation is measured by the amount of pain associated with the current level of activity, which determines whether advancement to a higher level or a period of rest is needed (72). The rehabilitation may be long and frustrating, and if the athlete's compliance is a problem, immobilization with a cast might be considered. In general, good cardiovascular conditioning can be maintained with non-weight-bearing cross-training, at first swimming or pool running, then bicycling.

REFERENCES

1. Keifhaber T, Stern P: Upper extremity tendonitis and overuse syndromes in the athlete. Clin Sports Med 11:39, 1992

2. Renstrom P, Johnson R: Overuse injuries in sports. Sports Med 2:316, 1985

3. Hart L: Exercise and soft tissue injury. Baillieres Clin Rheumatol 8:137, 1994

4. Fu FH, Harner CD, Klein AH: Shoulder impingement syndrome. Clin Orthop 269:162–173, 1991

5. Neer CS II: Impingement lesions. Clin Orthop 173:70, 1983

6. Miniaci A, Fowler PJ: Impingement in the athlete. Clin Sports Med 12:91–111, 1993

7. Jobe FW, Kvitne RS: Shoulder pain in the overhand or throwing athlete: the relationship of anterior instability and rotator cuff impingement. Orthop Rev 18:963, 1989

8. Kibler WB, Chandler TJ: Functional scapular instability in throwing athletes. Paper presented at the American Orthopaedic Society for Sports Medicine 15th Annual Meeting, Traverse City, MI, June 19–22, 1989

9. Neer C: Anterior acromioplasty for chronic impingement syndrome in the shoulder. J Bone Joint Surg 54A:4, 1972

10. Jobe F, Bradley J: The diagnosis and non-operative treatment of shoulder injuries in the athlete. Clin Sports Med 8:419, 1989

11. Beach W, Caspari R: Arthroscopic management of rotator cuff disease. Orthopedics 6:1007, 1993

12. Bonutti P, Hawkins R: Rotator cuff disorders. Baillieres Clin Rheumatol 3:535, 1989

13. Kibler W: Pathophysiology of overload injury around the elbow. Sports Med 14:447, 1995

14. Roetert E, Brody H, Dillman C: The biomechanics of tennis elbow: an integrated approach. Clin Sports Med 14:47, 1995

15. Field L, Althcheck D: Elbow injuries. Clin Sports Med 14:59, 1995

16. Mattalino A, Deese J, Campbell E: Office evaluation and treatment of lower extremities in the runner. Clin Sports Med 8:461, 1989

17. Steindler A: Kinesiology of the Human Body. Springfield, IL, Charles C Thomas, 1955

18. Jacobson K, Flandry F: Diagnosis of anterior knee pain. Clin Sports Med 8:179, 1989

19. Fu FD, Maday MG: Arthroscopic lateral release and the lateral patellar compression syndrome. Orthop Clin North Am 23:601–612, 1992

20. Wertheimer C: Patello-femoral mechanics as a cause of anterior knee pain. Your Patient and Fitness 9:19, 1995

21. Fulkerson J: Evaluation of peripatellar soft tissue and retinaculum in patients with patello-femoral pain. Clin Sports Med 8:197, 1989

22. Galea A, Albers J: Patello-femoral pain. Physician and Sports Medicine 22(4):48, 1994

23. Kelly M, Insall J: Historical perspectives of chondromalacia patellae. Orthop Clin North Am 23:517, 1992

24. Host J, Craig R, Lehman R: Patello-femoral dysfunction in tennis players. Clin Sports Med 14:177, 1995

25. Rintala P: Patello-femoral pain syndrome and its treatment in runners. Athletic Training 25:2, 1990

26. Fulkerson J, Schutzer S: After failure of conservative treatment for painful patello-femoral malalignment: lateral release or realignment? Orthop Clin North Am 17:283, 1986

27. Nichols CE: Patellar tendon injuries. Clin Sports Med 11:807–813, 1992

28. Martens M, Wouters P, Burssens A, Muller JC: Patellar tendonitis: pathology and results of treatment. Acta Orthop Scand 53:445–450, 1982

29. Davies SG, Baudouin CJ, King JB, Perry JD: Ultrasound, computed tomography and magnetic resonance imaging in patellar tendonitis. Clin Radiol 43:52–56, 1991

30. Bodne D, Quinn SF, Murray WT, et al: Magnetic resonance images of chronic patellar tendonitis. Skeletal Radiol 17:24–28, 1988

31. Alexeeff M: Ligamentum patellae rupture following local steroid injection. Aust N Z J Surg 56:681–683, 1986

32. Orava S, Osterback L, Hurme M: Surgical treatment of patellar tendon pain in athletes. Br J Sports Med 20:167–169, 1986

33. Tindel NL, Nisonson B: The plica syndrome. Orthop Clin North Am 23:613–618, 1992

34. Hardaker WT, Whipple TL, Bassett FH: Diagnosis and treatment of the plica syndrome of the knee. J Bone Joint Surg 62A:211, 1980

35. Barber FA, Sutker AN: Iliotibial band syndrome. Sports Med 14:144–148, 1992

36. Ekman EF, Pope T, Martin DF, Curl WW: Magnetic resonance imaging of iliotibial band syndrome. Am J Sports Med 22:851–854, 1994

37. Messier SP, Edwards DG, Martin DF, et al: Etiology of iliotibial band friction syndrome in distance runners. Med Sci Sports Exerc 27:951–960, 1995

38. Pinshaw R, Atlas V, Noakes TD: The nature and response to therapy of 196 consecutive injuries seen at a runner's clinic. S Afr Med J 65:291–298, 1984

39. Sutker AN, Barber FA, Jackson DW, Pagle JW: Iliotibial band friction syndrome in distance runners. Sports 2:447–451, 1985

40. McKenzie DC, Clement DB, Tauton JE: Running shoes, orthotics, and injuries. Sports Med 2:334–347, 1985

41. Noble CA: The treatment of iliotibial band friction syndrome. Br J Sports Med 13:51–54, 1979

42. Soma C, Mandelbaum B: Achilles tendon disorders. Clin Sports Med 13:811, 1994

43. DeMaio M, Paine R, Drez D: Achilles tendonitis. Orthopedics 18:195, 1995

44. Scioli M: Achilles tendonitis. Orthop Clin North Am 25:177, 1994

45. Kvist M: Achilles tendon injuries in athletes. Sports Med 18:173, 1994

46. Galloway M, Jokl P, Dayton O: Achilles tendon overuse injuries. Clin Sports Med 11:771, 1992

47. Williams J: Achilles tendon lesions in sport. Sports Med 3:114, 1986

48. Barry NN, McGuire JL: Acute injuries and specific problems in adult athletes. Rheum Dis Clin North Am 22:531–549, 1996

49. Clanton T, Solcher B: Chronic leg pain in the athlete. Clin Sports Med 13:743, 1994

50. Detmer D: Chronic shin splints: classification and management of medial tibial stress syndrome. Sports Med 3:436, 1986

51. Black K, Taylor D: Current concepts in the treatment of common compartment syndrome in athletes. Sports Med 15:408, 1993

52. Karr S: Subcalcaneal heel pain. Orthop Clin North Am 25:161, 1994

53. Schepsis A, Leach R, Gorzyca J: Plantar fasciitis: etiology, treatment, surgical results and review of literature. Clin Orthop 266:185, 1991

54. Jackson D, Haglund B: Tarsal tunnel syndrome in runners. Sports Med 13:146, 1992

55. Jackson D, Haglund B: Tarsal tunnel syndrome in athletes. Am J Sports Med 19:61, 1991

56. Edwards W, Lincoln C, Bassett F, et al: The tarsal tunnel syndrome: diagnosis and treatment. JAMA 207:77, 1969

57. Estwanik JJ, Sloane B, Rosenberg MA. Groin strain and other possible causes of groin pain. Physician and Sportsmedicine 18:59–65, 1990

58. Balduini FC: Abdominal and groin injuries in tennis. Clin Sports Med 7(2):349–357, 1988

59. Karlsson J, Sward L, Kalebo P, Thomee R: Chronic groin injuries in athletes. Sports Med 17:141–148, 1994

60. Speer K, Lohnes J, Garrett W: Radiographic imaging of muscle strain injury. Am J Sports Med 21:89–96, 1993

61. Kalebo P, Karlsson J, Sward L, Peterson L: Ultrasonography of chronic tendon injuries in the groin. Am J Sports Med 20:634–639, 1992

62. Van Holsbeek M, Introcaso J: Musculoskeletal ultrasonography. Radiol Clin North Am 30:907–925, 1992

63. Middleton R, Carlile R: The spectrum of osteitis pubis. Compr Ther 19:99, 1993

64. Harris N, Murray R: Lesions of the symphysis pubis in athletes. Br Med J 4:211, 1974

65. Gamble J, Simmons S, Freedman M: The symphysis pubis: anatomic and pathologic considerations. Clin Orthop 203:261–272, 1986

66. Fricker P, Taunton J, Ammann W: Osteitis pubis in athletes: infection, inflammation, or injury? Sports Med 12:266, 1991

67. Vincent C: Osteitis pubis. J Am Board Fam Pract 6:492, 1993

68. Grace J, Sim F: Wedge resection of the symphysis pubis for the treatment of osteitis pubis. J Bone Joint Surg 71A:358, 1989

69. Pavlov H, Nelson T, Warren R, et al: Stress fractures of the pubic ramus. J Bone Joint Surg 64A:1020, 1982

70. Wiley J: Traumatic osteitis pubis: the gracilis syndrome. Am J Sports Med 11:360, 1983

71. Noakes T, Smith J, Lindenberg G, et al: Pelvic stress fractures in long distance runners. Am J Sports Med 13:11, 1982

72. Sallis RE, Jones K: Stress fractures in athletes. Postgrad Med 89:185, 1991

73. Meyer SA, et al: Stress fractures of the foot and leg. Clin Sports Med 12:395, 1993

74. Matheson GO, Clement DB, McKenzie DC, et al: Stress fractures in athletes. Am J Sports Med 15:46, 1987

75. Paty J: Diagnosis and treatment of musculoskeletal running injuries. Semin Arthritis Rheum 18:48, 1988

76. Hershman EB, Mailly T: Stress fractures. Clin Sports Med 9:183, 1990

Chapter 9

THE OLDER AND
YOUNGER ATHLETE

OLDER ATHLETES

The number of athletes over the age of 45 has increased dramatically in the past twenty-five years. Many of these athletes have been exercising, often running, since the exercise boom of the 1970s. As increasing numbers of studies demonstrate the multiple benefits of exercise, regardless of the age at which the person begins, more individuals are embarking on regular exercise later in life (1).

Many organ systems undergo changes with age, a process that was once thought to occur at a fixed, unalterable rate. The cardiovascular system functionally declines as maximal heart rate, stroke volume, and cardiac output decline, and blood pressure increases. The Vo_{2max} decreases also, and vital lung capacity and expiratory flow diminish. Some studies have estimated that a normal adult loses 10% of aerobic power with each decade after the age of 30 (2). Motor response, proprioception, and balance also decrease, as do the average strength and flexibility of muscles. Some of these changes seem to be potentiated by medications that older athletes may require for various health problems.

The concept of an unavoidable and irreversible aging process has recently been challenged. Many studies have demonstrated that regular aerobic exercise can minimize, if not prevent, the decrease in aerobic power shown in earlier studies (3). The gain in aerobic power is probably related to the intensity and duration of training. Exercise performed regularly helps athletes to avoid weight gain and to lower their blood pressure and cholesterol levels, improve glucose tolerance, and minimize the risk of osteoporosis (2). The risk of cardiovascular disease is also minimized, because exercise contributes to a lower hematocrit, low fibrinogen, normal platelets, and brisk fibrinolysis. Athletes who continue to exercise into their later years have a 23% lower risk of death and cardiac-related causes of death than their inactive age-matched peers. The so-called aging process may actually be the result of inactivity (2).

Everyone should be encouraged to participate in regular aerobic exercise, regardless of age. Before beginning a new exercise program, individuals should have a screening exam similar to the athlete's preparticipation exam. The exam should include a detailed medical history; a review of systems, specifically including risk factors for cardiac disease; and an exploration of previous difficulties during exercise or problems with imbalance and gait. The recommended contraindications to beginning an exercise program include the following:

–severe coronary disease
–decompensated congestive heart failure
–uncontrolled atrial arrhythmia
–severe valvular heart disease
–uncontrolled hypertension
–severe cardiomyopathy
–acute myocarditis or infectious illness with fever
–recent pulmonary embolism or deep venous thrombosis (2)

Medications need to be reviewed and discussed in detail. Hypnotics, tranquilizers, and antihistamines may alter mentation and blunt response time or may contribute to orthostatic hypotension (2). Certain antihypertensives may decrease performance or exercise tolerance. Diuretics significantly increase the risk of dehydration and coupled with the use of an NSAID place the athlete at a higher risk for renal injury; they also may decrease serum potassium. Insulin decreases blood glucose. Other medications may be substituted for those known to impede exercise tolerance. Individuals' need for some of these medications may also change with regular exercise. Athletes taking medication should be counseled on the effects of the medications on exercise so that they can select an appropriate form and level of activity.

Appropriate tests include an ECG, complete blood count (CBC), urinalysis, and screening for diabetes, cholesterol, and renal disease in adults over the age of 35 years. Screening tests for adults between 30 and 35 years of age should be individualized, based on the individual's previous medical history, findings on physical examination, and risk factors (2). When to obtain an exercise stress test remains controversial. The American College of Sports Medicine and most cardiologists recommend a stress test before starting an exercise program for men over the age of 40 and women over the age of 50 who have no cardiac risk factors, for any individual with risk factors, or for individuals with an abnormal ECG (2). The choice, however, should be individualized. Some physicians consider a stress test unwarranted for healthy individuals who plan to participate in moderate exercise, such as walking (2,4).

Recommendations for an appropriate exercise program depend upon the findings of the preparticipation exam, any medications being taken, and any medical problems. Individuals should be encouraged to select a form of exercise that they will enjoy enough to continue regularly. Exercising in groups or as a class can help maintain participation, as the exercise becomes a social activity. The athlete should start exercising slowly and for short periods, then increase the duration. The intensity of the exercise is also important. The best way to monitor intensity is by heart rate, and athletes should be encouraged to either monitor their pulse regularly or use a heart-rate monitor. In order to benefit from aerobic exercise, the athlete must increase his pulse rate at least 50%, but 70–80% is better. A rough estimate of maximal heart rate is 220 – age. Raising the heart rate to at least 60% of this number is a reasonable goal to improve cardiovascular fitness.

The composition of collagen in various tissues, such as the nucleus pulposus and meniscus, begins to change before the age of 45. Although aging is inevitable, the rate and extent of these changes seem to vary (5). Sports injuries and overuse syndromes in older athletes are more likely to have a greater impact than similar injuries in younger athletes. Injuries in older individuals who exercise require more care and attention in order to allow the athlete to continue exercising, which should always be the goal. Most connective tissue becomes less compliant and less resilient with age. In general, acute injuries to connective tissues in older athletes require longer periods of rest to allow adequate healing. During the recovery period, the athlete needs to balance rest with some active movement to minimize loss of motion (6). The rehabilitation should emphasize stretching and strengthening. Older athletes usually require a longer period of rehabilitation before returning to their previous level of activity, but restoration of strength and complete range of motion is critical to minimize loss of joint function and risk of re-injury (5,6). Like their younger counterparts, older athletes often try to return to their sport too quickly; but, again, older athletes are at higher risk for re-injury and require an even longer recovery period. They need to be reminded that return to activity should be gradual and that proper rehabilitation is critical.

Most athletic injuries in the older population are due to chronic overuse, as the potential for chronic injury increases with the aging of tissues and the duration of participation in a particular sport. Older athletes are also more likely to suffer injuries or problems related to a previous injury incurred years earlier. For example, an older athlete with symptomatic osteoarthritis of the knee most likely has a history of ligamentous or meniscal injury (or meniscectomy). In addition, some injuries, such as meniscal tears, may occur more easily in all older athletes, even those without a history of significant trauma. It is important to rule out the presence of any possible soft tissue injury in an older athlete before attributing activity-related pain in or around a joint to degenerative arthritis. Degenerative changes evident on a radiograph do not always correlate with the level of pain an individual is experiencing (7). Athletes with symptomatic degenerative arthritis should be encouraged to exercise, and they may find that strengthening the muscles surrounding and supporting the affected joint alleviates some of the discomfort and allows increased activity. Cross-training or other activities for cardiovascular fitness that are not weight bearing, such as swimming, bicycling, or pool running, may be reasonable alternatives to running or walking daily (5). One of the newer management options for degenerative arthritis, viscosupplementation, may play a role in pain management and allow older athletes to participate in their sports more comfortably.

Given older athletes' higher risk of injury and longer recovery time, prevention of injury is most important. Adequate warm-up periods before exercise to increase mobility, along with stretching exercises, can help prevent muscle and joint injuries. Resistance exercises to build and

maintain muscle strength can help protect joints from injury and minimize strains and tears. Older athletes may tolerate exercise better if they
alternate days of more intense physical activity with days of lighter exercise, since recovery from intense exercise may take longer than 24
hours (6).

Whether exercise causes osteoarthritis is still under debate. Presently,
no data exist that directly attribute arthritis to exercise alone, without a
history of some degree of injury. Every sport has its associated injuries,
even minute injuries that may go unnoticed, which may contribute to
osteoarthritis. Some retrospective studies have demonstrated a higher
incidence of osteoarthritis in elite or higher-level competitive athletes;
however, the history of injury in these athletes was not usually evaluated (8). Some injuries can be directly related to the development of
arthritis, such as a torn meniscus in the knee. Before 1980, a complete
meniscectomy was the preferred treatment for a partially torn meniscus. Unfortunately, it became evident that removal of the entire
meniscus led to a rapid development of cartilage degeneration and osteoarthritis in a high percentage of patients (9). In addition, recent
long-term studies on the incidence and development of osteoarthritis of
the knee in runners have found that runners who do not have a previous injury tend to develop arthritis at a slower rate than non-runners.
Athletes with a history of injury, biomechanical malalignment, or preexisting osteoarthritis in a weight-bearing joint may accelerate the development of further degeneration with repetitive-impact exercise,
such as running, especially if overweight (1).

The benefits of regular exercise are innumerable throughout the life-
time of every individual. The special care and attention required to allow older athletes to continue to exercise is certainly justified and
should be provided by all heath care professionals.

YOUNGER ATHLETES

The number of children and adolescents involved in sports is also growing at a rapid rate. Physicians dealing with young athletes should be familiar with pediatrics, since many injuries deserve special consideration
because of the patient's immature physique. Pediatric sports medicine is
not covered in detail here; however, a few important, more common in-

juries will be mentioned. It is critical that the physician caring for adolescents (i.e., high school students), some of whom may not be skeletally mature, should be aware of injuries particular to this population. In addition, some injuries incurred as a child can have long-term effects on an athlete's future performance.

Epiphyseal Fractures

Approximately one-third of fractures in children are associated with some level of disruption of the epiphyseal growth plate (10), the site of skeletal maturation located between the epiphysis and metaphysis. The growth plate contains four cell layers, or zones: the resting, proliferation, hypertrophy, and mineralization zones. The weakest portion of the epiphyseal plate is the zone of hypertrophy, and this is the site of most epiphyseal fractures. Adolescents have the highest risk of an epiphyseal fracture, because the epiphysis may be weaker than the surrounding ligaments during the growth spurt. Traumatic dislocations tend to be less common in this age group because the epiphysis is weaker than the capsular ligaments (11).

The Salter-Harris classification system helps in the description and prognosis of epiphyseal fractures (12):

–type I: fracture resulting from shearing or torsional force; radiographic findings often negative; diagnosis often based on tenderness over the epiphyseal plate; heals well, usually in 3 weeks.
–type II: fracture resulting from lateral force rupturing the periosteum on one side with an intact metaphyseal fragment on the opposite side, forming a periosteal hinge; growth arrest is possible, depending on the location of the fracture.
–type III: intra-articular injury through the physis and epiphysis; rarely leads to growth arrest, but high risk of articular incongruity, so requires anatomical reduction.
–type IV: intra-articular fracture extending through the metaphysis, across the physis, through the epiphysis; high risk of bony bridging through the epiphysis to the metaphysis, which leads to growth arrest; also risk of intra-articular incongruity; requires open reduction and internal fixation to minimize complications.

–type V: fracture resulting from crushing axial load; radiographic findings may be normal; high risk of growth abnormalities (12).

Some of these injuries, then, are associated with growth disturbances or angular deformities. Tension or compression of the physis may stimulate growth, whereas excessive force results in cessation of growth— both of which may lead to disabling deformities (13). Therefore, potential fractures in young athletes should be managed with caution to minimize any stress that may further injure the growth plate. On-site manipulation of an injured appendage should be avoided unless no tenderness is present over the epiphyseal plate. If any suspicion of fracture exists, the limb should be immobilized and evaluated by x-ray immediately.

Osteochondritis Dissecans

Osteochondritis dissecans (OD) is a separation of a segment of cartilage and subchondral bone from an articular surface. It is most often encountered in the knee, ankle, and elbow. OD should not be confused with chondral delamination, a condition in which cartilage "peels" away from the underlying surface of the joint leaving large areas of denuded bone, which tends to occur in individuals in their 20s and 30s (14). There are two distinct types of OD, depending on the stage of the epiphysis. The juvenile form is associated with an open physis, usually in individuals younger than 15 years. The adult form occurs when the physis is closed. Young male athletes are most often affected, and the knee is involved in more than 75% of cases (15,16).

The exact etiology of OD remains unclear, although many hypotheses exist. Direct trauma has been proposed as one cause, but given the predilection for OD to occur in specific locations rather than randomly, trauma is not considered a major factor (17). Repetitive mictrotrauma coupled with some other factor may play a role. Ischemia or a vascular mechanism has also been proposed; this hypothesis has recently been questioned, however, because the condylar region of the femur has a rich supply of blood vessels with numerous anastomoses, rendering ischemia unlikely (18). Osteonecrosis of the knee may result in a lesion similar in appearance to OD, but histological examination of an OD lesion does not show any evidence of osteonecrosis (19). Another hypothesis suggests defects in ossification during growth so that fragments are easily detached with repetitive trauma (20,21). This mechanism has also been questioned.

The symptoms of OD initially tend to be a diffuse pain involving the entire joint, without any specific location, possibly associated with swelling. As the fragment begins to detach, catching and locking may begin. Symptoms tend to be intermittent and usually are associated with activity. Entirely detached fragments cause more constant pain and swelling. Physical examination reveals diffuse tenderness during the early stages but a well-defined area of tenderness in the later stages. An effusion may be present during all stages. An athlete with OD may walk with a limp. Wilson's sign for OD in the knee is elicited by flexing the knee to 90 degrees and internally rotating the tibia. A positive sign is elicited when the knee is passively extended and pain occurs at 30 degrees of flexion, which is then relieved with external rotation of the tibia (22).

In the knee, the medial femoral condyle is affected in up to 85% of cases (depending on the study), and mostly the lateral aspect of the condyle (23). Lesions involving the medial femoral condyle tend to occur anteriorly and face obliquely away from the tibiofemoral articular surface; in this location, the lesion affects both tibiofemoral and patellofemoral articulation. The average size is 2 cm in diameter. Lesions on the lateral condyle are usually located farther posteriorly and thus mostly affect only the tibiofemoral articular surface. Lateral lesions are usually larger, averaging 3–4 cm in diameter, more symptomatic, and prone to rapid degeneration (24).

On plain radiographs, OD usually appears as an area of sclerotic subchondral bone, separated by what can sometimes be a subtle radiolucent line. A lateral radiograph is often the most helpful. MRI is perhaps the most useful diagnostic tool, since it allows visualization of the entire bone and articular surface. The size and depth of the lesion, degree of displacement, and any loose bodies or fragmentation are easily evaluated, providing critical information for the appropriate treatment. MRI arthrography adds even more information on the integrity of the surface of the lesion and interface (25–27). Serial MRIs can be helpful to follow the healing and revascularization of the lesion (14).

Treatment of OD depends primarily on the age of the patient. In most cases of juvenile OD the lesion heals spontaneously. Long-term complications and failure to heal are most often related to continued activity and lack of sufficient rest (28). Three to 6 months of rest and avoidance of any activity that produces symptoms is usually advised. Serial radiographs are usually sufficient to follow healing. In cases of persistent pain, serial MRIs are more helpful. Arthroscopy is usually not necessary unless symptoms are present for longer than 3–6 months or the lesion is located on the face of the femoral condyle (24).

The adult form of OD, in which the physis is closed, is more worrisome. It has a much poorer chance of healing spontaneously. As the bone fragment separates from the underlying bone, the articular cartilage tends to soften, leading to detachment with even minor trauma. A "crater" remains in the articular cartilage, which eventually may fill with fibrocartilage rather than the more highly resilient hyaline cartilage. The fibrocartilage eventually degenerates at a higher rate than the surrounding hyaline cartilage, resulting in early osteoarthritis (29). Operative management for adult OD is usually recommended. Every attempt is made to restore congruity of the articular surface by fixing the unstable fragment(s), usually with a screw, which also enhances the blood supply to the fragment and increases the chance of healing. Strict limitation of weight bearing postoperatively until healing has been documented is recommended. The use of allogenic and autogenous osteochondral grafts to repair or "fill in" the defects resulting from OD is gaining popularity as research continues. Results are mixed but promising as techniques improve (30).

Avulsion Fractures

The weakest component in the musculotendinous unit in skeletally immature individuals is at the insertion of the unit on the bone, so avulsion fractures are more common in young athletes than in adults participating in strenuous activities (31,32). These fractures usually occur at an apophysis, an insertion of a major muscle that is nonarticular and does not contribute to bone growth. Examples include the greater and lesser trochanters, medial epicondyle, and iliac spines. Most avulsion fractures are the result of a sudden, forceful, eccentric or concentric muscle contraction without direct external trauma (33). Chronic avulsion injuries with gradual onset may also occur, most likely the result of chronic traction (34,35).

Athletes with avulsion fractures complain of localized pain. Physical examination reveals tenderness in the area of the avulsion and limited motion of the closest joint(s). The physician must have a high index of suspicion in order to make the correct diagnosis in these cases, and thus a low threshold for obtaining an x-ray. The correct diagnosis is critical for proper treatment. Conservative treatment has proved quite successful for avulsion fractures (31,32). Some physicians advocate surgical intervention, especially for fractures of the ischial tuberosity or for a displacement of the fragment of more than 2 cm, since some long-term disability has been associated with conservative treatment in such cases (35–37). Conservative treatment of avulsion fractures includes relative rest and maintenance of motion and conditioning (38). The treating physician needs to remember that bone malignancies, such as osteosarcoma and Ewing's sarcoma, which may also be associated with local bone pain, have a higher incidence in children and adolescents.

Osgood-Schlatter Disease

Osgood-Schlatter disease (OSD) is an apophysitis of the tibial tubercle. Apophysitis is an inflammation at the attachment of a tendon to an apophysis, which occurs in skeletally immature individuals. In young athletes, apophysitis rather than tendonitis is seen in overuse syndromes. It is the result of repetitive stress and traction at the apophysis and is associated with exercise and participation in sports (39). With avoidance of the activities producing repetitive traction the inflammation resolves without any longstanding disability (40).

The apophysitis of OSD occurs in young athletes during the growth spurts in early adolescence, usually at the age of 12 years in girls and 13 years in boys (24); boys seem to be affected more often than girls. OSD occurs bilaterally in 50% of cases. The patellar tendon grows longitudinally at the site of insertion and develops small areas of ossification (41). The apophysis then develops as these ossification centers fuse with the tibial tuberosity at the insertion site (42). Repetitive loading of the patellar tendon at the insertion during the phase of growth and ossification, as in kicking or running sports, can lead to inflammation at the insertion around the apophysis, and thus OSD.

The diagnosis of OSD is primarily based on the clinical findings of pain, tenderness, heat, and local swelling in the area of the tibial tuberosity. The pain is exacerbated with extension of the knee against resistance (43). Radiographs demonstrate soft tissue swelling just anterior to the tibial tuberosity and possibly a separate area of ossification in the same area. In MRI studies, T1- and T2-weighted images have shown thickening and increased signal intensity at the insertion of the patellar tendon, consistent with inflammation within the tendon (44). An infrapatellar bursa with high signal intensity has been demonstrated in 75% of cases. The patient may also have an ossicle located anterior to the tibial tuberosity, which in some cases fuses to the tubercle, as found on follow-up (45).

Treatment is usually conservative: avoidance of symptomatic activities and perhaps NSAIDs for the inflammation. Resolution of symptoms occurs in 3 months in the majority of cases treated conservatively (24). The use of local corticosteroid injection into the infrapatellar bursa is controversial and has been associated with subcutaneous atrophy (24, 45). A focus of ossification within the infrapatellar tendon is the most common long-term complication of OSD. These ossified regions do not need to be surgically removed unless symptoms persist after ossification of the tibial tuberosity is complete, although this approach is somewhat controversial as well (46,47). Long-term (up to 30 years) follow-up in one study showed no limitation on activities associated with a history of OSD in 75% of cases (48). Interestingly, in 60% of these cases the individual reported persistent discomfort on kneeling. In most cases, OSD heals leaving an asymptomatic prominence of the tibial tuberosity.

The rising incidence of anterior cruciate ligament tears and the need for reconstruction has led to the question of whether to use an autogenous bone–patellar tendon–bone graft in an athlete with a history of OSD. According to one study, the use of these grafts is not associated with an increased incidence of complications or delayed return to competition. The study emphasized the importance of recognizing an Osgood-Schlatter ossicle, which was then removed after harvest, prior to placement (49).

Slipped Capital Femoral Epiphysis

Slipped capital femoral epiphysis (SCFE) is the most common disorder of the hip in adolescents. It is not a sports injury, but it may present in the context of exercise and sports, and therefore the sports physician needs to be familiar with SCFE as a possible diagnosis in adolescent athletes with hip pain. The etiology has yet to be determined. It tends to occur in males between the ages of 11 and 15 years. Obesity is a common associated condition (50).

The most common symptom is hip pain, usually located in the groin but sometimes referred to the thigh or knee. The discomfort may be enough to cause the athlete to limp. Symptoms may appear acutely, with a sudden onset of pain and difficulty walking, or may arise more gradually. Active and passive range of motion of the hip is limited, especially internal rotation. If the symptoms are chronic, the physical exam may reveal quadriceps atrophy and a leg length discrepancy (33).

Diagnosis requires plain radiographs, usually an anteroposterior view of the pelvis and lateral view of the hip. Because SCFE occurs bilaterally in up to 40% of cases, evaluation of the opposite hip should always be performed to detect a possible "silent" lesion (51). The slip is graded by measuring the percentage of epiphyseal displacement relative to the diameter of the femoral neck on the lateral radiograph (52). A grade 1 slip is less than 30% displacement on the femoral neck; grade 2, between 30% and 50% displacement; and grade 3, greater than 50% displacement (53).

An SCFE is also described as acute or chronic: acute if the pain has been present for less than 3 weeks—often a type 1 physeal fracture; chronic if the symptoms have been present for more than 3 weeks (54). Surgery is usually required in both types of SCFE in order to prevent further progression of the slip, promote epiphysiodesis, and minimize the risk of a second slip (33). Long-term complications include avascular necrosis and chondrolysis.

REFERENCES
1. Ting A: Running and the older athlete. Clin Sports Med 10:319, 1991
2. Eichner ER: Exercise and aging: getting McTuff off his duff. Senior Patient 43–47, 1989

3. Pollock ML, Foster C, Knapp D, et al: Effect of age and training on aerobic capacity and body composition in master athletes. J Appl Physiol 62:725–731, 1987

4. Wheat ME: Exercise in the elderly. West J Med 147:477–480, 1987

5. Leach R, Abramowitz A: The senior tennis player. Clin Sports Med 10:283, 1991

6. Brown M: The older athlete with tennis elbow. Clin Sports Med 14:267, 1995

7. Matheson GO, MacIntyre JG, Taunton JE, Clement DB, Lloyd-Smith R: Musculoskeletal injuries associated with physical activity in older adults. Med Sci Sports Exerc 21:379–385, 1989

8. Lequesne MG, Dang N, Lane NE: Sport practice and osteoarthritis of the limbs. Osteoarthritis Cartilage 5:75–86, 1997

9. Dorr L: Arthritis and athletics. Clin Sports Med 10:343, 1991

10. Rang M: Children's Fractures. Philadelphia, JB Lippincott, 1974

11. Gill TJ IV, Micheli LJ: The immature athlete. Clin Sports Med 15:401–423, 1996

12. Salter RB, Harris WR: Injuries involving the epiphyseal plate. J Bone Joint Surg Am 45:587–622, 1963

13. Bright RW, Burstein AH, Elmore EM: Epiphyseal plate cartilage—a biomechanical and histological analysis of failure modes. J Bone Joint Surg Am 56:668–703, 1974

14. Schneck RC Jr, Goodnight JM: Osteochondritis dissecans. J Bone Joint Surg 78A:439–456, 1998

15. Clanton TO, DeLee JC: Osteochondritis dissecans: history, pathophysiology, and current treatment concepts. Clin Orthop 167:50–64, 1982

16. Pappas AM: Osteochondrosis dissecans. Clin Orthop 158:59–69, 1981

17. Mubarak SJ, Carroll NC: Juvenile osteochondritis dissecans of the knee: etiology. Clin Orthop 157:200–211, 1981

18. Rogers WM, Gladstone H: Vascular foramina and arterial supply of the distal end of the femur. J Bone Joint Surg 32A:867–874, 1950

19. Chiroff RT, Cooke CP III: Osteochondritis dissecans: a histologic and microradiographic analysis of surgically excised lesions. J Trauma 15:689–696, 1975

20. Barrie HJ: Hypothesis—a diagram of the form and origin of loose bodies in osteochondritis dissecans. J Rheumatol 11:512–513, 1984

21. Langer F, Percy EC: Osteochondritis dissecans and anomalous centres of ossification: a review of 80 lesions in 61 patients. Can J Surg 14:208–215, 1971

22. Wilson JN: A diagnostic sign in osteochondritis dissecans of the knee. J Bone Joint Surg 49A:477–480, 1967

23. Aichroth P: Osteochondritis dissecans of the knee: a clinical survey. J Bone Joint Surg 53B:440–447, 1971

24. Kujala UM, Kvist M, Heinonen O: Osgood-Schlatter's disease in adoles-

cent athletes: retrospective study of incidence and duration. Am J Sports Med 13:236–241, 1985

25. Kramer J, Stiglbauer R, Engel A, Prayer L, Imhof H: MR contrast arthrography (MRA) in osteochondrosis dissecans. J Comput Assist Tomog 16:254–260, 1992

26. DeSmet AA, Fisher DR, Burnstein MI, Graf BK, Lange RH: Value of MR imaging in staging osteochondral lesions of the talus (osteochondritis dissecans): results in 14 patients. Am J Roentgenol 154:555–558, 1990

27. Wojtys E, Wilson M, Buckwalter K, Braunstein E, Martel W: Magnetic resonance imaging of knee hyaline cartilage and intraarticular pathology. Am J Sports Med 15:455–463, 1987

28. Cahill BR: Osteochondritis dissecans of the knee: treatment of juvenile and adult forms. J Am Acad Orthop Surg 3:237–247, 1995

29. Landells JW: The reactions of injured human articular cartilage. J Bone Joint Surg 39B:548–562, 1957

30. Garrett JC: Treatment of osteochondral defects of the distal femur with fresh osteochondral allografts: a preliminary report. Arthroscopy 2:222–226, 1986

31. Metzmaker JN, Pappas AM: Avulsion fractures of the pelvis. Am J Sports Med 13:349–358, 1985

32. Sundar M, Carty H: Avulsion fractures of the pelvis in children: a report of 32 fractures and their outcome. Skeletal Radiol 23:85–90, 1994

33. Paletta GA Jr, Andrish JT: Injuries about the hip and pelvis in the young athlete. Clin Sports Med 14:591–628, 1995

34. Cossi CG, Cossi A, Colavita S, Barile L: Apophyseolysis and osteochondrosis of the ischial tuberosity: criteria of differential diagnosis. Ital J Orthop Traumatol 12:515–524, 1986

35. Winkler AR, Barnes JC, Ogden JA: Break dance hip: chronic avulsion of the anterior superior iliac spine. Pediatr Radiol 17:501–502, 1987

36. Wootton JR, Cross MJ, Holt KW: Avulsion of the ischial apophysis: the case for open reduction and internal fixation. J Bone Joint Surg 72B:625–627, 1990

37. Weiker GC: How I manage hip and pelvis injuries in adolescents. Physician and Sportsmedicine 21(12):72–82, 1993

38. Marder RA, Chapman MW: Principles of management of fractures in sports. Clin Sportsmed 9(1):1–11, 1990

39. Krahl H, Steinbruck K: Apophysenverletzungen in Wachstumsalter. Therapiewoche 29:3091–3105, 1979

40. Larson RL: Physical activity and growth and development of bone and joint structures. In Lorenz E, Rarick GL (eds): Physical Activity, Human Growth, and Development. New York, Academic Press, 1973, 32–59

41. Viderman T: An experimental study of the effects of growth on the rela-

tionship of tendons and ligament to bone at the site of diaphyseal insertion. Ann Chir Gynaecol Fenn Suppl 59:35–41, 1970

42. Ehrenborg G: The Osgood-Schlatter lesion: a clinical and experimental study. Acta Chir Scand Suppl 288:1–36, 1962

43. Cahill RB: Chronic orthopaedic problems in the young athlete. J Sports Med 1:36–39, 1973

44. Rosenberg AS, Kawelblum M, Cheung YY, Beltran J, Lehman WB, Grant AD: Osgood-Schlatter lesion: fracture or tendonitis? Scintigraphic, CT, and MR imaging features. Radiology 185:853–858, 1992

45. Rostron PKM, Calver RF: Subcutaneous atrophy following methyl prednisolone injection in Osgood-Schlatter epiphysis. J Bone Joint Surg 61A:627–628, 1979

46. Mital MA, Matza RA, Cohen J: The so-called unresolved Osgood-Schlatter lesion. J Bone Joint Surg 62A:732–739, 1980

47. Wray DG, Muddu BN: Operative treatment for longstanding Osgood-Schlatter's disease. J R Coll Surg Edinb 27:200–203, 1982

48. Krause BL, Williams JPR, Catterall A: Natural history of Osgood-Schlatter disease. J Pediatr Orthop 10:65–68, 1990

49. McCarroll JR, Shelbourne KD, Patel DV: Anterior cruciate ligament reconstruction in athletes with an ossicle associated with Osgood-Schlatter's disease. Arthroscopy 12:556–560, 1996

50. Stanitski CL: Acute slipped capital femoral epiphysis. J Am Acad Orthop Surg 2:96–106, 1994

51. Klein A, Joplin R, Reidy J, et al: Management of the contralateral hip in slipped capital femoral epiphysis. J Bone Joint Surg 35A:81, 953

52. Butler JE, Eggert AW: Fracture of the iliac crest apophysis: an unusual hip pointer. J Sports Med 3:192–193, 1975

53. Wilson PD, Jacobs B, Schecter L: Slipped capital femoral epiphysis: an end-result study. J Bone Joint Surg 47A:1128–1145, 1965

54. Fahey J, O'Brien E: Acute slipped capital femoral epiphysis. J Bone Joint Surg 47A:1105, 1965

THE FEMALE ATHLETE

PREGNANCY AND EXERCISE

Throughout history, girls and women have been discouraged from exercising, for a variety of reasons. The most common fear was a possible irreversible detrimental effect on reproduction. Beginning in the twentieth century, however, the number of women and girls exercising regularly and participating in sports increased exponentially. As more young women began exercising, the issue arose of the risks of continuing or even starting to exercise during pregnancy. Even as recently as 1984, pregnant women were advised to severely limit their participation in daily exercise, based on pulse rate and body temperature. These recommendations have come under greater scrutiny as more female athletes exercise and compete at levels above those previously recommended, without any apparent negative effect and possibly with some benefit.

Pregnancy is associated with numerous physiological changes, and the additional changes associated with exercise further complicate the issue of acute or chronic effects on the course and outcome of the pregnancy, for the athlete and her offspring. The cardiovascular system adapts to the demands of aerobic exercise with vasoconstriction of the splanchnic circulation (in direct proportion to the intensity and duration of the exercise) and vasodilation of the vessels supplying the skin and muscles. As a result, splanchnic circulation may decrease to about 50% of the resting level, and possibly more in the presence of further demands such as competition, dehydration, and a hot environment (1). Because blood flow to the uterus is also provided by the splanchnic bed, the concern arises that exercise could result in decreased blood flow to the uterus, especially during endurance activities such as running, cross-country skiing, and aerobics (2). The decreased blood flow not only might limit nutrient and oxygen supply to the fetus but also could increase the risk of preterm labor. In addition, cardiac output and blood volume are increased during pregnancy, each by 30–45% (3).

The elevated progesterone level during pregnancy causes a resting hypocapnia and increased baseline oxygen consumption due to an increased minute ventilation. Further hyperventilation occurs with strenuous aerobic exercise, so less oxygen is available for aerobic exercise and the athlete's maximal exercise performance decreases (4).

Exercise normally produces a rise in the athlete's rectal temperature, which is proportional to the intensity of exercise, extent of dehydration, and environmental factors impairing dissipation of heat (5,6). Some teratogenesis has been associated with a rectal temperature above 39.2°C; the evidence is primarily derived from the observation of increased congenital anomalies with the use of hot tubs early in pregnancy (4). For women who are already cardiovascularly fit, the increase in thermal temperature during pregnancy and the resulting stress on the embryo or fetus may not be as great. No increase in congenital anomalies in the children of women who participate in vigorous exercise throughout their pregnancies has been demonstrated (4).

Metabolic changes during moderate exercise include an increased mobilization of fat and carbohydrates for energy. Pregnant athletes should keep in mind that pregnancy increases the metabolic requirement by over 300 calories daily, and exercise further increases the need for calories. In addition, glucose supplies the majority of fetal energy requirements, and the amount available to the fetus during exercise may be limited as glucose is rapidly absorbed by muscle tissue (7,8). Pregnant women tend to utilize carbohydrates at a higher rate than nonpregnant women, which increases the risk of hypoglycemia in all states—resting, fasting, and exercise (4).

Concerns have been expressed about other physiological and anatomical changes in the pregnant athlete. Joint and ligament laxity increase during pregnancy, but no increase in the incidence of injury due to ligamentous laxity has been documented (4). A woman's center of gravity alters significantly during pregnancy, secondary to enlargement of the breasts and uterus and an increase in weight. This may impede balance, agility, and coordination, especially during the second and third trimester. Pregnant athletes should be aware of these changes and alter their exercise activities to sports that do not require these skills. The impact forces of weight-bearing activities and shearing force produced by sudden lateral movement may also affect the enlarged, mobile uterus and thus increase the risk of membrane rupture, entanglement of the umbilical cord, and placental separation (9).

All reports indicate that the risk of spontaneous abortion is not increased in runners who continue to run during early pregnancy (10–12). A more recent study of women who train vigorously (>50% Vo_{2max}) in endurance exercise (running) for longer than 30 minutes at least 3 days a week demonstrated no difference in the incidence of infertility or, in pregnant women, of congenital anomalies or placental anomalies compared with age-matched controls (9). Increased fatigue, however, whether related to workload or other factors, has been associated with an increased risk of premature labor (13). The possible association between increased risk of preterm labor and exercise has been examined. No increase in uterine activity has been associated with brisk walking and cycling at moderate to high intensities (14,15). Continued exercise does not induce preterm labor, but it does seem to be associated with delivery at an earlier full term (>260 days).

One study has shown that regular aerobic exercise seems to decrease the need for medical intervention during labor, such as the use of oxytocin (Pitocin) or cesarean section, to less than 50% of that in nonexercising women. More than 85% of these active women are able to undergo a normal vaginal delivery. The length of labor, during both the active first stage (4 cm to full cervical dilation) and the second stage (pushing), is also shorter (9). Other studies, however, have not shown such a significant reduction in length of labor with exercise (11,16,17). The incidence of low Apgar score, abnormal fetal heart rate patterns, cord entanglement, and meconium-stained amniotic fluid was significantly less for pregnant women who exercised (9).

Multiple environmental factors influence birth weight, so it cannot be used as a sole indicator of the effect of exercise. Pregnant women who begin to exercise aerobically during their pregnancy (in the first trimester) do not give birth to infants of abnormally low birth weight (18,19). However, women who continue to participate in endurance exercise at a higher and more intense level seem to deliver infants with lower birth weights, in proportion to the intensity of exercise during the last trimester (20,21). A similar association is found between birth weight and physically demanding work (22,23). Women who exercise at more than 50% of their preconceptual level (of intensity or duration) deliver infants with birth weights more than 400 g lower than the infants of nonexercising controls. The primary difference between the two groups of infants is in fat mass, no more than 220 g—the significance of which has yet to be determined (9). High-intensity exercise, above the preconceptual level, is associated with a lower birth weight due to a shorter gestation period and less fat growth. No difference in linear growth, head circumference, or lean body mass was demonstrated (24). Follow-up of the children of the women who exercised vigorously during pregnancy, at both 1 and 5 years of age, showed normal neurodevelopment and morphology.

Exercise can be beneficial for women who are pregnant and healthy. It reduces many of the common musculoskeletal complaints associated with pregnancy, such as low-back aches (24,25). Continued exercise also maintains aerobic capacity despite a perceived decrease in overall performance during pregnancy. Even women who are sedentary before becoming pregnant may gain increased aerobic fitness with exercise during pregnancy, which continues into the postnatal period (18,26–28). Certain medical conditions are considered absolute contraindications to exercise during pregnancy (table 10.1).

Recent studies have begun to show the safety of vigorous exercise and question the previous recommendations of limited exercise during pregnancy. Vigorous exercise produces physiological changes that are fetoprotective and enhance many of the adaptations accompanying pregnancy. For example, the ability to reduce body heat is improved in pregnancy by endurance exercise, thus reducing the risk of thermal injury to the fetus (5). In fact, core temperature and the temperature at which sweating begins tend to fall as the pregnancy progresses, to close to 70% of baseline in the last trimester (9). Regular exercise also decreases the use of glucose by muscles as they become more efficient, stabilizing the blood glucose level and its availability to the fetus (7,16). The increase in plasma volume in pregnancy, added to a greater volume already resulting from pre-pregnancy endurance exercise, tends to allow adequate fetal blood flow during strenuous exercise, thus minimiz-

Table 10.1. Contraindications to Exercise during Pregnancy

Absolute
   Severe cardiovascular disease
      History of myocardial infarction
      History of cardiomyopathy
      History of pulmonary edema
      Thrombophlebitis
   Conditions secondary to the pregnancy
      Vaginal bleeding
      Possible membrane rupture
      Hypertension
   Any documented fetal complications
      Fetal distress
      Abnormal growth
Relative
   Mild cardiovascular disease
      Preexisting or controlled hypertension
      Well-controlled cardiac disease
      Mitral valve prolapse
   Medical complications
      Diabetes mellitus (especially if pregnancy induced)
      Anemia
      Thyroid dysfunction
   Fetal complications
      Breech
      Multiple fetuses

---

ing the effect of exercise-induced shunting of blood to muscles and skin (29,30). The placentas of pregnant athletes contain a higher volume of blood than those of sedentary women, which provides further fetal protection during exercise and against other stresses such as maternal hemorrhage, hypoxia, and hypoglycemia (31).

Advice to pregnant athletes should always include education about the effects of pregnancy on the body. The physician should assess the woman's preconceptual fitness level and assist her in setting reasonable training goals to maintain and possibly increase cardiovascular fitness. The athlete needs to be aware that the decreased oxygen levels during pregnancy will begin to limit her aerobic tolerance level and performance. Her perceived level of fatigue is a good indicator for determining when to discontinue activity. The athlete should be advised not to exercise to exhaustion. She should avoid situations that may add to body temperature; adequate hydration and exercise in cool environments are critical. Some physicians recommend that pregnant athletes monitor their rectal temperature before and after exercise and alter training as necessary to keep temperatures below 38.7°C. Weight gain and body fat percentage are also important to help monitor training levels and adequate nutritional intake. Increasing the intake of complex carbohydrates will help maintain blood glucose and replace glycogen used during exercise.

Most aerobic exercise can be continued during pregnancy and should be performed regularly, at least three times a week, rather than intermittently. Again, exercise above 50% of Vo_{2max} for longer than 30 minutes at a time is not associated with complications of pregnancy, as long as the above-mentioned precautions are followed (31). Water exercise is appropriate, but it is associated with diuresis, dehydration, and significant increases in rectal temperature (in heated pools especially). Increased fluid intake is essential for these athletes. Any exercise or sports associated with a risk of falling or of abdominal trauma (especially after the 16th week of pregnancy) should probably be avoided. Exercise in the supine position is not recommended after the first trimester, since it is associated with decreased cardiac output, as is prolonged standing. Weight lifting and breath holding, and scuba diving, should probably be avoided, although no data exist to support this recommendation.

The physiological changes associated with pregnancy continue for 4–6 weeks postnatally, and resumption of exercise to the pre-pregnancy level of intensity and duration should occur gradually.

EXERCISE AND AMENORRHEA

The passing of Title IX, which legislated equal funding for women's sports in college athletics, was a major factor contributing to the exponential rise of women's and girls' participation in sports, especially at the competitive and elite levels. For most female athletes, exercise provides numerous health benefits and contributes significantly to improved physical fitness and emotional well-being (32). However, women who exercise and participate in organized sports are at risk for certain medical problems that may have a profoundly adverse impact on performance and quality of life.

Intense and excessive exercise and training can cause amenorrhea, delayed menarche, anovulation, and infertility. Amenorrhea is defined as the absence of three consecutive menstrual periods in women who have already begun menstruating, in the absence of pregnancy. Athletic amenorrhea is amenorrhea secondary to exercise. This condition is not uncommon and is most often associated with particular activities such as long-distance running, gymnastics, cheerleading, and ballet. The risk of athletic amenorrhea increases with increasing intensity, duration, and frequency of training. One study found an incidence of amenorrhea of 6% in runners totaling 10 miles per week compared with 43% in runners totaling 80 miles per week (33). Amenorrheic runners tend to run farther distances, although some studies suggest that a higher pace is a more significant factor in the development of amenorrhea (34).

The intensity of gymnastic, ballet, and cheerleading training may be difficult to quantify, but athletes participating in these activities have reported an incidence of amenorrhea (at some point in their athletic career) of close to 40% (35). Nutrition certainly plays a role in the development of amenorrhea. Many female endurance athletes are thin and seem to have a lower caloric intake than might be expected for their level of competition and training. Trained female athletes with amenorrhea consume fewer daily calories than normally menstruating (eumenorrheic) athletes at the same level of competition (36). Protein consumption is significantly reduced among the amenorrheic athletes. Vegetarian diets and low red-meat intake are also contributing factors. Though some of the poorly balanced diets may be unintentional, many female athletes strive to maintain a low body fat level, falsely believing that it will enhance their performance. This misconception may lead to eating disorders (discussed below).

The specific mechanism relating intense exercise to amenorrhea is still unclear. Athletic amenorrhea is related to impairment of the release of gonadotropin-releasing hormone (GnRH) by the hypothalamus, or "hypothalamic amenorrhea." The lack of sufficient GnRH results in low levels of gonadotropins (luteinizing and follicle-stimulating hormones), progesterone, and estrogen (37,38). Multiple hypotheses have been proposed to explain the apparent relationship between exercise and suppression of GnRH, including the transient increase in cortisol, prolactin, and endogenous opioids, or a decrease in the basal metabolic rate (32,39).

Percentage of body fat was once considered a crucial factor in influencing the onset of amenorrhea: 17% body fat required for the onset of puberty and 22% for the maintenance of regular menses (40). This hypothesis has been questioned as more accurate methods of measuring body composition have become available. Various studies have found both amenorrheic and eumenorrheic athletes with body fat percentages below 22% (37,41,42). As has become apparent, each individual athlete has a threshold of body fat for the maintenance of menses, and this level depends on multiple factors, such as genetics, energy balance, and metabolism (37).

Although most athletes consider amenorrhea and the lack of ovulation "convenient," the associated hypoestrogenemia can be detrimental, especially in the teenage years. Women accumulate bone mass rapidly during their teen years and slightly during their 20s. Bone loss normally begins sometime in the early 30s. The rate of bone loss before menopause is minimal, increases to 5% each year in the peri- to postmenopausal years, for 10 years after menopause, and then begins to slow (43). The changes in bone density in a normal woman are primarily related to estrogen levels and the subsequent hypoestrogenic state of menopause. Weight-bearing exercise augments bone formation, although the beneficial effects of exercise on bone density are negated once athletic amenorrhea occurs.

Amenorrheic athletes lose bone mass at a rate comparable to that in early postmenopausal women (32,44,45). The loss of bone density can be even more significant if amenorrhea occurs during the teens or early 20s, before the young woman has acquired maximum bone density. This premature osteoporosis may be irreversible to some extent, depending on the age of the athlete and the length of amenorrhea. Osteoporosis secondary to amenorrhea lasting for more than 3 years has been shown to be irreversible, despite estrogen replacement and calcium supplementation (46). Resumption of menses in amenorrheic athletes may lead to an increase in bone density of up to 6% during the first year and 3% during the following year, but then tends to stabilize (47). In general, women with a history of irregular menses will most likely have a lower bone density than women who have had regular menses (43). Thus it is critical to restore the menstrual cycle or at least replace estrogen in amenorrheic athletes as early as possible to prevent the possibly devastating effects of premature osteoporosis.

Amenorrhea also places the athlete at a much higher risk for stress fractures. The incidence of stress fractures in runners with irregular menses approaches 45%, compared with 29% in runners with normal menses (37). A similar pattern of stress fractures has been demonstrated in ballet dancers, primarily in the lower extremities, with an incidence of stress fractures approaching 60% in amenorrheic dancers (48). In managing stress fractures in young women, the physician should always include an evaluation of their menstrual function and restoration of their menses (or at least estrogen replacement) if found to be abnormal. The physician should also consider the possibility of an eating disorder. If the athlete is amenorrheic or if she has a history of stress fractures, a bone-density measurement should be considered.

Estrogen has been shown to influence blood flow by relaxation of arterioles. Decreases in estrogen level can affect blood-flow control mechanisms and thus decrease the flow of oxygen and glucose to the exercising muscles. This decrease may be subtle but enough to be relevant to elite athletes, whose performance is often measured in intervals of milliseconds to seconds (49).

The diagnosis of athletic amenorrhea is one of exclusion. An extensive history can be very helpful (table 10.2). A complete physical exam and subsequent blood tests are necessary to rule out other causes of amenorrhea, including pituitary tumors (especially prolactinomas), thyroid dysfunction, polycystic ovary disease, premature ovarian failure, and, of course, pregnancy (50,51). The need for bone mineral density (BMD) measurement is debatable but is probably warranted for an athlete with a history of a stress fracture; the test should be repeated yearly after treatment is initiated.

The treatment of amenorrhea involves, first, a search for the underlying cause and subsequent correction of the primary problem. Treatment begins with educating the athlete about the detrimental effects of amenorrhea and its consequences, both short and long term. The physi-

Table 10.2. Medical History for Evaluating the Female Athlete

Past medical history
  Congenital anomalies (that may interfere with performance)
  Chronic diseases
  Previous surgeries
  Previous or chronic injuries (including management)
  Any medications taken regularly *or* intermittently
  History of fractures
  History of concussions (including severity, date, any post-concussive symptoms)
Menstrual history
  Age of menarche
  Frequency and duration of menstruation
  Date of last two periods (if possible)
  Any dysmenorrhea or problems during menstruation
  Form of birth control
  Obstetric history
Social history
  Alcohol or drug abuse (present or past)
  Smoking (present or past)
  Use of any supplements, ergogenic agents, or herbs and any over-the-counter
    medications
  Type of sport
  Training history
General review of systems
  Calorie and calcium intake
  Dieting or recent changes in weight; include questions on the athlete's percep-
    tion of her body type
  History of headaches (including management)
  Recent visual changes
  Gastrointestinal and neurological symptoms

cian should evaluate the athlete's nutritional status and diet and recommend appropriate changes, including the use of calcium supplements. Convincing her about the benefits of weight gain may be difficult; close monitoring and support are crucial, especially by the coach.
The athlete must also reduce her training schedule, in both intensity
and duration. The extent of reduction will vary with the individual, but

if menses do not resume after 2 months, further reduction should be implemented. (The physician also needs to scrutinize the athlete's compliance with the reduced training schedule.)

If the athlete is unable to reduce training, or refuses to do so, or if menses do not resume after 3–6 months of lifestyle change, alternative treatment is recommended (52). Estrogen and progesterone therapy administered cyclically help to maintain bone mass and produce regular menstruation (50). The minimal estrogen dose required to prevent loss of bone mass in postmenopausal women is 0.625 mg daily (39); the recommended schedule, at least to start, is 0.625 mg of conjugated estrogen daily for days 1 to 25, with 10 mg of medroxyprogesterone acetate on days 16 to 25. Progesterone is important to avoid the risks of unopposed estrogen. The estrogen dose may need to be increased to 1.25 mg daily for the amenorrheic athlete in order to stimulate the resumption of menses. Whether the level of estrogen required to stimulate menstruation is the same level needed to prevent loss of bone density is unclear. It is generally accepted that the female athlete with amenorrhea should receive estrogen replacement at a higher dose than the typical hormone replacement used for postmenopausal women. Birth control pills are best, if possible. Athletes who do not wish to menstruate can use daily combined hormonal replacement therapy (42). Another approach may be to cycle the estrogen with progesterone every 3 months, so that the athlete only menstruates every third month. Some women prefer this approach because it allows them to avoid menstruating "in season." Hormone therapy should continue at least until the athlete has improved diet, weight, and possibly BMD measurements. At that point, a trial without hormone therapy may be attempted to evaluate the possible return of regular menstruation. Absolute contraindications for hormone therapy are a history of breast, uterine, or cervical cancer, liver disease, cerebrovascular accident, or deep vein thrombosis.

Side effects from hormone therapy are a major concern to athletes. Some athletes may notice lethargy or bloating with the medroxyprogesterone; the dose may be reduced to 5 mg a day with a reduction in symptoms. Mild weight gain or fluid retention sometimes occurs initially but usually stabilizes, or it can be diminished by reducing the progesterone or estrogen. Side effects are more common with hormone therapy at higher doses, such as those used for contraception. Trying some of the different contraceptives will often allow the athlete to find the one with fewest side effects. Athletes' use of oral contraceptives has not been shown to have any significant deleterious effects on performance or strength. In fact, combined oral contraceptives tend to increase cardiac output and stroke volume, which may potentiate oxygen delivery to tissues. The reduction in overall menstrual blood loss may be beneficial as well (53).

EATING DISORDERS AND THE FEMALE TRIAD

Society itself places an emphasis on thinness as being attractive, an image that all too many young women take to heart. The pressure to maintain a low body weight is even greater for athletes. In some sports, such as long-distance running, figure skating, and ballet, the benefits of low body fat for performance have become greatly exaggerated, by both athletes and coaches. Few, if any, studies support their claims. In addition, in such sports as diving and gymnastics, appearance itself is a component of overall scoring, which places further stress on the female athlete to become and remain thin. A low body weight is also almost "required" for activities that involve throwing and jumping maneuvers, such as ballet, pairs figure skating, and cheerleading. The association between improving performance and maintaining low body fat has placed all female athletes at a high risk for developing eating disorders. The association between eating disorders, amenorrhea, and, ultimately, osteoporosis has been referred to as the "female triad."

The prevalence of eating disorders among female athletes is difficult to determine. Most studies depend on self-reporting by athletes, which tends to underestimate the incidence. Even by this method, however, incidences of up to 60% are reported for some sports (32). *Disordered eating* is actually a better term to describe unhealthy eating and exercise habits, since these are not limited to anorexia or bulimia. Excessive exercise, such as an extra 5-mile run after a 2-hour soccer practice, can be a strategy to maintain an abnormally low and unhealthy body weight but does not technically fit into the strict category of anorexia or bulimia. Many athletes with disordered eating are not strictly anorexic, and they may ingest a few thousand calories a day, but if their energy output exceeds their input daily they are at a high risk of developing significant problems, including increased risk of injuries and poor healing rates. Detecting disordered eating in an athlete as early as possible greatly improves her chances of recovery. Education of everyone involved with athletes is critical, including the athletes themselves, who will then be more willing to help a teammate or friend. Coaches and trainers are in a good position to pick up on clues of disordered eating or weight issues.

The preparticipation physical provides an opportunity for the physician to screen for possible problems. Specific questioning of the athlete on her eating patterns, recent diets or attempts at weight loss, and what she considers her ideal body weight are important means of exploring her perception of her body image and its influence on her performance. It is also a good time to educate the athlete on her possible misconceptions and answer any of her questions.

The physical examination itself may provide some clues. Body weight is not always helpful, since athletes who binge and purge are usually of normal weight or slightly heavy. A low pulse rate is one physiological response to abnormal eating, especially a rate below 50. Hypotension and orthostasis resulting from dehydration or electrolyte imbalance may be noted. Hypothermia also is seen in individuals with disordered eating. More extreme eating disorders can be suggested by other findings on examination, such as "lanugo" hair (light hair growth), which is encountered in severe anorexia. Parotid gland swelling and erosions of tooth enamel are often encountered in bulimic individuals. A history of a stress fracture can be a tip-off, suggestive of osteoporosis (53). Diagnosis based on examination can be difficult. Most often the possibility of disordered eating is raised by the athlete's behavior or comments, noted by friends, trainers, parents, and coaches.

Treatment of disordered eating is difficult in general, and particularly when the athlete is driven by the pressure to perform. Sports medicine physicians are only now beginning to deal with this extremely difficult problem, on multiple levels. Preventive measures, by education of athletes, coaches, trainers, and parents, are strongly encouraged. Once the diagnosis of disordered eating is suspected or established, a multidisciplinary approach seems to be most successful. This approach might start with a written agreement between the athlete and the team physician on the requirements she must meet in order to continue participating in the sport. The contract should focus on regaining optimal health and performance, without loss of her player status. It may need to include specific weight-gain goals, such as one-half pound per week, and a total-weight goal (54). The rapidity of the weight gain can be tailored to the situation, but it is important to keep in mind that these individuals have an abnormal concept of weight. Weight gained slowly is more likely to be comfortable for the athlete and thus more likely to be maintained. Another helpful approach is to emphasize the gain of muscle, strength, and endurance with the increase in weight, rather than a gain in fat.

A psychologist or counselor experienced with eating disorders plays a key role in the multidisciplinary approach. Disordered eating is associated with complicated psychological issues that need to be addressed. Regular (weekly) meetings with the psychologist should be part of the contract agreement. Of note, selective serotonin reuptake inhibitors can be very useful in conjunction with therapy in bulimic individuals. An experienced nutritionist is also quite helpful, to discuss specific food issues, set up meal plans, and gradually increase the athlete's food intake (54). Prognosis is improved with this intensive approach, but successful treatment may require years of therapy. Support by teammates, coaches, family members, and friends is always important. As with any disorder, prevention by education is the best treatment.

MENOPAUSE

The changes associated with menopause can affect many organ systems. Psychological issues also arise, including dealing with the process of aging. Exercise may help minimize some of the changes and stresses associated with menopause.

The cessation of regular menstruation and the decrease in serum estrogen level have a significant effect on the cardiovascular system. Lowered estrogen levels influence the relaxation potential of arterioles, increasing resistance to blood flow and possibly blunting the response of blood vessels to normal control mechanisms (49). Hypoestrogenemia is also associated with an increase in serum triglycerides and cholesterol. The potential hypercholesterolemia and hypertriglyceridemia contribute to and may accelerate arteriosclerosis (55,56). Aerobic fitness tends to fall after menopause; this change is presently considered to be a result of decreased activity and general aging rather than a direct consequence of hypoestrogenemia (57). Peri- and postmenopausal women are capable of improving their cardiovascular fitness level with regular aerobic exercise, almost as much as sedentary premenopausal women (58,59). In addition to improving cardiovascular fitness, postmenopausal women can exercise to lower their cholesterol level and weight, both of which are considered major risk factors for cardiac disease (60). Hormone replacement therapy is another means of minimizing the effects of menopause on the cardiovascular system, an effect that is certainly potentiated by regular exercise.

Before embarking on an exercise program, a previously sedentary woman older than 35 should consult her physician, and a woman who has two or more risk factors for heart disease or any cardiopulmonary symptoms should be considered for an exercise stress test. A good cardiovascular maintenance program requires aerobic activity for 20 minutes or longer at least 3 days a week. The intensity of the exercise should increase the heart rate by 60–80% of the resting heart rate (see Chapter 2). The woman should monitor her heart rate, by a manual pulse or a heart-rate monitor, in order to obtain maximum benefit (61).

Hypoestrogenemia is a major risk factor for osteoporosis, as are early menopause, smoking, low calcium intake, family history of osteoporosis, excessive alcohol or caffeine use, and sedentary lifestyle (62,63). The accelerated loss of bone density in the first few years following menopause is reduced with regular weight-bearing exercise. It is important to note, however, that exercise cannot completely negate the loss of bone density associated with hypoestrogenemia (63). Two recent studies have demonstrated the osteogenic effect of the combined use of hormone replacement therapy and exercise (64,65).

Many other symptoms can occur during menopause, with varying frequency: hot flashes, fatigue, sweating, depression, insomnia, myalgias, and dizziness (63). Regular aerobic exercise in middle-aged adults tends to reduce anxiety, tension, depression, and fatigue (66). In fact, strenuous exercise produces a greater improvement of symptoms in depressed women than do relaxation exercises or no exercise (67). Another benefit of exercise is a decrease in psychosocial stress response

(68). All these benefits can minimize the various adverse effects of menopause.

ANTERIOR CRUCIATE LIGAMENT INJURIES

Women's participation in competitive team sports, most of which were previously considered "men's sports," has been increasing significantly over the past twenty years. The level and intensity of competition has risen as women have demonstrated the ability to play with speed, precision, power, and finesse as never before. This increased participation and intensity of play has led to higher injury rates. In fact, compared with male athletes participating in the same sport at the same levels of play, female athletes have a higher injury rate, especially in basketball, alpine skiing, volleyball, and gymnastics (69–71).

Most studies rank the knee and the ankle as the most commonly injured joints during exercise and sports (71–73). Injuries to the anterior cruciate ligament have become one of the most common knee injuries in athletes (74,75) (see the discussion in Chapter 7). Interestingly, the ACL is most often injured in noncontact situations, with planting of the foot and cutting, landing on an extended knee, and pivoting with sudden deceleration (74,76). The highest rates of ACL injuries are found in basketball, soccer, snow skiing, and volleyball across most age groups. Running and gymnastics also have significant rates of ACL injuries (70,73,77). Injuries are also more likely to occur in games rather than during practices (74,78).

The National Collegiate Athletic Association, which has been compiling data on injuries in female athletes since 1982, reports that female athletes have a higher rate of knee injuries in general. The NCAA data also reveal an ACL injury rate for female soccer players that is more than twice that for male soccer players (0.31 vs. 0.13 occurrences per 1,000 athlete exposures) (79). Female basketball players have an ACL injury rate four times that of the male players (0.29 vs. 0.07) (79).

Various factors have been proposed to account for the significantly higher rate of ACL injuries in female athletes. Gender-related anatomical differences may play a role. The width of the intercondylar notch has been suggested as a possible factor, but the study results are contradictory and inconclusive. Some studies have demonstrated that a smaller intercondylar notch is associated with a higher rate of ACL injury (80–82). Whether women have a smaller notch-width index, as reported by one study (82), remains a subject of debate and requires further research (81). An inherent hypermobility of joints is another possible factor, but a definite association between ACL injuries and joint laxity has yet to be demonstrated (83,84). The influence of alignment differences between women and men, including the wider female pelvis and the greater incidence of femoral anteversion, genu valgum, and external tibial torsion in women, all of which alter biomechanics, has yet to be clarified.

Extrinsic factors may contribute to the propensity for female athletes to injure the ACL. Certain sports seem to be associated with a higher ACL injury rate. The imbalance between quadriceps and hamstring strength has also been examined as a possible cause of gender differences in ACL injury rates. The quadriceps muscle, an ACL antagonist, is considered the primary knee-stabilizing muscle in women, whereas the hamstrings are the more important stabilizing muscles in men (85). The hamstring-to-quadriceps strength ratios are lower in most women, but an association between knee injuries—and specifically ACL injuries in women—and strength ratios has not been established (86,87). Many universities are now instituting training programs for female athletes that focus on balance of hamstring and quadriceps strength, as well as retraining techniques for jumping and landing. The success of these new approaches remains to be seen. The etiology of the higher rate of ACL injuries in female athletes, then, is still unclear, but it certainly warrants more extensive investigation, given the rapidly rising number of competitive athletes who are at risk.

MIGRAINE HEADACHES

Migraine headaches have been estimated to affect up to 10% of the general population, the majority of migraine sufferers being women. A headache that is new in onset should be evaluated as any new headache, but many athletes will be able to give a history of a typical migraine. Whether exercise induces a migraine is unclear and most likely depends upon the individual. Certainly, an athlete who complains of a migraine headache should be removed from active play, since the distraction caused by the pain, as well as the possible associated symptoms (such as weakness, visual changes, vertigo, aphasia), places the athlete at risk of injury. Treatment is individualized and in most cases the athlete will know which abortive medication is the most effective.

Various medications have been used to treat migraine headaches. The type of medication the athlete uses, as well as how often she requires treatment, is an important issue since the medication may negatively affect her level of training and performance. For example, the use of prophylactic beta-blockers or clonidine has been shown to decrease performance, especially at the elite level (see the discussion of hypertension in Chapter 2). Calcium channel blockers may be a better alternative for these athletes. Tricyclic antidepressants, such as amitriptyline, may also have sedating effects that should be evaluated. Even the intermittent use of narcotics or caffeine-based medication should be monitored, since both the NCAA and the USOC have limits on the allowed level of caffeine ingested and the use of narcotics. If the athlete uses NSAIDs regularly, she should be aware of the potential side effects and should keep well hydrated. The effect of the serotonin receptor agonists (sumatriptan, rizatriptan) has yet to be evaluated.

The "acute-effort migraine" is a recently described form of headache that occurs in athletes performing short, vigorous, and often anaerobic activity (88). It is not necessarily more common in female athletes. The etiology is thought to be related to a decrease in cerebral PCO_2 (due to hyperventilation), leading to vasoconstriction followed by vasodilation (the typical events occurring in a migraine). Effort migraines have been described in runners (88), weight lifters (89), and swimmers (90). These headaches tend to be brief and may be exacerbated by dehydration, caffeine, heat, hypoglycemia, and the use of alcohol (88). Other more common causes of headaches should be ruled out, as acute-effort migraine is more a diagnosis of exclusion and can be treated like a common migraine. Interestingly, these headaches tend to improve with better overall conditioning and a regular pre-activity warm-up session (88).

BENIGN HYPERMOBILITY SYNDROME

Generalized joint hypermobility due to ligamentous laxity can be present in up to 10% of the general population. Benign hypermobility syndrome, more common in women than men, is joint laxity, without any other symptoms of Marfan's syndrome or Ehlers-Danlos syndrome, accompanied by arthralgias without any evidence of other etiology (91). Individuals with this syndrome can hyperextend their elbows and knees, touch the floor with their hands while their knees are extended, and hyperflex the wrist to touch the thumb to the forearm. Hypermobility and flexibility can be advantageous in certain activities such as ballet dancing and gymnastics (92).

Unfortunately, hypermobile joints tend to be unstable and thus at higher risk of injury due to overuse, tendonitis, and dislocation (92). Some risk of injury can be minimized, such as by taping unstable ankles, but the laxity of some joints may lead to chronic problems such as tendonitis. The recent development of capsulorrhaphy performed arthroscopically has allowed many athletes with chronic dislocations and instability to return to play; this procedure should be considered in athletes with symptomatic joint laxity.

REFERENCES

1. Rowell LB: Cardiovascular aspects of human thermoregulation. Circ Res 52:367–379, 1983

2. Clapp JF, Little KD, Capeless EL: Fetal heart rate response to various intensities of recreational exercise during mid and late pregnancy. Am J Obstet Gynecol 168:198–206, 1993

3. Araujo D: Expecting questions about exercise and pregnancy? Physician and Sportsmedicine 25(4):85–93, 1997

4. American College of Obstetricians and Gynecologists: Technical Bulletin 189. Washington, DC, American College of Obstetricians and Gynecologists, Feb. 1995

5. Clapp JF: The changing thermal response to endurance exercise during pregnancy. Am J Obstet Gynecol 165:1684–1689, 1991

6. Clapp JF, Wesley M, Sleamaker RH: Thermoregulatory and metabolic responses to jogging prior to and during pregnancy. Med Sci Sports Exerc 19:124–130, 1987

7. Bonen A, Campagna P, Gilchrist L, et al: Substrate and endocrine responses during exercises at selected stages of pregnancy. J Appl Physiol 73:134–142, 1992

8. Ingermann RI: Control of placental glucose transfer. Placenta 8:557–571, 1987

9. Clapp JF III: A clinical approach to exercise during pregnancy. Clin Sports Med 13:443–458, 1994

10. Cohen GC, Prior JC, Vigna Y, et al: Intense exercise during the first two trimesters of unapparent pregnancy. Physician and Sportsmedicine 17:87–94, 1989

11. Dale E, Mullinax KM, Bryant DH: Exercise during pregnancy: effects on the fetus. Can J Sports Sci 7:98–102, 1982

12. Hansen KA: Exercise and pregnancy. Swim Magazine, May–June, 12–15, 1989

13. Mamelle N, Laumon B, Lazar P: Prematurity and occupational activity during pregnancy. Am J Epidemiol 119:309–322, 1984

14. van Doorn MB, Lotgering FK, Strujik PC, et al: Maternal and fetal cardiovascular responses to strenuous exercise. Am J Obstet Gynecol 166:854–859, 1992

15. Vielle JC, Hohimer AR, Burry K, et al: The effect of exercise on uterine activity in the last eight weeks of pregnancy. Am J Obstet Gynecol 151:729–733, 1985

16. Lokey EA, Tran ZV, Wells CL, et al: Effects of physical exercise on pregnancy outcomes: a meta-analytic review. Med Sci Sports Exerc 23:1234–1239, 1991

17. Sternfield B, Sidney S, Eskenazi B: Patterns of exercise during pregnancy and effects on pregnancy outcome. Med Sci Sports Exerc 24:S170, 1992

18. Collings CA, Curet LB, Mullen JP: Maternal and fetal responses to a maternal aerobic exercise program. Am J Obstet Gynecol 146:702–707, 1983

19. Webb KA, Wolfe LA, Trammer JE, et al: Pregnancy outcome following physical fitness training. Can J Sport Sci 13:93–94, 1994

20. Clapp JF, Capeless EL: Neonatal morphometrics following endurance exercise training during pregnancy. Am J Obstet Gynecol 163:1805–1811, 1990

21. Clapp JF, Dickstein S: Endurance exercise and pregnancy outcome. Med Sci Sports Exerc 16:56–62, 1984

22. Manshande JP, Eeckels R, Manshande-Desmet V, et al: Rest versus heavy work during the last weeks of pregnancy: influence on fetal growth. Br J Obstet Gynaecol 94:1059–1067, 1987

23. Naeye RL, Peters EC: Working during pregnancy: effects on the fetus. Pediatrics 69:724–727, 1982

24. Clapp JF: Exercise in pregnancy: good, bad, or indifferent? In Lee RV, Cotton DB, Barron W, et al (eds): Current Obstetric Medicine, vol 3. Chicago, CV Mosby, 1993, 24–48

25. Wallace AM, Boyer DB, Dan A, et al: Aerobic exercise, maternal self-esteem, and physical discomforts during pregnancy. J Nurse Midwifery 31:255–262, 1986

26. Sibley L, Ruhling RO, Cameron-Foster J, et al: Swimming and physical fitness during pregnancy. J Nurse Midwifery 26:3–12, 1981

27. Wolfe LA, Ohtake PJ, Mottola MF, et al: Physiological interactions between pregnancy and aerobic exercise. Exerc Sports Sci Rev 17:295–351, 1989

28. Wong SC, McKenzie DC: Cardiorespiratory fitness during pregnancy and its effects on outcome. Int J Sports Med 8:79–83, 1987

29. Astrand PO, Rodal K: Textbook of Work Physiology: Physiological Basis of Exercise, ed 3. New York, McGraw Hill, 1986

30. Clapp JF, Capeless EL, Little KD: The effect of sustained exercise on follicular phase levels of estradiol-17ß in recreational athletes. Am J Obstet Gynecol 168:581–584, 1993

31. Clapp JF III: The effect of continuing regular endurance exercise on the physiologic adaptations to pregnancy and pregnancy outcome. Am J Sports Med 24:S28–S29, 1996

32. Nattiv A, Argostini R, Drinkwater B, et al: The female triad: the interrelatedness of disordered eating, amenorrhea, and osteoporosis. Clin Sports Med 13:405, 1994

33. Feicht CB, Johnson TS, Martin BS, et al: Secondary amenorrhea in athletes (correspondence). Lancet 2:1145–1146, 1978

34. Gray DP, Dale E: Variables associated with secondary amenorrhea in women runners. J Sports Sci 1:55–67, 1983

35. Hershman E, Mailly T: Stress fractures. Clin Sports Med 9:183, 1990

36. Nelson ME, Fisher EC, Catsos PD, et al: Diet and bone status in amenorrheic runners. Am J Clin Nutr 43:910–916, 1986

37. Constatini N, Warren M: Special problems of the female athlete. Baillieres Clin Rheumatol 8:199, 1994

38. McArthur JW, Bullen BA, Betens IZ, et al: Hypothalamic amenorrhea in runners of normal body distribution. Endocr Res Commun 7:13–25, 1980

39. Ding JH, Scheckter CB, Drinkwater BL, et al: Higher serum cortisol levels in exercise associated amenorrhea. Ann Intern Med 108:530–534, 1988

40. Frisch R, McArthur J: Menstrual cycles: fatness as a determinant of minimum weight for height necessary for their maintenance or onset. Science 185:949, 1974

41. Cohen JL, Chung SK, May PB Jr, et al: Exercise, body weight and amenorrhea in professional ballet dancers. Physician and Sportsmedicine 10(4):92–101, 1982

42. White CM, Hergenroeder AC: Amenorrhea, osteopenia, and the female athlete. Pediatr Clin North Am 37:1125–1141, 1990

43. Drinkwater B, Breumner B, Chestnut C: Menstrual history as a determinant of current bone density in young athletes. JAMA 263:545, 1990

44. Drinkwater BL, Nelson K, Chestnut CH, et al: Bone mineral content of amenorrheic and eumenorrheic athletes. N Engl J Med 311:277–281, 1984

45. Cann CE, Martin MC, Genant HK: Detection of premenopausal women at risk for development of osteoporosis (abstract). Athletic Amenorrhea Bull 1:3, 1982

46. Cann CE, Cavanaugh DJ, Schnurpfel K, et al: Menstrual history is the pri-

mary determinant of trabecular bone density in women runners (abstract). Med Sci Sports Exerc 20:S59, 1988

47. Clanton T, Solcher B: Chronic leg pain in the athlete. Clin Sports Med 13:743, 1994

48. Warren M, Brooks-Gunn J, Hamilton L, et al: Scoliosis and fractures in young ballet dancers: relation to delayed menarche and secondary amenorrhea. N Engl J Med 314:1348, 1986

49. Collins P: Estrogen and cardiovascular dynamics. Am J Sports Med 24:S30–S32, 1996

50. Shangold MM, Rebar RW, Wentz AC, Schiff I: Evaluation and management of menstrual dysfunction in athletes. 263:1665–1669, 1990

51. Emans SJ: The adolescent athlete with amenorrhea. Pediatr Ann 13:605–612, 1984

52. Prior CP, Vigna Y: The therapy of reproductive systemic changes associated with exercise training. In Puhl JL, Brown CH (eds): The Menstrual Cycle and Physical Activity. Champaign, IL, Human Kinetics Publishers, 1986, 105–113

53. Nattiv A, Lynch L: The female athlete triad: managing an acute risk to long-term health. Physician and Sportsmedicine 22(1):60–68, 1994

54. Joy E, Clark N, Ireland ML, Martire J, Nattiv A, Varechok S: Team management of the female athlete triad. Physician and Sportsmedicine 25(4):55–69, 1997

55. Johansson S, Vedin A, Wilhelmsson C: Myocardial infarction in women. Epidemiol Rev 5:67–95, 1983

56. Matthews KA, Meilahn E, Kuller LH, et al: Menopause and risk factors for coronary heart disease. N Engl J Med 321:641–646, 1989

57. Wells CL, Boorman MA, Riggs DM: Effect of age and menopausal status on cardiorespiratory fitness in master women athletes. Med Sci Sports Exerc 24:1147–1154, 1992

58. White MK, Yeater RA, Martin RB, et al: Effects of aerobic dancing and walking on cardiovascular function and muscular strength in postmenopausal women. J Sports Med Phys Fitness 24:159–166, 1984

59. Cowan MM, Gregory LW: Responses of pre- and post-menopausal females to aerobic conditioning. Med Sci Sports Exerc 17:138–143, 1985

60. Wood PD, Haskell WL: The effect of exercise on plasma high density lipoproteins. Lipids 14:417–427, 1979

61. American College of Sports Medicine Preventive and Rehabilitative Exercise Committee: Guidelines for Exercise Testing and Prescription, ed 4. Philadelphia, Lea & Febiger, 1991, 100

62. U.S. Dept of Health and Human Services: Osteoporosis: Cause, Treatment, Prevention. U.S. Dept of Health and Human Services publication no. (NIH) 86–2226. Bethesda, MD, National Institute of Arthritis and Musculoskeletal and Skin Diseases, 1986

63. Hargarten KM: Menopause: how exercise mitigates symptoms. Physician and Sportsmedicine 22(1):49–58, 1994

64. Notelovitz M, Martin D, Tesar R, McKenzie L, Fields C: Estrogen therapy and variable resistance weight training increases bone mineral in surgically menopausal women. J. Bone Miner Res 6:583–590, 1991

65. Prince R, Smith M, Dick IM, et al: Prevention of osteoporosis: a comparative study of exercise, calcium supplementation, and hormone-replacement therapy. N Engl J Med 325:1189–1195, 1991

66. Blumenthal JA, Williams RS, Needels TL, et al: Psychological changes accompany aerobic exercise in healthy middle-aged adults. Psychosom Med 44:529–536, 1982

67. McCann IL, Holmes DS: Influence of aerobic exercise on depression. J Pers Soc Psychol 46:1142–1147, 1984

68. Crews DL, Landers DM: A meta-analytic review of aerobic fitness and reactivity to psychosocial stressors. Med Sci Sports Exerc 19(5, suppl):S114–S120, 1987

69. Moeller JL, Lamb MM: Anterior cruciate ligament injuries in female athletes: why are women more susceptible? Physician and Sportsmedicine 25(4):31–48, 54, 1997

70. de Loes M: Epidemiology of sports injuries in the Swiss organization, Youth and Sports, 1987–1989: injuries, exposure, and risks of main diagnosis. Int J Sports Med 16:134–138, 1995

71. Zelisko JA, Noble HB, Porter M: A comparison of men's and women's professional basketball injuries. Am J Sports Med 10(5):297–299, 1982

72. Backx FJG, Beijer HJM, Bol E, et al: Injuries in high-risk persons and high-risk sports: a longitudinal study of 1818 school children. Am J Sports Med 19(2):124–130, 1991

73. Tenvergert EM, Ten Duis HJ, Klasen HJ: Trends in sports injuries, 1982–1988: an in-depth study on four types of sport. J Sports Med Phys Fitness 32:214–220, 1992

74. Ferretti A, Papandrea P, Conteduca F, et al: Knee ligament injuries in volleyball players. Am J Sports Med 20(2):203–207, 1992

75. Natri A, Jarvinen M, Kannus P, et al: Changing injury pattern in acute anterior cruciate ligament tears treated at Tampere University Hospital in the 1980s. Scand J Med Sci Sports 5:100–104, 1995

76. Daniel DM, Stone ML, Dobson BE, et al: Fate of the ACL-injured patient: a prospective outcome study. Am J Sports Med 22(5):632–644, 1994

77. Chan KM, Yuan Y, Li CK, et al: Sports causing most injuries in Hong Kong. Br J Sports Med 27:263–267, 1993

78. DeLee JC, Farney WC: Incidence of injury in Texas high school football. Am J Sports Med 20(5):575–580, 1992

79. Arendt E, Dick R: Knee injury patterns among men and women in colle-

giate basketball and soccer: NCAA data and review of literature. Am J Sports Med 23(6):694–701, 1995

80. Anderson AF, Lipscomb AB, Liudahl KJ, et al: Analysis of the intercondylar notch by computed tomography. Am J Sports Med 15(6):547–552, 1987

81. LaPrade RF, Burnett QM II: Femoral intercondylar notch stenosis and correlation to anterior cruciate ligament injuries: a prospective study. Am J Sports Med 22(2):198–203, 1994

82. Souryal TO, Freeman TR: Intercondylar notch size and anterior cruciate ligament injuries in athletes: a prospective study. Am J Sports Med 21(4):535–539, 1993

83. Grana WA, Moretz JA: Ligamentous laxity in secondary school athletes. JAMA 240:1975–1976, 1978

84. Moretz JA, Walters R, Smith L: Flexibility as a predictor of knee injuries in college football players. Physician and Sportsmedicine 10(7):93–97, 1982

85. Huston LJ, Wojtys EM: Neuromuscular performance characteristics in elite female athletes. Am J Sports Med 24(4):427–436, 1996

86. Moore JR, Wade G: Prevention of ACL injuries. Nat Strength Condit Assoc J 11:35–40, 1989

87. Grace TG, Sweetser ER, Nelson MA, et al: Isokinetic muscle imbalance and knee-joint injuries. J Bone Joint Surg Am 66:734–740, 1984

88. Dimeff RJ: Headaches in the athlete. Clin Sports Med 11(2):339–349, 1992

89. Poweel B: Weightlifter's cephalalgia. Ann Intern Med 11:449–451, 1992

90. Pestronk A, Pestronk S: Goggle migraine. N Engl J Med 308:226–227, 1983

91. Larsson L, Baum J, Mudholkar GS: Hypermobility: features and differential incidence between the sexes. Arthritis Rheum 30:1426–1430, 1987

92. Larsson L-G, Baum J, Mudholkar GS, et al: Benefits and disadvantages of joint hypermobility among musicians. N Engl J Med 329:1079–1082, 1993

Chapter 11

ENVIRONMENTAL CONDITIONS
AND EXERCISE

Exercising in extreme temperatures or at high altitudes can have detrimental effects. Athletes need to be aware of these effects and should try to avoid environment-related complications (e.g., by dressing appropriately). The physician caring for athletes or covering athletic events should not only be attuned to the influence of the environment but also make sure that facilities for appropriate management of environmentally caused injuries are available.

A collapsed athlete must be evaluated quickly; treatment should not begin until evaluation is complete and the most likely diagnosis made. Even management of life-threatening conditions such as heatstroke and hypothermia can be delayed for a minute or two while the athlete's temperature is taken (1). Treatment with rehydration, even administration of intravenous (IV) fluids, is very often started before a diagnosis is made. The widely accepted belief that all collapse must be associated with dehydration and that treatment should be started immediately is unsubstantiated (2,3).

Initial evaluation of the collapsed athlete is best made on the basis of his level of consciousness. Obviously, the athlete who is unconscious or has an altered mental state requires priority treatment. The point at which he collapsed is important information, since more seriously ill athletes tend to experience an altered level of conscious before the end of a longstanding or endurance event. The other critical information is the rectal temperature, blood pressure, and heart rate. A quick measurement of serum glucose should also be possible at endurance or prolonged events (1).

The best method of determining body temperature, or at least one as close as possible to the core body temperature, is rectally (4). Even in an open environment, rectal temperature can be measured in a discrete manner under a blanket. If the athlete is unconscious, determination of the rectal temperature is crucial. Other medical conditions that may not be directly associated with exercise and environment, such as a myocardial infarction, grand mal seizure, or subarachnoid hemorrhage, should be considered in the diagnosis. Otherwise, the most likely exercise-related diagnosis is heatstroke or hypothermia. Severe hypoglycemia is also possible, but it is not a common cause of coma in nondiabetic athletes (1).

Unconsciousness and a rectal temperature higher than 41°C (106°F) is most consistent with heatstroke; cooling should begin immediately. Hypotension and tachycardia are usually present with heatstroke (1). A rectal temperature of less than 40°C, along with a relatively normal blood pressure and heart rate, should be treated as a case of exercise-associated hyponatremia. Once other medical conditions have been eliminated, the definitive diagnosis of hyponatremia can be made only by measuring serum sodium, but treatment with IV fluid with high sodium content (3–5%), administered slowly (<50 mL/hour), can be initiated while the athlete is transferred to an emergency room as soon as possible (5). Because symptomatic hyponatremia is presently considered to be associated with overhydration by at least 2–6 L, a large volume of IV fluid should not be given to an unconscious athlete without proper evaluation (1).

HYPERTHERMIA (HEATSTROKE)

Heatstroke occurs when the body's thermoregulatory mechanism fails and more heat is produced than the body can eliminate (6). The increased metabolic rate of exercise leads to a greater production of heat: at least 70% of the energy produced during exercise is given off as heat (7). In order to prevent a lethal rise in core temperature, the heat needs to be dissipated (8). Although humans can tolerate external temperatures from –88°C to 58°C (for limited periods), the body can only tolerate core temperatures in a much smaller range, 35–41°C, before significant morbidity and mortality occur (9). Heat is primarily lost by evaporation of sweat. The ability of the body to lose heat energy by sweat evaporation is significantly diminished in hot and humid weather when skin temperature is elevated. The situation is further complicated because in a hot environment heat production is also increased by an increased cardiac workload (6).

Before loss of consciousness, the athlete on the verge of heatstroke suffers from vomiting and diarrhea, hypotension, and mental status changes: lethargy and obfuscation (6). Blood tests may demonstrate abnormal LFTs and elevated creatinine kinase, and urinalysis may show red blood cells, casts, and myoglobin. Rhabdomyolysis and acute renal failure have been reported as complications (10).

There are no studies demonstrating that dehydration is a critical factor in the development of heatstroke, although it does play a role (3). The physician must keep in mind, therefore, that anhydrosis is not always present in heatstroke and absence of dehydration should not influence the diagnosis. IV fluids should be administered to normalize the level of hydration and help stabilize the hypotension and tachycardia; approximately 1–1.5 L of 0.5% or 0.9% normal saline is appropriate (1). For an athlete with a rectal temperature higher than 41°C, cooling should take precedence. Various methods have been used, but a bath of ice water for no longer than 5–10 minutes seems to work well and is easy to set up in a medical tent (11,12). If a tub is used, keep in mind that the rectal temperature lags behind the core temperature, so immersion (and active cooling) should be ended before the rectal temperature reaches normal body temperature. Shivering occurs when the core temperature is below 37°C. The temperature should be measured every 5 minutes until it has reached 38°C (100°F), when cooling should be discontinued. It is important to continue to monitor the temperature frequently until it stabilizes, since it may continue to drop below normal even after treatment (1,13). Application of icepacks to the face and neck, axilla, and groin is an alternative method of cooling. Icepacks in these areas induce heat exchange at the sites of greatest heat loss from the body (14). The mortality from heatstroke, which can be as high as 80%, is directly proportional to both the duration and severity of hyperthermia (15).

The physician responsible for medical management at the event should plan ahead, deciding on the method of cooling to be used and making preparations in order to avoid any delay in treatment and to optimize the prognosis for any athlete with heatstroke. A written log of rectal temperature, time of measurement, and mental status on presentation and during treatment is very helpful to keep track of the athlete's progress and assist in the decision for further treatment. Admission to a hospital should be initiated if the athlete does not regain consciousness in 20–30 minutes (at the most) or if body temperature rises within an hour after active cooling has been discontinued (1).

Evaluation of the collapsed athlete who remains conscious should include measurement of blood pressure and heart rate when the athlete is supine. Postural hypotension is not an uncommon occurrence after prolonged exercise in the heat and is a likely mechanism in a large number of post-event collapses (16). The temperature will be normal, with a normal mental status (while supine).

The most common cause of collapse at endurance athletic events, especially in hot and humid temperatures, has been described as "exercise-associated collapse" (EAC) (17). It differs from heatstroke in that the affected athlete has a rectal temperature of less than 39°C (and in some cases lower than normal) (18), is sweating, and does not demonstrate significant mental status changes, such as confusion, irritability, or extreme lethargy. The athlete is often unable to walk, even assisted, and experiences nausea, vomiting, and muscle cramps. Heart rate may be elevated, as is normal for a period after exercise lasting longer than 2 hours (1). Because the signs and symptoms can be nonspecific, it is helpful to divide EAC into classes based on temperature and the mental status of the athlete (table 11.1). Severe hyperthermia with mental status changes is considered heatstroke and should be managed as such.

The exact mechanism of EAC is unknown. It most likely is a form of postural hypotension resulting from multiple factors, including increased blood flow to the peripheral blood vessels (for regulation of body temperature), loss of the calf muscle pump when exercise stops (so that blood pools in dilated capacitance veins of the lower extremities), and alterations in the autonomic nervous system that are a training adaptation but diminish vasoconstrictor response to hypotensive stress (16,19,20). Depleted energy reserves may also play a role. Severe dehydration as the primary cause is unlikely, since evidence now shows that dehydration is no more prevalent in collapsed athletes than in other athletes (18,21). In addition, the levels of dehydration most usu-

Table 11.1 Classification of Exercise-Associated Collapse

| Class | Subdivision of Classes According to Severity | | |
	Mild	Moderate	Severe
Hyperthermic	Temp ≥ 39.4°C (103°F); CNS, normal; walk with or without assistance	Temp ≥ 40.5°C (105°F); CNS, normal; or no oral intake; or extra fluid loss; or unable to walk; or severe muscle spasm	Temp ≥ 41.1°C (106°F); or CNS changes
Normothermic	Temp < 39.4°C (103°F) and > 36.1°C (97°F); CNS, normal; walk with or without assistance	Temp < 39.4°C (103°F) and > 36.1°C (97°F); CNS, normal; no oral intake; or extra fluid loss; or unable to walk; or severe muscle spasm	Temp < 39.4°C (103°F) and > 36.1°C (97°F); CNS changes
Hypothermic	Temp ≤ 36.1°C (97°F); CNS, normal; walk with or without assistance	Temp ≤ 35°C (95°F); CNS, normal; or no oral intake; or extra fluid loss; or unable to walk; or severe muscle spasm	Temp ≤ 32.2°C (90°F); or CNS changes

Source: Used with permission of McGraw-Hill, Inc., from: Roberts WO: Exercise-associated collapse in endurance events: a classification system. Physician and Sportsmedicine 17(5):49–55, 1989.

ally encountered in long-distance runners, between 1% and 4%, may impair performance but do not seem to pose a significant risk to health (22,23).

The physician should begin management of EAC by placing the athlete supine and elevating his legs and pelvis. In mild cases and many moderate cases, the athlete can take fluids orally and should be encouraged to do so. Sports drinks with 5–10% glucose are the best, since they also replenish carbohydrates (1). IV fluids are not really necessary unless the athlete cannot tolerate oral fluids or is persistently tachycardic (heart rate >100) or hypotensive (systolic blood pressure <110 mm Hg). IV fluids of 5% dextrose in 0.5N saline are recommended, up to 4 or 5 L as needed (17). Keep in mind that athletes who do not seem to be responding to fluid replacement and cooling may require carbohydrate replacement, which may be delivered quickly with a 50 mL bolus of 50% dextrose in water, if necessary (17).

Exercise-associated collapse may also be associated with leg cramps, especially in runners. These may resolve with fluid replacement, but in severe cases may be treated with IV 50% dextrose in water (17). Massaging muscles is best avoided until the athlete is well hydrated. Cramps lasting more than 1 hour can be treated with IV diazepam (in 1 mg doses) (24). Any seizures associated with EAC or heatstroke can also be treated with IV diazepam; this is an important medication to have available at all endurance athletic events.

Most athletes with EAC respond well to basic management and are able to stand and walk within 10–30 minutes (1). Once their temperature has stabilized and mental and physical findings are normal, they can be released. It is always advisable to release the athlete in the company of another person and to advise her to continue fluid replacement and consult a physician if symptoms reoccur. If an athlete with EAC has not responded to the basic management techniques, or if certain treatments, such as IV fluids, are not available, transfer to a hospital should occur sooner rather than later. The availability of an emergency facility and the means of notifying an ambulance should be reviewed before the event (13).

Heatstroke can occur even in cool or moderate environments (temperatures of 13–28°C), which suggests individual susceptibility probably is a factor (25,26). Certain risk factors seem to be associated with a higher incidence of heat-related illness, such as prior or concurrent illness (especially if associated with vomiting, diarrhea, or fever), skin disease or sunburn, alcohol or drug use, obesity, sleep deprivation, or advanced age (25,26). Some medications may also increase the risk of heatstroke, because of increased heat production (thyroid hormones, amphetamines) or decreased sweat production (antihistamines, anticholinergics, and phenothiazines) (6). Sedatives and haloperidol may increase the incidence of heat-related illness by diminishing the athlete's ability to recognize thirst.

One important method to prevent or at least minimize the occurrence of heat-related illness and EAC is acclimatization, the physiological adaptation to exercise and heat stress. This includes increased blood volume and, during intense exercise, a decreased heart rate and cardio-vascular demand compared with the nonacclimatized state. An in-creased ability to sweat, including faster onset at lower core tempera-ture, an increased rate of sweating, and a greater distribution of sweat over the body surface all increase the dissipation of heat. The sodium content of sweat is also reduced to conserve extracellular fluid (27). Plasma volume can expand by 10–25% (28). Regular exposure to hot and humid environments during moderate exercise can produce these adaptations to heat stress. Optimal acclimatization requires at least 7–14 days (29). Training in a cool climate while wearing extra clothing may lead to some degree of adaptation, but exercise in a hot and humid en-vironment produces acclimatization more effectively (30). In fact, the best method for acclimating to competition in hot and humid environ-ments is to train in a climate similar to that of the event, regardless of the temperature during nontraining hours. Training in artificial cli-mates is just as effective as living in a climate for a prolonged period of time (27).

Training intensity and volume need to be reduced for the first few sessions during acclimatization, since exercise capacity is lower in hot and humid environments. If the athlete uses two training sessions per day, the session of higher intensity should be performed first. The length of the sessions should be shorter than in normal training, then gradu-ally increased (27). Interestingly, the type of exercise for heat adapta-tion is not critical, as long as the sessions are moderately strenuous and last between 60 and 100 minutes; there is no advantage in longer peri-ods of exercise in hot and humid environments (31). The response of each athlete and her ability to adapt will vary.

Warm-up sessions also must be modified to some extent in warmer conditions. A longer and more intense warm-up, as well as avoidance of direct sunlight, helps prevent any additional heat stress before the competition. Rest breaks should be more frequent and last longer, and fluid loading should be encouraged (27). A common misconception of acclimatization is that the requirement for fluids will decrease. Athletes should drink more in hot and humid environments; the need for fluid actually increases because of the enhanced sweating response in the ac-climatized athlete. If the athlete does not replenish fluids appropriately, the advantage gained from acclimatization is forfeited because he will not adapt to dehydration (32).

Although dehydration is not the primary cause of EAC or heatstroke, adequate hydration does play an important role in maintaining thermoregulation. Exercise-associated dehydration results in hypertonicity of body fluids, which may reduce the sweating rate and thus limit dissipation of heat through evaporation (33). Dehydration (>3% body weight loss) can also lead to a reduction in cardiac stroke volume and therefore a reduction in cardiac output, since at the same point, the increase in heart rate will not be enough to compensate for the volume reduction (34,35). Adequate fluid replacement can offset an excessive increase in body heat and thus core temperature, or at least delay it, decreasing the risk of heat-related illness (36).

Athletes tend to have difficulty replacing water lost as sweat during exercise. Humans do not drink a volume of water equal to that lost as sweat during exercise; one study showed subjects voluntarily replacing only two-thirds (at most) of body water lost as sweat (37). Athletes can lose 2–6% of body weight in water, even when fluid is available for rehydration (38,39). Thirst does not reflect the degree of fluid lost and should not be used as an indication of adequate rehydration. Athletes need to be aware of this fact and should employ other means of monitoring their fluid status to provide and maintain adequate rehydration. Monitoring body weight and taking in fluid to restore weight to its pre-exercise level is a fairly reliable method. One commonly used estimate is a pint of fluid for each pound of body weight lost (33). An easier method is to monitor the color of urine. The darker the urine, the more concentrated it is, reflecting the body's attempt to conserve fluid. Athletes should always try to keep their urine as clear in color (and thus dilute) as possible to ensure adequate hydration.

Replenishing fluid loss from sweating during exercise can also be made difficult by gastrointestinal upset, especially with intakes of more than 1 L/hour. This response tends to be individual: some athletes can tolerate a greater intake of fluid while exercising than others. Athletes should be encouraged to drink as much fluid as tolerated both during and after exercise. Using flavored and chilled drinks seems to increase palatability and thus tolerance of a greater intake. Exercise intensity that exceeds 80% of maximal capacity may slow gastric emptying and delay absorption of fluids (40). A fluid with more than 8% glucose can also slow gastric emptying (41,42).

Sports drinks to replenish both carbohydrates and electrolytes lost during exercise have gained popularity over the last ten years. The addition of sodium to oral rehydration solutions is not necessary for either enhancing intestinal absorption of water or replacing sodium lost as sweat (32). The amount of sodium in a normal diet is adequate for both (43).

Carbohydrates in a sports drink or oral rehydrating solution increase the rate of absorption of water from the intestine (44). Maintenance of blood glucose concentration is critical for optimal exercise performance. The influence of carbohydrates in rehydrating solutions on exercise lasting less than 1 hour is still debatable (45–47). However, for exercise performed at greater than 65% Vo_{2max} for more than 1 hour, the benefit on performance by delaying the onset of fatigue has been demonstrated (48,49).

Glucose, sucrose, and complex carbohydrates in oral rehydrating solutions are equally effective in increasing carbohydrate oxidation, delaying fatigue and thus improving performance (48–52). Fructose, however, should be avoided; it is not readily oxidized, owing to its slow conversion to glucose, and thus does not improve performance (53–55). Fructose has also been associated with a high incidence of GI upset (56).

HYPOTHERMIA

Hypothermia occurs when the core body temperature is below 35°C (6); the environmental temperature must be less than the core body temperature, allowing heat loss from the body to exceed heat production. The risk of hypothermia is highest in outdoor activities such as hiking, skiing, scuba diving, mountaineering, sailing, and swimming. Marathons held in cool or cold weather can also create an environment conducive to the development of hypothermia, especially when the distance runner slows down during the second half of the race (57). Cooling from evaporation and radiation of heat increases when wet skin (due to sweat, rain, or snow) and clothing are exposed to a higher wind speed while the production of metabolic heat diminishes.

Hypothermia can occur over a short or long period. Acute hypothermia is most often the result of submersion in cold water. Subacute hypothermia results from exposure to cold environments for a few hours, and chronic hypothermia takes place over a few days, often with exposure to milder temperatures. The primary physiological difference is in the athlete's fluid status—more chronic hypothermia allows a longer period of time for the development of peripheral vasoconstriction, resulting in a greater fluid shift and subsequent diuresis, and thus larger volumes of fluid are necessary for resuscitation (6).

The stages of hypothermia are defined by core body temperature: mild (32–36°C), moderate (28–32°C), and severe (<28°C). Mild hypothermia is typically characterized by shivering, tachycardia, tachypnea, diuresis, and cyanosis. Ataxia and amnesia may also occur. An ECG will demonstrate sinus tachycardia. In moderate hypothermia, the shivering reflex is lost and the individual may become confused and try to undress. Muscles become rigid and pulses are difficult to palpate and may be absent. The ECG finding is distinctly abnormal, with sinus bradycardia (refractory to atropine), prolonged PR/QRS/QT waves, and a J wave at 30°C. Atrial fibrillation may also develop. Severe hypothermia may actually protect the body from anoxic injury, the result of a progressive decrease in cellular metabolism (58). At 28°C the basal metabolic rate is decreased by 50% (58). Symptoms are distinct, with loss of reflexes, fixed and dilated pupils, and probable coma. Ventricular fibrillation is a significant risk. Although the patient may appear nonviable, the usual criteria for death (i.e., Glasgow coma score, ECG, EEG) are invalid with core temperatures below normal (59). Multiple cases of successful resuscitation after prolonged periods of severe hypothermia with nonperfusing cardiac rhythms have been reported (60).

The "best" method, rate, and setting for rewarming are still under debate, but some basic techniques can be employed. Rewarming can be either passive (with warm blankets in a sheltered environment) or active (addition of hot packs, heat lamps, and possibly hot bath immersion). Core rewarming is invasive and involves warm IV fluids, hollow viscous lavage, and pleural or peritoneal lavage with fluids warmed to 40–42°C (6). Hollow viscous lavage has been shown to have minimal benefit.

For the hypothermic athlete, simple rewarming techniques should be initiated as soon as possible, including removing his cold wet clothing and surrounding him with warm and dry blankets, even before measuring his body temperature. The administration of warm IV fluids is helpful to decrease the hypotension usually encountered with rewarming. As the core temperature increases, vasoconstriction diminishes and blood pressure drops. Lactated Ringer's solution should be avoided, since the hypothermic liver cannot metabolize lactate to bicarbonate as easily (6). The rate of rewarming should not exceed 1–2°C per hour, in order to avoid any severe cardiovascular instability (61). Avoiding any rough movements or jolting of the individual is recommended, since sudden movements have been documented to precipitate arrhythmias (6).

Athletes exercising in cold environments, or at cooler temperatures for prolonged periods, need to prepare themselves and dress appropriately. To minimize heat loss, athletes can protect themselves from moisture, wind, and cold air by layering light loose clothes that insulate the body with trapped warm air (62). The outermost layer should be windproof and water-resistant but still allow moisture to escape (such as Gore-Tex) (58). Wool and polyester fabrics can still be protective when wet, but cotton and goose down cannot (58). Athletes should cover areas of the body associated with the greatest amount of heat loss, such as head, neck, legs, and hands (62). Proper nutrition and hydration, with avoidance of alcohol, are also important (6).

HIGH-ALTITUDE ILLNESS

High-altitude illness (HAI) includes various symptoms related to the stress of exposure to high altitude. Symptoms begin at altitudes above 8,000 feet. Altitude illness becomes more severe at higher altitudes, most serious between 10,000 and 18,000 feet (63). Although many ski resorts are located above 8,000 feet, only 25% of skiers develop any altitude-related illness, because most skiers sleep at lower altitudes, decreasing the amount of time spent at the higher altitude and thus reducing the risk of developing HAI (64).

The partial pressure of oxygen (Po_2) in the atmosphere decreases as altitude increases; the low Po_2 at high altitudes results in hypoxia. In an attempt to restore the oxygen pressure within tissues to its sea-level value and maintain it at that level—another type of acclimatization—

minute ventilation increases (6) and respiratory alkalosis results. Other physiological changes include increased heart rate, sympathetic nervous system activity, and cerebral blood flow (64). Pulmonary artery vasoconstriction also occurs. Interestingly, the individuals least affected by altitude symptoms are those who can maintain a higher minute ventilation. Therefore, pulmonary function is probably the limiting factor determining exercise tolerance at high altitudes (65). The effect of altitude on oxygen dissociation from hemoglobin also plays an important role, since above 8,000 feet even small increases in altitude result in a significant decrease in oxygen saturation (66). The process of acclimatization is a function of an individual's physiology, the rate of altitude change, the altitude reached, and the intensity of exercise—all of which vary to some degree. Acclimatization also requires time. HAI results if the change in altitude happens too quickly to allow acclimatization or the individual's system simply cannot adjust to the lower Po_2. HAI is divided into three types of reactions: acute mountain sickness (AMS), high-altitude pulmonary edema (HAPE), and high-altitude cerebral edema (HACE) (6). These are most likely related on a continuum, based on the same underlying pathophysiological process.

Acute mountain sickness is the most frequent and first group of symptoms encountered when ascending above 8,000 feet for longer than 24 hours. The most common symptom is a headache, which is throbbing and is worse in the morning, with exercise, and while supine. Other symptoms include nausea, vomiting, fatigue, difficulty concentrating, insomnia, and declining exercise performance. These symptoms are self-limiting and resolve in a few days after staying at a constant altitude (6). Individuals in good physical condition are not immune to the development of AMS or the intensity of symptoms.

High-altitude pulmonary edema is the most frequent cause of death among the altitude illnesses (67). It can occur at any altitude above 8,000 feet but is usually associated with higher altitudes, a too rapid ascent, cold temperature, and an increased level of exertion. The exact etiology is not known but may be related to an intense pulmonary vasoconstriction in response to alveolar hypoxia (6). Symptoms include excessive fatigue, generalized weakness, dyspnea on exertion, dry cough, decreased exercise tolerance, and possibly confusion, all of which increase during sleep. An elevated temperature up to 38.5°C, tachycardia, tachypnea, rales on auscultation, and pink or frothy sputum are found on clinical exam. Chest x-ray often reveals fluffy or patchy infiltrates around peripheral borders, unilateral or bilateral (67). A diagnosis of HAPE requires two of the following symptoms: dyspnea at rest, cough, and weakness; and two or more of the following findings during exercise: rales or wheezing in more than one lung field, cyanosis, tachypnea, and tachycardia (68). The earliest sign of developing HAPE is often decreased exercise tolerance and a prolonged recovery period (69). The death rate due to HAPE can be as high as 44% in the absence of appropriate management, but is 11% overall (70). Interestingly, the recurrence rate can be up to 66%, suggestive of a predisposition in some individuals (which is not seen with AMS) (71).

High-altitude cerebral edema occurs less commonly than HAPE and is not usually encountered below 12,000 feet (72). It occurs at a mean altitude of 15,500 feet, somewhat higher than HAPE. The mortality rate is 13%, just slightly higher than for HAPE. HACE is typically associated with headache, severe lethargy, altered mental status, and ataxia, although focal neural deficits, seizures, and papilledema may also be found on examination (6). The skin may be gray or cyanotic secondary to pulmonary edema, which is often present to some degree (67). The diagnosis is based on evidence of mental status changes or ataxia occurring at an altitude above 8,000 feet (6). It has been suggested that ataxia may be the most sensitive finding for HACE, which suggests a cerebellar sensitivity to hypoxia (69). Lethargy and mental status changes precede coma, which is an ominous development since the mortality rate increases to 60% once coma occurs (66).

Acute mountain sickness may progress to HACE, if acclimatization does not occur and ascent to higher altitude continues. Progression usually occurs within 1–3 days but may occur within 12 hours. Therefore, treatment should begin as soon as symptoms appear, making early recognition critical. The most important component of management is descent, as quickly as possible. For milder cases of AMS, immediate descent may not be necessary but close monitoring of symptoms for further deterioration is important to avoid serious illness (6). Time for further acclimatization is necessary, so further ascent must be delayed.

Individuals with any signs of AMS (or HAPE or HACE) should keep warm, since the stress of lower temperatures exacerbates the symptoms of high-altitude illness by increasing pulmonary artery pressure (73). Any activity worsens symptoms because it increases oxygen consumption and causes greater hypoxia.

If supplemental oxygen is available, it can also be helpful to decrease hypoxia, but its use should not delay descent. Even descents of 1,000 feet may produce dramatic improvement in HAPE or HACE (6). Pharmacological agents as adjunctive treatments have been used as well. Acetazolamide can help with AMS symptoms, since its metabolic effect of stimulating excretion of bicarbonate induces a mild metabolic acidosis, which results in an increase in ventilation (similar to acclimatization). It does have side effects, however, including polyuria, nausea, and mild paresthesias. The usual dose is 250 mg every 8 hours; this has produced significant improvement in symptoms of AMS in some studies (74,75). Of note, acetazolamide should not be given to pregnant women or to individuals with sulfa allergy.

For the more severe HAPE and HACE, nifedipine and dexamethasone may be helpful. Nifedipine is thought to reverse pulmonary hypertension, decrease pulmonary edema, and thus improve oxygenation in HAPE. Again, the use of nifedipine should not take the place of timely descent (70). Dexamethasone has not been shown to reduce symptoms of AMS. Any symptoms improved by this drug (with AMS) usually recur once it is discontinued (76). Used as adjunctive treatment for HACE, however, dexamethasone may decrease cerebral edema and lower intracranial pressure—two important components of the development of HACE (76). Any narcotics or sedatives may worsen symptoms by depressing ventilation and should be avoided.

REFERENCES

1. Holtzhausen L-M, Noakes TD: Collapsed ultraendurance athlete: proposed mechanisms and an approach to management. Clin J Sports Med 7:292–301, 1997

2. Noakes TD: Dehydration during exercise: what are the real dangers? Clin J Sports Med 5:123–128, 1995

3. Noakes TD: Fluid and electrolyte disturbances in heat illness. Int J Sports Med 19(suppl 2):S146–149, 1998

4. Roberts WO: Assessing core temperature in collapsed athletes: what's the best method? Physician and Sportsmedicine 22(8):49–55, 1994

5. Noakes TD: The hyponatremia of exercise. Int J Sport Nutr 2:205–228, 1993

6. Tom PA, Garmel GM, Auerbach PS: Environmental-dependent sports emergencies. Med Clin North Am 78:305–325, 1994

7. Sawka MN: Physiological consequences of hypohydration: exercise performance and thermoregulation. Med Sci Sports Exerc 24:657–670, 1992

8. Nadel ER: Control of sweating rate while exercising in the heat. Med Sci Sports Exerc 11:31–35, 1979

9. Sawka MN, Wenger CB: Physiological responses to acute exercise-heat stress. In Pandolf KB, Sawka MN, Gonzalez RR (eds): Human Performance Physiology and Environmental Medicine at Terrestrial Extremes. Indianapolis, Benchmark Press, 1988, 97–153

10. Pattison ME, Logan JL, Lee SM, Ogden DA: Exertional heat stroke and acute renal failure in a young woman. Am J Kidney Dis 9:184–187, 1988

11. Armstrong LE, Hubbard RW, Kraemer WJ, de Luca JP, Christensen EL: Signs and symptoms of heat exhaustion during strenuous exercise. Ann Sports Med 3:182–189, 1987

12. Costrini A: Emergency treatment of exertional heatstroke and comparison of whole body cooling techniques. Med Sci Sports Exerc 22:15–18, 1990

13. Roberts WO: Managing heatstroke: on-site cooling. Physician and Sportsmedicine 20(5):17–28, 1992

14. Hayward JS, Collis M, Eckerson JD: Thermographic evaluation of relative heat loss areas of man during cold water immersion. Aerospace Med 44:708–711, 1973

15. Hubbard RW, Armstrong LE: Hyperthermia: new thoughts on an old problem. Physician and Sportsmedicine 17(6):97–113, 1989

16. Holtzhausen L-M, Noakes TD: The prevalence and significance of post-exercise (postural) hypotension in ultramarathon runners. Med Sci Sports Exerc 27:1595–1601, 1995

17. Roberts WO: Exercise-associated collapse in endurance events: a classification system. Physician and Sportsmedicine 17(5):49–55, 1989

18. Hotlzhausen L-M, Noakes TD, Kroning B, De Klerk M, Roberts M, Emsley R: Clinical and biochemical characteristics of collapsed ultramarathon runners. Med Sci Sports Exerc 26:1095–1101, 1994

19. Myrhe L, Lutt UC, Venters MD: Responses of athletes and non-athletes to lower body negative pressure and acute dehydration (abstract). Med Sci Sports Exerc 8:53–54, 1976

20. Smith ML, Graitzer HM, Hudson DL, Raven PB: Baroreflex function in endurance- and static-exercise trained men. J Appl Physiol 64:585–591, 1988

21. Noakes TD, Berlinski N, Solomon E, Weight LM: Collapsed runners: blood biochemical changes, after IV fluid therapy. Physician and Sportsmedicine 19(7):70–81, 1991

22. Noakes TD: Fluid replacement during exercise. Exerc Sports Sci Rev 12:297–330, 1993

23. Noakes TD, Myburgh KH, Du Plessis JH, Lang L, van der Riet C, Schall R: Metabolic rate, not % dehydration, predicts rectal temperature in marathon runners. Med Sci Sports Exerc 23:443–449, 1991

24. Krochel JP: Heat stroke and related heat stress disorders. Dis Mon 35:301–377, 1989

25. Armstrong LE, De Luca JP, Hubbard RW: Time course of recovery and heat acclimation ability of prior exertional heatstroke patients. Med Sci Sports Exerc 22:36–48, 1990

26. Epstein Y: Heat intolerance: predisposing factor or residual injury? Med Sci Sports Exerc 22:29–35, 1990

27. Maughan RJ, Shirreffs SM: Preparing athletes for competition in the heat: developing an effective acclimatization strategy. Sports Sci Exchange 10(2), 1997

28. Appenzeller O: Temperature regulation and sports. *In* Appenzeller O (ed): Sports Medicine. Baltimore, Urban & Schwarzenberg, 1988, 11–35

29. Montain SJ, Maughan RJ, Sawka MN: Heat acclimatization strategies for the 1996 summer Olympics. Athl Ther Today 1:42–46, 1996

30. Dawson B: Exercise training in sweat clothing in cool conditions to improve heat tolerance. Sports Med 17:233–244, 1994

31. Lind AR, Bass DE: Optimal exposure time for development of heat acclimation. Fed Proc 22:704–708, 1963

32. Sawka MN, Pandolf KB: Effects of body water loss on physiologic function and exercise performance. *In* Gisolfi CV, Lamb DR (eds): Perspectives in Exercise and Sports Medicine. Vol 3: Fluid Homeostasis during Exercise. Indianapolis, Benchmark Press, 1990, 1–38

33. Convertino VA, Armstrong LE, Coyle EF, et al: Exercise and fluid replacement. Med Sci Sports Exerc 28:i–vii, 1996

34. Montain SJ, Coyle EF: Fluid ingestion during exercise increases skin blood flow independent of increases in blood volume. J Appl Physiol 73:903–910, 1992

35. Sawka MN, Knowlton RG, Critz JB: Thermal and circulatory responses to repeated bouts of prolonged running. Med Sci Sports 11:177–180, 1979

36. Hubbard RW, Armstrong LE: The heat illness: biochemical, ultrastructural, and fluid-electrolyte considerations. *In* Pandolf KB, Sawka MN, Gonzalez RR (eds): Human Performance Physiology and Environmental Medicine at Terrestrial Extremes. Indianapolis, Benchmark Press, 1988, 305–360

37. Hubbard RW, Maller O, Sawka MN, Francesconi RN, Drolet L, Young AJ: Voluntary dehydration and allesthesia for water. J Appl Physiol 57:868–875, 1984

38. Greenleaf JE, Sargent F II: Voluntary dehydration in man. J Appl Physiol 20:719–724, 1965

39. Greenleaf JE, Brock PJ, Keil LC, Morse JT: Drinking and water balance during exercise and heat acclimation. J Appl Physiol 54:414–419, 1983

40. Costill DL: Gastric emptying of fluids during exercise. *In* Gisolfi CV, Lamb DR (eds): Perspectives in Exercise Science and Sports Medicine. Vol. 3: Fluid Homeostasis during Exercise. Indianapolis, Benchmark Press, 1990, 97–128

41. Costill DL, Saltin B: Factors limiting gastric emptying during rest and exercise. J Appl Physiol 37:679–683, 1974

42. Hunt JN, Knox MT: Regulation of gastric emptying. *In* Handbook of Physiology, vol IV. Washington, DC: American Physiological Society, 1969, 1917–1935

43. National Research Council: Recommended Dietary Allowances, ed 10. Washington, DC, National Academy Press, 1989, 250–255

44. Gisolfi CV, Summers RW, Schedl HP: Intestinal absorption of fluids during rest and exercise. *In* Gisolfi CV, Lamb DL (eds): Perspectives in Exercise Science and Sports Medicine. Vol. 3: Fluid Homeostasis during Exercise. Indianapolis: Benchmark Press, 1990, 129–180

45. Ball TC, Headley S, Vanderburgh P: Carbohydrate-electrolyte replacement improves sprint capacity following 50 minutes of high-intensity cycling (abstract). Med Sci Sports Exerc 26:S196, 1994

46. Below PR, Coyle EF: Fluid and carbohydrate ingestion individually benefit intense exercise lasting one hour. Med Sci Sports Exerc 27:200–210, 1995

47. Millard-Stafford M, Rosskopf LB, Snow TK, Hinson BT: Pre-exercise carbohydrate-electrolyte ingestion improves one-hour running performances in the heat (abstract). Med Sci Sports Exerc 26:S196, 1994

48. Coggan AR, Coyle EF: Carbohydrate ingestion during prolonged exercise: effects on metabolism and performance. Exerc Sport Sci Rev 19:1–40, 1991

49. Mitchell JB, Costill CL, Houmard JA, Flynn MG, Fink WJ, Beltz JD: Effects of carbohydrate ingestion on gastric emptying and exercise performance. Med Sci Sports Exerc 20:110–115, 1988

50. Coyle EF: Timing and method of increased carbohydrate intake to cope with heavy training, competition and recovery. J Sports Sci 9:29–52, 1991

51. Saris WHM, Goodpaster BH, Jeukendrup AE, Brouns F, Halliday D, Wagenmakers AJM: Exogenous carbohydrate oxidation from different carbohydrate sources during exercise. J Appl Physiol 75:2168–2172, 1993

52. Wagenmakers JM, Brouns F, Saris WHM, Halliday D: Oxidation rates of orally ingested carbohydrate during prolonged exercise in men. J Appl Physiol 75:2774–2780, 1993

53. Massicottie D, Perronnet R, Allah C, Hillaire-Marcel C, Ledoux M, Brisson G: Metabolic response to [^{13}C]glucose and [^{13}C]fructose ingestion during exercise. J Appl Physiol 61:1180–1184, 1986

54. Massicottie D, Perronnet F, Brisson G, Bakkouch K, Hillaire-Marcel C: Oxidation of glucose polymer during exercise: comparison of glucose and fructose. J Appl Physiol 66:179–183, 1989

55. Bjorkman OK, Sahlin L, Hagenfeldt L, Wahren J: Influence of glucose

and fructose ingestion on the capacity for long-term exercise. Clin Physiol 4:483–494, 1984

56. Murray R, Paul GL, Seifert JG, Eddy DE, Halaby GA: The effects of glucose, fructose, and sucrose ingestion during exercise. Med Sci Sports Exerc 21:275–282, 1989

57. Maughan RJ, Light IM, Whiting PH, Miller JDB: Hypothermia, hyperkalemia, and marathon running. Lancet 11:1336, 1982

58. Bangs C, Hamlet MP, Mills WJ: Help for the victim of hypothermia. Patient Care 12:46–50, 1977

59. Corneli HM: Accidental hypothermia. J Pediatr 120:671–679, 1992

60. Michenfelder JD, Milde JH: The effect of profound levels of hypothermia (below 14°C) on canine cerebral metabolism. J Cerebral Blood Flow Metab 12:877–880, 1992

61. Elder PT: Accidental hypothermia. In Shoemaker W et al (eds): Textbook of Critical Care, ed 2. Philadelphia, WB Saunders, 1989, 101–109

62. Buckley RL, Hostetler R: The physiologic impact and treatment of hypothermia. Med Times 118:38–44, 1990

63. Yaron M, Honigman B: High-altitude illness. In Rosen P, Baker FJ, Barkin RM, et al (eds): Emergency Medicine: Concepts and Clinical Practice, ed 3. Boston, Mosby–Year Book, 1992, 994–1009

64. Alexander JK, Hartley LHH, Modelski M, et al: Reduction of stroke volume during exercise in men following ascent to 3100 m altitude. J Appl Physiol 23:849, 1967

65. Houston CS: Operation Everest II: man at extreme altitude. J Appl Physiol 63:877, 1987

66. Hultgren HN: High altitude medical problems. Sci Am 9:1–16, 1992

67. Klocke DL, Decker WW, Stepanek J: Altitude-related illnesses. Mayo Clin Proc 73:988–993, 1998

68. Sutton JR, Coates G, Houston CS (eds): The Lake Louise Consensus on the Definition and Quantification of Altitude Illness: Hypoxia and Mountain Medicine. Burlington, VT, Queen City Printers, 1992, 237

69. Hackett PH, Roach RC, Sutton JR: High altitude medicine. In Auerbach PS, Geehr EC (eds): Management of Wilderness and Environmental Emergencies, ed 2. St Louis, CV Mosby, 1989, 1–29

70. Oelz O, Ritter M, Jenni R: Nifedipine for high altitude pulmonary edema. Lancet 2:1241–1244, 1989

71. Kawashima A, Kubo K, Kobayashi T, et al: Hemodynamic responses to acute hypoxia, hypobaria, and exercise in subjects susceptible to high-altitude pulmonary edema. J Appl Physiol 67:1982–1989, 1989

72. Houston CS: High altitude illness. JAMA 236:2193, 1976

73. Hackett PH: High altitude medical problems. In Tintinalli JE, Krome RL, Ruiz E (eds): Emergency Medicine: A Comprehensive Study Guide, ed 3. San Francisco, McGraw-Hill, 1992, 670–677

74. Grisson CK, Roach RC, Sarnquist FH, et al: Acetazolamide in the treatment of acute mountain sickness: clinical efficacy and effect on gas exchange. Ann Intern Med 116:461–465, 1992

75. Tso E: High-altitude illness. Emerg Med Clin North Am 10:231–247, 1992

76. Hackett PH, Roach RC, Wood RA, et al: Dexamethasone for prevention and treatment of acute mountain sickness. Aviat Space Environ Med 59(10):950–954, 1988

Chapter 12

MEDICAL COVERAGE OF
ATHLETIC EVENTS

The medical coverage of an athletic event can be relatively straightforward if the personnel, equipment, and available transportation reflect the injury potential of the particular sport within the particular venue. The contents of the sports medicine physician's medical bag usually reflect the sports injury profile and the complement of professionals on the supporting medical team. For sports such as football, the trainer attending the event usually has his own medical bag. If the physician is working without a trainer, then her supplies should include items such as splints, tourniquets, and airways. On the other hand, if the trainer and a full medical team are present, including an orthopedist, physiatrist, and internist, specific responsibilities and equipment need to be delineated (how to respond to an on-field injury and the "waves" of backup, depending upon the need for physician support or items from the medical bag). The trainer usually wears a medical and appliance pack that includes tourniquet, gloves, gauze, pliers, and tape. The trainer's bag usually contains more instruments, such as airways, splints, neck braces, bandages, and other immobilizers to be used in potential back and neck injuries (a back board and stretcher are usually available on the ambulance, should these become necessary), as well as intravenous fluid and a few medicines, including "smelling salts." The physician's bag should reflect the medical side of a potential examination: stethoscope, a large blood-pressure cuff, reflex hammer, gloves, Kelly clamp, Swiss army knife, gauze, bandages, ophthalmoscope and light source, and medicines such as analgesics and epinephrine for bee stings—all of which are not usually part of the trainer's bag. Table 12.1 lists the items in the optimal trainer's and M.D.'s medical bags.

Table 12.1. Trainer's Bag and Physician's Bag

Trainer's Bag _____

Gauze (various sizes)*
Tape*
Band-aids*
Antibiotic ointment*
Splints
Tourniquet*
Surgical gloves*
NSAIDs
Cough drops
Sterile saline
Steri-Strips and benzoin
Drops for contact lens wearers
Sunblock
Equipment for suturing
Ace-wraps*
Neck immobilizer*
Spine board
Sling
Alcohol wipes
Cooler with many already-prepared
  icepacks*
A few syringes (helpful for flushing
  eyes, wounds)

Flashlight*
Fluorescein strips and portable UV
  penlight
Second Skin
Blanket
Few sterile containers
Nasal tampons and ointment
Q-Tips
Tongue blades

Physician's Bag _____

Stethoscope
Ophthalmoscope
Blood-pressure cuff
Cell phone (if trainer does not have
  access)*
Reflex hammer
Epi-Pen (for possible anaphylactic
  reactions)
Sutures

Note: The bare essentials are indicated by an asterisk. Optional additions to the physician's equipment are walkie-talkie, IV materials, portable table (to set up on sideline).

Depending on the size of the physician team, the primary responsibility for head injury, back and neck injury, and cardiovascular events should be clear. For acute musculoskeletal injuries in the extremities, the orthopedic surgeon is in charge of the coordination of assessment, diagnosis, and transportation. When the internist is the sole physician on the sideline, she should carefully review information on head injury protocol, spinal immobilization, internal medicine aspects (including cardiac rhythms and volume), and the physical examination and assessment of the most common injuries expected from that particular sport.

In football, head injuries are not uncommon. The assessment of whether a player can return to the game should be made only after asking the following five questions and completing a neurological exam, including pupil assessment:

1. Did the player lose consciousness?
2. Does he have retrograde amnesia?
3. Does he have a headache?
4. Does he have nausea?
5. Does he have blurring of vision?

Before a final decision to allow the athlete to reenter the game, his pupils should be checked, although this can be difficult using a weak light source on a bright day. Any injury to the head may involve the cervical spine. The neck should be evaluated as well, even if just by asking, "How does your neck feel?" As a rule of thumb, when treating an athlete with a head injury, keeping him out of play for at least 5 or 10 minutes allows for more complete evaluation and observation. Although frustrating for the athlete who feels fine and thinks the team needs him, it gives the physician more opportunity to reevaluate and ensure that the decision to return to play is the correct one.

The various approaches to acute injuries to the extremities have been described in earlier chapters. For injuries incurred during a sporting event, even the most attentive physician and trainer see only 80% of them as they occur in real time. The use of replay on television has been helpful in some cases to assess the severity of the injury, though this has not yet been translated to the field management of an injury. The physician should ask three general questions about peripheral injuries before addressing the injury itself:

1. Can the athlete move the extremity distal to the injury?
2. Is there evidence of soft tissue bleeding?
3. Are the pulses intact? (Usually, movement of a distal part replaces the need for evaluation of tendon reflexes.)

The trainer and physician who are first on the scene play a critical role in obtaining valuable history and physical exam information before the inevitable swelling that may prevent an optimal exam for several days. Questions about the history should reflect the athlete's perception of what happened: "Did you feel or hear a pop or a snap?" starts the localization process when an athlete is experiencing acute pain. Even the initial observations of the physical exam can be critical. For instance, the athlete with a complete tear of the ACL has no effusion in the first 5 minutes, but may have a large one by 15 minutes after injury. Another athlete with a torn meniscus may have no effusion until the next day when she awakes from sleep. In both cases, on day 2 following a knee injury, if the athlete has a large effusion accompanied by diffuse pain, the temporal appearance of the effusion is a helpful differentiating factor.

Physicians who provide on-site coverage of multiple sports events should review the list of most likely injuries for the specific sport:

–football: ankle, knee, neck
–soccer: ankle, knee
–gymnastics: ankle, wrist, spine
–basketball: ankle, knee
–volleyball: ankle, shoulder
–hockey: knee, spine
–wrestling: neck, knee, shoulder
–skiing: knee, hand (thumb), lower leg

This list covers approximately 90% of the acute injuries seen at sporting events. By reviewing the management of these injuries just before the event, the physician will have the confidence to reassure the athlete and family that the first assessment of the injury is correct. Moreover, she will more easily recognize nontypical findings, allowing the early search for an appropriate alternative.

The sports venue itself is another critical factor. Most large stadiums have a first-aid area and training facilities for the athletes, and many have extensive first-aid facilities and staff for fans attending the game, which can be called on as a resource for the athletes if necessary. At many professional sports stadiums, the fans' first-aid room has an entire nursing staff, hospital beds, ECG machines, cardiac-support devices, and an ambulance waiting in a nearby bay. Other large stadiums have plain x-ray facilities (fixed or mobile equipment). Turnaround times for test results can be under ten minutes, and these facilities should be used when assessing a possible fracture. Players with major injuries are transported directly to a hospital facility, whereas a minor injury such as a potential metatarsal fracture, caused by being stepped on during a football game, can be readily detected by x-ray with a minimal loss from playing time.

Weather conditions should be part of the pregame assessment so that the medical team can anticipate issues of hyperthermia, hypothermia, and potential fluid requirements (see Chapter 11). Body heat increases with vigorous exercise, and massive amounts of fluid may be lost. Weight losses of up to twenty pounds have been observed in some interior football linemen. The loss of fluid and electrolyte accounts for most of this, and the loss threatens intravascular volume. The physician, especially if IV fluids are unavailable, must be vigilant in looking for any erratic behavior in a perspiring athlete. Beginning in the pregame warm-up and continuing throughout the game, the physician should insist on every athlete drinking water or athletic formulas at each transition. Intravascular volume can drop by several liters. The adverse effects on mental status and strength and the accompanying cramps can be reversed very quickly by the administration of IV fluid through a large-gage needle inserted in the antecubital fossa. The trainer's medical bag should be prepared for this intravenous support.

Sideline coverage has the medical team dispersed over forty yards in some sports. Frequent communication through check-ins with the training staff is mandatory. Each physician should write down a player's number and injury, no matter how trivial it seems at the time. A quick follow-up during halftime or a period break with the athlete and the training staff gives maximal reassurance and optimizes communication. Ideally, all covering physicians should be on the sidelines during the event. The physicians on the medical team should dress appropriately and professionally. A layered approach is wise, such as a jacket, sweater, and short-sleeved shirt (depending on the temperature), and appropriate footwear should be worn. All-weather gear should be available. The sidelines often have no protection from the sun, so sunblock, sunglasses, and a baseball cap from the team are handy. Trainers usually dress more functionally and casually, carrying their medical packs and tools around their waists—a reflection of their triage duties.

Physicians on the sports medical team must convey professionalism at every opportunity. It is essential to maintain the physician-patient relationship; the importance of this is stressed by coaches who want to know when an athlete can return to play and family members who appropriately want to know the extent of a player's injuries. No matter how tempting it is to cheer for your team, a professional demeanor should be maintained. This is especially true for an on-site physician covering both teams.

Following a game, physicians should review their lists of players and injuries with the trainers and assign responsibility for follow-up. Especially on weekends, when medical cross-coverage might well be tested, careful instructions and phone numbers should be given to the athlete and family so that they can get in touch with a physician if a condition worsens. Team physicians should call the local hospital emergency room to alert the staff of an athlete's condition if transportation to the ER is needed. The physician who is covering a team at an away event should check with the head coach and injured players before departure, especially when the distance to home is over an hour. This simple courtesy provides reassurance and is good medicine. Providing simple instructions as necessary, from the use of ice to information about the location of local medical facilities should problems arise, can be helpful to a traveling team. In the days of cellular telephones, the physician should not hesitate to call a family member or medical facility to alert them of potential concerns, especially on weekends and nights, the most common times for major sporting events.

Appendix A

ALGORITHMS FOR
DECISION MAKING IN
MANAGEMENT OF INJURIES

Appendix A.1. Decision Making in Head Injury

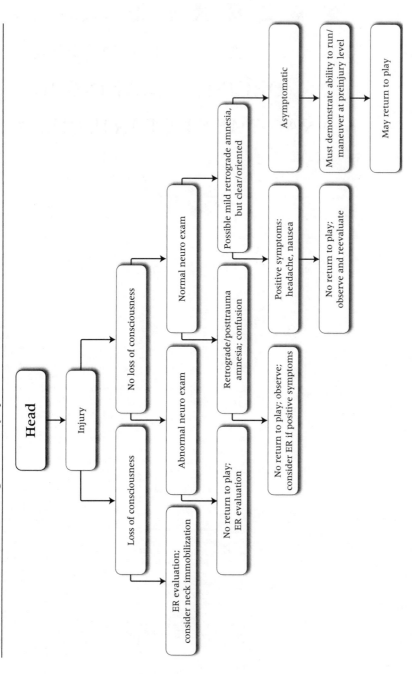

Note: Monitor for headache, nausea, unequal pupils, level of consciousness.

Abbreviations: ER = emergency room; neuro = neurological

Appendix A.2. Decision Making in Neck Injury

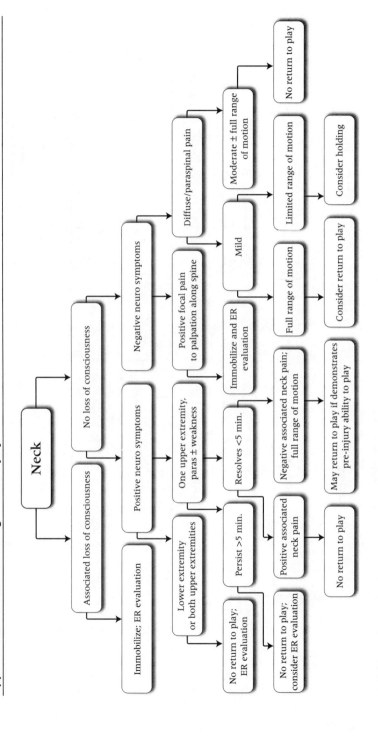

Abbreviations: Paras = Paresthesias; neuro = neurological

Appendix A.3. Decision Making in Shoulder Injury

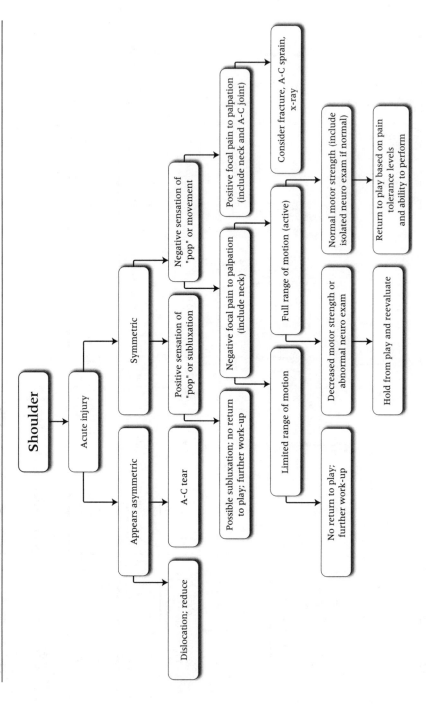

Abbreviations: A-C = acromioclavicular; neuro = neurological

Appendix A.4. Decision Making in Knee Injury

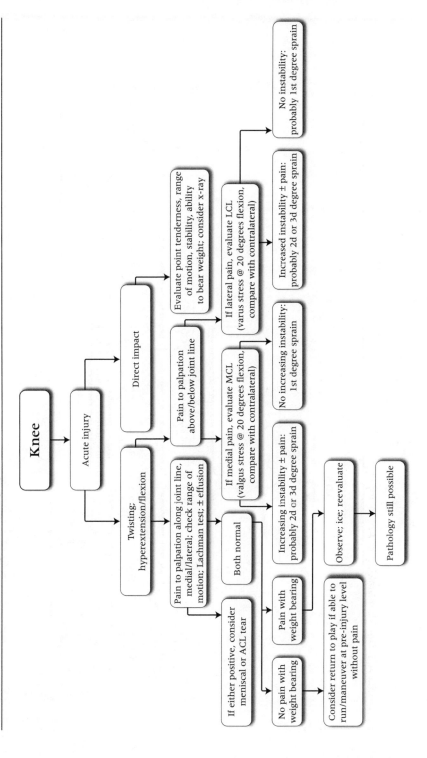

Note: Athlete may have more than one injury present in same knee from one event.

Abbreviations: ACL = anterior cruciate ligament; MCL = medial collateral ligament; LCL = lateral collateral ligament

Appendix A.5. Decision Making in Ankle Injury

Ankle → **Acute injury mechanism**

Direct impact:
- Positive focal pain to palpation, including tibia/fibula and foot; x-ray
  - Positive pain with weight bearing
    - X-ray
- Negative focal pain to palpation
  - No pain to mild pain with weight bearing
    - Return to play if able to demonstrate pre-injury running/maneuvering ability

Twisting:
- Focal increasing pain to palpation; x-ray
  - Limited range of motion or positive anterior drawer test or pain to palpation along fibula (Maissoneuve); immobilize; x-ray
- Diffuse pain to palpation above/below joint line
  - No pain to mild pain with weight bearing; no swelling
    - Consider return to play
  - Increasing pain with weight bearing
    - No return to play

MOST COMMON
INJURIES, BY SPORT

Appendix B. Most Common Injuries, by Sport

Sport	Most Commonly Injured Joints	Comments
Football	Knee, neck, foot, ankle	Collision/head injuries: no helmet removal
Rugby	Knee, shoulder, neck	Ear injury and scrum burn
Soccer	Knee, ankle	
Field hockey	Knee, ankle	
Running	Knee, ankle, foot	Overuse versus injury
Swimming	Shoulder, knee	
Diving	Neck, back	
Basketball	Knee, ankle	Sport with highest rate of ankle sprain and instability
Volleyball	Shoulder, ankle	Shoulder laxity
Gymnastics	Spine, wrist, hand, knee	Spondylolisthesis; also consider osteoporosis
Bicycling	Knee	Biker's palsy
Baseball	Shoulder, elbow	Overuse in pitching
Racquet sports	Shoulder, elbow	
Skiing	Knee, hand, wrist	Anterior cruciate ligament tears common
Ice hockey	Neck, knee	
Wrestling	Spine, knee, shoulder	

INDEX